Sensory Mechanisms
of the Spinal Cord

Sensory Mechanisms of the Spinal Cord

W. D. Willis
and
R. E. Coggeshall

University of Texas Medical Branch
Galveston, Texas

Plenum Press · New York and London

Library of Congress Cataloging in Publication Data

Willis, William D 1934-
  Sensory mechanisms of the spinal cord.

  Bibliography: p.
  Includes index.
  1. Spinal cord. 2. Senses and sensation. 3. Afferent pathways. 4. Spinal cord —
Localization of functions. I. Coggeshall, Richard E., 1932-   joint author. II.
Title.
QP374.W54   612′.8   78-15764
ISBN 0-306-40083-9

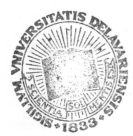

QP
374
.W54

© 1978 Plenum Press, New York
A Division of Plenum Publishing Corporation
227 West 17th Street, New York, N.Y. 10011

Printed in the United States of America

To the Beginning Student of the Nervous System

Preface

The goal of this monograph is to provide an overview of current thought about spinal cord mechanisms for sensory processing. We hope that the book will be useful both to basic neuroscientists and to clinicians.

Some historical aspects of the problem and a few definitions are treated in the first chapter. The second chapter reviews the organization of the peripheral nervous system from the standpoint of sensory receptors and primary afferent axons. The third chapter is concerned with what is known about the structure of the dorsal horn, while the fourth chapter considers the activity of dorsal horn interneurons. The clinical, behavioral, and neurophysiological evidence for what parts of the cord white matter contain particular sensory pathways is discussed in Chapter 5, and details about the various pathways in the dorsal columns, the dorsolateral fasciculus, and the ventral quadrant form the subject matter of Chapters 6 through 8. The final chapter is an attempt to summarize what is presently known about the receptors and the spinal cord pathways responsible for the sensations of touch–pressure, flutter–vibration, pain, temperature, position sense and visceral sensation and about descending control systems.

The authors wish to thank the following publishers and journals for permission to reproduce illustrations: *Acta Physiologica Scandinavica,* Raven Press Publishers, *The American Journal of Psychology, Anatomical Record, Archives of Neurology & Psychiatry, Archives of Surgery,* Hart-Davis Educational Limited (Granada Publishing, Limited), *Brain, Brain Research, British Medical Bulletin, Experimental Brain Research, Experimental Neurology,* Springer-Verlag, Consejo Superior de Investigaciones Cientificas, Instituto Ramon y Cajal, *Journal of Anatomy, The Journal of Comparative Neurology, Journal of Neurophysiology, Journal of Neurocytology, Journal of Physiology,* Williams & Wilkins Publishing Co., International Publishers in Science & Medicine, *Neuroscience, Neuroscience Letters, Pain,* Charles C. Thomas, Publisher, *Physiological Reviews, Proceedings of the Japan Academy, Quarterly Journal of Experimental Physiology, Ltd. & Cognate Medical Sciences, Research in Physiology, Science,* Pergamon Press, Ltd., and Georg Thieme Verlag.

We would also like to acknowledge the considerable and unfailing efforts of Gail Silver (photography), Elizabeth Perez (bibliography), Phyllis Waldrop, Pat Williamson, and Carolyn Holt (typing).

Contents

Chapter 4

Functional Organization of Dorsal Horn Interneurons 129

Chapter 5

Ascending Sensory Pathways in the Cord White Matter...... 167

Chapter 6

Sensory Pathways in the Dorsal Columns 197

Chapter 7

Sensory Pathways in the Dorsolateral Fasciculus 261

Chapter 8

Sensory Pathways in the Ventral Quadrant 301

Chapter 9

The Sensory Channels 363

1   Introduction

SPECIFICITY VERSUS PATTERN THEORIES OF SENSATION

The way in which the nervous system differentiates between the various forms of sensory experience has been a central issue since the beginnings of sensory physiology. A brief history of the major theories is given by Sinclair (1967). The notion of specificity of cutaneous sensation can be attributed to Bell (1811), and the idea was forwarded by Müller's doctrine of specific nerve energies (Müller, 1840–1842). However, Müller had in mind the Aristotelean five senses and lumped together the sensations derived from the body surface under the category of "touch." According to Sinclair (1967), Volkmann extended the specificity concept in 1844 to include the postulate of separate nerve endings for each variety of sensation arising from cutaneous stimulation.

Evidence supporting the notion that the doctrine of specific nerve energies applied to the different cutaneous senses came from the observations of Blix (1884), who discovered that stimulation of separate localized points on the skin give rise to distinct sensations of touch, warmth, cold or pain. This observation was confirmed by numerous other investigators, including Goldscheider and Donaldson (Donaldson, 1885). Specificity was shown by the fact that a cold spot, for instance, could be stimulated by cold, but not by heat, and that even if it were stimulated by an electric current, the sensation aroused was still of cold. Mapping of marked areas of skin proved that the sensory spots were in fixed positions that could be identified on subsequent days with a high degree of accuracy (Fig. 1.1), provided that care was taken to avoid a number of sources of technical error (Dallenbach, 1927). The spotlike distribution of mechanically and thermally sensitive areas suggested that each spot was associated with a specific sen-

1

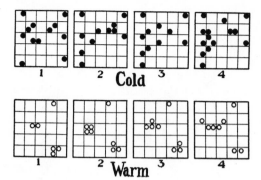

Fig. 1.1. Maps of the distribution of cold and warm spots within an area of 1 cm in a single subject. The maps were made on four different days (1–4). The cold spots were mapped first and then the warm spots during a given session. (From Dallenbach, 1927.)

sory receptor organ. Histologists had begun to describe a variety of cutaneous sense organs (Krause, 1859; Meissner, 1859; Ruffini, 1894), and so it was reasonable for von Frey (1906, 1910) to suggest that each type of sensory spot was associated with a particular kind of sense organ. From his knowledge of the distribution of the sense organs at that time, von Frey proposed that touch is produced by activation of hair follicles in hairy skin and by Meissner's corpuscles in glabrous skin, cold by Krause's end-bulbs, warmth by Ruffini endings, and pain by free endings.

The match suggested by von Frey between particular sensory receptors and the sensory spots was shown to be incorrect in the cases of Ruffini endings and Krause's end-bulbs (Donaldson, 1885; Dallenbach, 1927; Weddell, 1941; 1955; Weddell and Sinclair, 1953; Lele and Weddell, 1956, 1959; Weddell and Miller, 1962). The function of the Ruffini endings of the skin is now known to be tactile, since these are equatable with type II slowly adapting receptors (M. R. Chambers, *et al.*, 1972). The function of Krause's end-bulbs has recently been clarified. These receptors are rapidly adapting mechanoreceptors (Iggo and Ogawa, 1977). It now appears that thermal sensibility, like pain, is due to activation of free endings, although the nature of the receptor membrane is different for the different kinds of free endings (Dallenbach, 1927; Andres and Düring, 1973; Burgess and Perl, 1973; Hensel, 1973a).

The criticisms by Weddell and his colleagues of von Frey's theory were directed not so much at the notion of sensory spots as at the histological correlations of the spots. But they point out that it is unlikely that a naturally occurring stimulus applied to a sensory spot activates only a single afferent fiber, since a stimulus to just 1 mm² of skin could affect more than one hundred underlying endings (Weddell and Miller, 1962). This criticism loses force if the differential sensitivity of the endings is taken into account. Recent evidence indicates that stimulation of individual sensory receptors, such as a Pacinian corpuscle or a type I (Merkel disk, touch corpuscle) ending can result in evoked potentials in the cerebral cortex, activation of spinal cord neurons, and behavioral responses (McIntyre *et al.*, 1967; Tapper and Mann, 1968; Tapper, 1970; Mann *et al.*, 1972; P. B. Brown *et al.*, 1973). On the other hand, it appears that single or even a few impulses in nociceptive afferents does not lead to the perception of pain in humans (Torebjörk and Hallin, 1974). Furthermore, the application of a stimulus of less than 100 mg by a probe with a diameter of 0.5–1 mm will excite ten to fifteen sensitive mechanoreceptor afferents in cat hairy skin (Burgess *et al.*, 1974). Thus, touch and pain spots are likely to be complex entities involving at least a small number of afferents, and touch spots are associated with a variety of receptor types in addition to those known to von Frey (see Burgess and Perl, 1973).

Another theory of cutaneous sensation is the pattern theory. Nafe (1927, 1929) suggested that a sensation results from a physiological pattern of input from the skin that is usually, but not necessarily always, associated with a particular kind of stimulus. Learning provides the name for the sensation associated with the stimulus. Specific sensory channels are not needed, just particular spatial and temporal patterns of nerve impulses in the central nervous system. This theory was supported by Sinclair (1955) and by Weddell (1955).

With the recent strengthening of the evidence that the sensory receptors are specific, a compromise theory has been proposed in which specific information from the sense organs generates a patterned activity centrally. The model of Melzack and Wall (1965) is known as the "gate theory" of pain. However, the details of the spinal cord gate circuit have been challenged, as discussed in Chapter 4.

Clinical evidence suggests that the sensory pathways in the central nervous system are specific, since dissociations of sensation can be produced either by disease processes such as the Brown–Sequard syndrome, or by therapeutic intervention, as in cordotomy for the relief of pain. However, Melzack and Wall (1962) point out that a lesion placed in the spinal cord white matter can affect sensory transmission in a number of ways in addition to the possible interruption of a specific sensory pathway. For example, a lesion will reduce the numbers of tract neurons capable of responding to sensory input; furthermore, the pattern of activity in the ascending pathways will be altered. Another important consideration is that descending pathways from the brain that control the activity of sensory pathways may be interrupted, with a consequent change in the operation of the sensory pathways.

EPICRITIC VERSUS PROTOPATHIC SENSATIONS

Brief consideration should be given to the proposal of Head and his colleagues (Head, 1920) that the cutaneous senses can be divided into two broad categories—protopathic and epicritic. The protopathic system, according to their view, mediates pain and the extremes of temperature sensation, while the epicritic system is responsible for touch, size discrimination, two-point discrimination, and also the detection of small thermal gradients. The experimental basis for the proposal was the introspective analysis of sensory changes in an area of skin after denervation and during regeneration of the cut nerve. Head himself was the experimental subject. Many of the observations and most of the interpretations of this experiment have been contested (Trotter and Davis, 1909; Boring, 1916; Walshe, 1942; Weddell *et al.* 1948), and the hypothesis should be laid to rest. However, perhaps because of the appeal of the terminology (cf. Walshe, 1942), the protopathic–epicritic dichotomy lingers. In fact, the terminology is sometimes applied to central nervous system pathways, such as the spinothalamic tract and the dorsal column pathway, despite the fact that Head clearly stated that the information conveyed by the two proposed systems in the periphery became intermingled centrally.

LEMNISCAL VERSUS NONLEMNISCAL SYSTEMS; LARGE- VERSUS SMALL-FIBER SYSTEMS

The notion of Head (Head, 1920) that somatic sensory functions can be described in terms of a dual system of epicritic and protopathic sensory mechanisms has been replaced more recently by two other dualities—lemniscal versus nonlemniscal systems and large- versus small-fiber systems.

The lemnsical versus nonlemniscal nomenclature was developed by Poggio and Mountcastle (1960, 1963) to describe the response properties of neurons in the thalamus to cutaneous stimulation. Lemniscal responses have the following attributes: the thalamic neurons have small, contralateral receptive fields; the kinds of effective stimuli are restricted, indicating that only one or a few kinds of sensory receptors are involved; and synaptic transmission is secure, so the cells can follow relatively high stimulus rates. Nonlemniscal responses have the following traits: the thalamic cells have large, often bilateral receptive fields; they receive convergent input from different kinds of receptors; and they are unable to follow repetitive stimulation well. The assumption was made that the lemniscal neurons of the thalamus, in recordings from the ventrobasal complex, were activated by the dorsal column-medial lemniscus pathway, whereas the nonlemniscal neurons, whose activity was recorded from other parts of the thalamus, including the posterior nuclear complex, were excited by the spinothalamic tract (Poggio and Mountcastle, 1960). This nomenclature has recently been criticized (Boivie and Perl, 1975), since the spinothalamic tract projects not only to the posterior nuclei, but also to the ventral posterior lateral nucleus (VPL), whereas the dorsal column nuclei project not only to VPL, but also to the posterior nuclei. Both the dorsal column path and the spinothalamic tract have neurons with response properties that will fit one category or the other (as do neurons in other sensory paths as well). Boivie and Perl (1975) suggest that the terms "lemniscal" and "nonlemniscal" be replaced by "specified" and "unspecified," although they warn that "unspecified" may simply reflect ignorance about the role of the neuron.

The other duality often cited in current literature is the notion of large-fiber versus small-fiber systems (Noordenbos, 1959; Melzack and Wall, 1965). The implication is that the large-fiber system has to do with innocuous forms of mechanoreception, whereas activation of the small-fiber system is required for pain. Interactions occur between inputs over large versus small fibers to central neurons, and the central nervous system determines from the outcome of the interactions whether or not a stimulus is painful. The difficulty with this nomenclature is that it tends to obscure the fact that both large- and small-fiber groups in cutaneous nerves contain the axons from a variety of receptors. Although most nociceptors have small axons, there are a number of kinds of receptors having small axons that are not nociceptors. These include sensitive mechanoreceptors and specific thermoreceptors (Burgess and Perl, 1973; Hensel, 1973a). Consequently, it is dangerous for experimenters to make the assumption that the results of stimulation of small fibers should necessarily be attributed to the activation of nociceptors.

SENSORY MODALITIES

According to Boring (1942), the term "sensory modality" was introduced by Helmholtz. A modality is a class of sensations connected by qualitative continua. Although Müller (1840–1842) regarded the general sense of "feeling" or "touch" derived from skin stimulation as an entity, following Aristole's classification of the five senses, most later investigators considered touch (or pressure), cold, warm, and pain as discrete modalities. A given sensory modality would have a number of characteristics or "attributes," such as quality, intensity, duration, and extension. On the basis of subjective awareness and also of clinical and psychophysical testing, a number of sensory modalities pertaining to the sensory experiences resulting from stimulation of the skin or of subcutaneous tissue may be recognized. These include touch, pressure, flutter, vibration, tickle, warmth, cold, pain, itch, position sense, and kinesthesia. Pain may be subdivided into several submodalities, including sharp or fast pain and burning, aching, or slow pain. More complicated somatic sensations, perhaps involving combinations of these modalities, are also of interest, especially in clinical testing. These include two-point discrimination, stereognosis, graphesthesia, and the abnormal sensations called paresthesias. Visceral sensations include the awareness of distention, hunger, nausea, and pain.*

SENSORY CHANNELS

The transmission of information that the brain interprets as a particular form of sensation is through neural discharges along one or more sensory pathways. Transection of the spinal cord completely abolishes any awareness of sensation from regions of the body below the transection. Interruption of one or more of the sensory pathways may partially or totally eliminate particular kinds of sensory experience.

The mechanism for transmission of information concerning a particular modality of sensation can be defined as a sensory channel. A sensory channel would include one or more sets of sensory receptors, one or more sensory pathways, and particular regions of the thalamus and cerebral cortex that are involved in receiving and processing the information. Activity in a sensory channel would be under the control of descending pathways.

The first part of this book will be concerned with the organization of the peripheral nervous system and spinal cord. Then, the sensory pathways in the spinal cord will be discussed, along with the kinds of information they carry. Their descending control will also be consid-

---

* Geldard (1953) cites Boring's list of sensory modalities—pressure, contact, deep pressure, prick pain, quick pain, deep pain, warmth, cold, heat, muscular pressure, articular pressure, tendinous strain, appetite, hunger, thirst, nausea, sex, cardiac sensation, pulmonary sensation—and adds itch, tickle, vibration, suffocation, satiety, and repletion.

ered. Portions of at least some sensory channels will be discussed in the last chapter.

CONCLUSIONS

1. The specificity theory of cutaneous sensation was originally based on the discovery of localized sensory "spots" that respond specifically to cold, warm, tactile, or painful stimuli.

2. The correlation of cold spots with Krause's end-bulbs and of warm spots with Ruffini endings proved to be incorrect. Krause's end-bulbs and Ruffini endings are tactile receptors, as are several other kinds of sensory endings. Specific thermoreceptors appear to have free endings with specialized membranes, as do nociceptors.

3. Stimulation of a sensory spot is likely to activate a number of sensory receptors, although it is true that in some instances a single afferent fiber can evoke behavioral or sensory events.

4. A pattern theory of cutaneous sensation does not require a high degree of specificity of sensory receptors or of central nervous system pathways. It is also possible to develop theories of sensation that accept an admixture of specific and nonspecific elements.

5. Lesions that affect sensory pathways can do so by reducing the total number of neurons conveying information to the brain, by altering the pattern of activity in ascending pathways, and by changing the operation of the control systems that originate in the brain and that regulate activity in sensory pathways.

6. Head's theory of the epicritic and protopathic divisions of the peripheral nervous system should be discarded.

7. The terms "lemniscal" and "nonlemniscal" should not be used to distinguish between activity evoked over the dorsal column pathway and that evoked by the spinothalamic tract. Better terms are needed to classify neurons that have the contrasting response properties that characterize many neurons in the somatosensory pathways (small, contralateral receptive fields; restricted convergence; secure synaptic coupling versus large, bilateral receptive fields; wide convergence; and weak synpatic coupling).

8. The subdivision of afferent fibers into large and small systems is misleading, since sensory receptors of a variety of types fall into each of these subdivisions. Small fibers, for example, are not equatable with pain afferents.

9. Sensory modalities are classes of sensation. A large number of

cutaneous, subcutaneous, and visceral sensory modalities can be recognized.

10. A sensory channel is the sensory mechanism responsible for conveying the information needed for recognition of a sensory modality. A sensory channel would include one or more sets of sensory receptors, one or more ascending pathways, regions of the thalamus and cerebral cortex, and also the descending pathways that modify the ascending activity.

2 Peripheral Nerves, Sensory Receptors, and Spinal Roots

COMPOSITION OF PERIPHERAL NERVES

Peripheral nerves are composed of the axons of sensory and motor neurons, along with the investing connective tissue sheaths (endoneurium, perineurium, and epineurium) (see Landon, 1976). The axons may be myelinated or unmyelinated. In cutaneous nerves, the largest axons belong to the A$\alpha\beta$ class (Erlanger and Gasser, 1937), while the small myelinated fibers belong to the Aδ group. A$\alpha\beta$ fibers conduct at 30–100 m/s, and Aδ fibers at 4–30 m/sec (Boivie and Perl, 1975). Unmyelinated afferents are often designated C fibers; they conduct at less than 2.5 m/s (Gasser, 1950). Joint and visceral nerves share the terminology of cutaneous nerve axons. However, a different terminology is used for muscle nerves. The myelinated fibers are subdivided into groups I, II, and III (Lloyd and Chang, 1948), conducting at 72–120, 24–71, and 6–23 m/s, respectively (Hunt, 1954). Muscle nerves also contain numerous unmyelinated, or group IV, afferents (Stacey, 1969), conducting at less than 2.5 m/s.

For at least the large myelinated fibers, it is possible to predict the conduction velocity in meters per second by multiplying the axon diameter (in micrometers), including the myelin sheath, by a factor of 6 (Hursh, 1939). A factor of 4.5 is more accurate for small myelinated fibers (Arbuthnott *et al.*, 1975).

ELECTRICAL STIMULATION OF PERIPHERAL NERVES

The threshold for exciting axons with an electrical stimulus is an inverse function of axonal diameter. The larger the fiber, the lower the threshold. In many experimental studies, advantage is taken of this property of axons to allow a selection of the population of axons that is activated by graded electrical stimuli. The strength of stimulation is commonly expressed as a multiple of the threshold of the largest axons of the nerve (e.g., 1.5T means one and a half times the threshold of the most excitable axon in the nerve).

In some nerves, it is possible to evoke a volley essentially in one class of afferent fibers by an electrical stimulus near threshold. For instance, stimuli below 1.3T applied to the sural nerve of the rabbit activate an almost pure population of axons belonging to type I slowly adapting receptors, and stimulation of the posterior tibial nerve of the same animal at strengths up to 1.5T will activate just guard-hair afferents (A. G. Brown and Hayden, 1971). Group Ia afferents from muscle spindle primary endings can often be activated essentially exclusively by weak stimuli applied to the nerves of the hamstring or quadriceps muscles in the cat (Bradley and Eccles, 1953; J. C. Eccles *et al.*, 1957). However, in general, electrical stimuli will coactivate afferents from more than one class of receptor. This is certainly the case when the "flexion reflex afferents" are stimulated. These include cutaneous afferents of all sizes, plus high-threshold muscle and joint afferents; such afferents tend to excite flexor motoneurons and to inhibit extensor motoneurons, the pattern of the flexion reflex (R. M. Eccles and Lundberg, 1959a).

Another approach to the use of electrical stimulation of cutaneous nerves is to excite either the $A\alpha\beta$ fibers alone, these plus the $A\delta$ fibers, or all of the A fibers plus the C fibers. The assumption often seems to be that the $A\alpha\beta$ fibers all belong to mechanoreceptors, whereas many of the $A\delta$ and C fibers connect with nociceptors, and any central effects may reflect activity either in the mechanoreceptive afferents or in the nociceptive ones. However, several reservations must be kept in mind about this approach. For example, some nociceptors have axons that conduct at velocities over 30 m/s (Burgess and Perl, 1967; Georgopoulos, 1976), and these may be included in an $A\alpha\beta$ volley. Small-fiber groups include mechanoreceptor and thermoreceptor afferents, as well as nociceptors, and care must be exercised before a central action can be attributed to just the nociceptors. Finally, activation of the whole spectrum of afferents is complicated by the fact that the volley in the largest fibers will reach the spinal cord before the volley in the smallest fibers. The central neural circuits activated by the largest fibers may cause an alteration of the effects that would otherwise have been produced by the smallest afferents. This problem can be circumvented by use of anodal blockade of the large-fiber volley (e.g., Brown *et al.*, 1975). However, the problem of the admixture of impulses in fibers of different function remains. This problem is usually dealt with by the use of more natural forms of stimulation to activate particular receptor types selectively in order to determine the central affects of specific classes of sensory receptors. The properties of the various types of somatic and visceral receptors will be discussed in the next section.

SENSORY RECEPTORS

Although the characteristics of sensory receptors of the body have been amply reviewed elsewhere (Matthews, 1972; Burgess and Perl, 1973; Hensel, 1973a, 1974; Boivie and Perl, 1975; Price and Dubner, 1977), it is necessary to provide a brief description of them here as background for later descriptions of the effects evoked by the different receptors in central neurons.

The sensory receptors can be grouped by their location—skin, skeletal muscles, joints, and viscera. The groups will be discussed in this order. A summary of the main types and their response properties is given in Table 2.1.

Cutaneous Receptors

Receptors in the skin (and the adjacent subcutaneous connective tissue) include mechanoreceptors, nociceptors, and thermoreceptors.

Mechanoreceptors. Cutaneous mechanoreceptors are most readily activated by mechanical changes in the skin. They are sometimes also affected by thermal changes, but the thermal responses are not appropriate to be significant in thermoreception (Werner and Mountcastle, 1965; Duclaux and Kenshalo, 1972). Noxious stimuli produce no greater excitation than do innocuous ones (Burgess and Perl, 1973).

The cutaneous mechanoreceptors can be classified in any of several ways. The adaptation rate to a maintained stimulus is one approach (Adrian and Zotterman, 1926a,b; Adrian, 1928). Slowly adapting receptors tend to continue discharging in a repetitive fashion so long as the stimulus is continued (Fig. 2.1). On the other hand, rapidly adapting receptors discharge only at the time that a stimulus is applied (or removed).

Another approach to the classification of mechanoreceptors is ac-

TABLE 2.1

Receptor type	Best stimulus	Signal	Background activity	Conduction velocity (m/s)
Cutaneous mechano-receptors Type I	Indentation of dome	Displacement and velocity	None	A. G. Brown and Iggo, 1967 Cat: 57.2 ± 0.99 (33–95) Rabbit: 47.3 ± 1.77 (16–96) Burgess et al., 1968 Cat: 65 (47–84) Tapper et al., 1973 Cat: 63.6 ± 2.3 Perl, 1968 Monkey: 46 ± 4, 51 ± 2 Knibestöl, 1975 Human: 58.7 ± 2.3
Type II	Skin deformation	Displacement and velocity	Sometimes	A. G. Brown and Iggo, 1967 Cat: 53.6 ± 2.21 (20–100) Rabbit: 31.4 ± 2.40 (24–45) Burgess et al., 1968 Cat: 54 (39–68) Perl, 1968 Monkey: 34 ± 12, 40 ± 10 Knibestöl, 1975 Human: 45.3 ± 3.6
G_2 (and T) hair	Movement of guard (or tylotrich) hair or of skin	Velocity	None	A. G. Brown and Iggo, 1967 Cat T: 68 ± 2.72 (44–72) Rabbit T: 35.6 ± 1.7 (8–53) Burgess et al., 1968 Cat G_2: 53 (39–73) Perl, 1968 Monkey G_2: 36 ± 14, 42 ± 16

D hair	Movement of down or guard hairs or skin	Velocity; very low threshold	None	A. G. Brown and Iggo, 1967 Cat: 17.9 ± 0.23 (15–24) Rabbit: 9 ± 0.2 (5–16) Burgess and Perl, 1967 Cat: 18.3 (11–30) Burgess et al., 1968 Cat: 21 (15–32) Perl, 1968 Monkey: 16 ± 6, 19 ± 6
Field	Skin indentation	Velocity; to some extent displacement	None	Burgess et al., 1968 Cat: 55 (36–72) Perl, 1968 Monkey: 39 ± 13, 39 ± 8
C mechanoreceptor	Skin indentation	Velocity (slow); to some extent displacement	None	Iggo, 1960 Cat: (0.55–1.25) Bessou et al., 1971 Cat: (0.5–1.0)
Meissner's corpuscle and Krause's end-bulb	Skin indentation	Velocity	None	Jänig et al., 1968a Cat: 50% >60 Iggo and Ogawa, 1977 Cat: 36.1 ± 6.2 Talbot et al., 1968 Monkey: (40–80) Knibestöl, 1973 Human: 55.3 ± 3.4 (26–91)
G_1	Rapid movement of guard hair or of skin	Transients	None	Burgess et al., 1968 Cat: 75 (56–85) Perl, 1968 Monkey: 47 ± 12, 49 ± 13
Pacinian corpuscle	Vibration	Transients	None	Hunt and McIntyre, 1960b Cat: (54–84) Burgess et al., 1968 Cat: 65 (54–82)

(continued)

TABLE 2.1. (*continued*)

Receptor type	Best stimulus	Signal	Background activity	Conduction velocity (m/s)
Cutaneous nociceptors				
Aδ mechanical	Damage to skin	Threat or damage	None	Jänig et al., 1968a Cat: 50% >57 Perl, 1968 Monkey: 41±8, 56±11 Knibestöl, 1973 Human 46.9±3.6 (34–61) Fitzgerald and Lynn, 1977 Rabbit: 15 (5–32.5) Cat: 27 (5.5–49) Burgess and Perl, 1967 Cat: (6–51) Burgess et al., 1968 Cat: (6–65) Perl, 1968 Monkey: 25±11, 21±13 Georgopoulos, 1976 Monkey: (4–44)
C mechanical	Damage to skin	Threat or damage	None	Bessou and Perl, 1969 Cat: (0.6–1.4) Georgopoulos, 1976 Monkey: (most 0.8–1)
Aδ heat	Noxious heat or mechanical damage	Threat or damage	None	Iggo and Ogawa, 1971 Monkey: (3.9–6.8) Georgopoulos, 1976 Monkey: (4–40)
Aδ and C cold	Severe cold; mechanical damage	Threat or damage	None	Georgopoulos, 1976 Monkey: (4–40, 0.8–1)

Receptor	Stimulus		Response	References

C polymodal	Noxious heat; sometimes severe cold; mechanical damage; algesic chemicals	Threat or damage	None	Bessou and Perl, 1969
				  Cat: (0.4–1.1)
				Beck et al., 1974
				  Cat: (0.4–1.8)
				Croze et al., 1976
				  Monkey: (0.6–1.1)
				Van Hees and Gybels, 1972
				  Human: 0.89 (0.66–1.1)

Cutaneous thermoreceptors
  Cold
	Reduced temperature	Cooling	Yes	Iriuchijima and Zotterman, 1960
				  Rat: (0.5–1.0)
				Hensel et al., 1960
				  Cat: (0.6–1.5)
				Perl, 1968
				  Monkey: 8 (4–14)
				Iggo, 1969
				  Monkey, baboon: (<1.5–15.3)
				  Dog (lip): (9–18)
				  Rat: (<1.5)
				Hensel and Iggo, 1971
				  Monkey: 5.8±2.5 (2.2–9.5),
				  0.7±0.3 (0.3–1.3)
				Darian-Smith et al., 1973
				  Monkey: 14.5 (5–31)
				R. R. Long, 1977
				  Monkey
				    Glabrous: 13.3±2.8
				    Hairy: 7.0±2.8
				    Junction: 10.8±3.1

Warm	Increased temperature	Warming	Yes	Iriuchijima and Zotterman, 1960
				  Rat: (0.7–1.5)
				Hensel et al., 1960
				  Cat: (0.84 for 1 fiber)

(continued)

TABLE 2.1.(*continued*)

Receptor type	Best stimulus	Signal	Background activity	Conduction velocity (m/s)
				Hensel and Iggo, 1971
				Monkey: 0.7 ± 0.2 $(0.4–0.9)$
				Duclaux and Kenshalo, 1978
				Monkey: (0.8 ± 0.09)
				Konietzny and Hensel, 1975
				Human: $(0.5–0.75)$
Muscle mechanoreceptors				
Muscle spindle primary ending	Change of spindle length and rate of change	Length and velocity	Sometimes	Hunt, 1954 Cat: 72–120
Muscle spindle secondary ending	Change of spindle length	Length	Sometimes	Hunt, 1954 Cat: 24–72
Golgi tendon organ	Change of muscle length or contraction	Tension	Sometimes	Hunt, 1954 Cat: 72–120
Pacinian corpuscle (see above)				
Muscle nociceptors				
Group III	Pressure; damage	Pressure; threat or damage	None or slight	Paintal 1960 Cat: (6–91, mostly 10–15) Mense and Schmidt, 1974 Cat: <2.5
Group IV	Pressure; damage	Threat or damage	Little	Franz and Mense, 1975 Cat: <2.5
Joint mechanoreceptors				
Ruffini ending	Flexion or extension (to extremes)	Joint pressure	Only at extreme positions	Burgess and Clark, 1969b Cat: (20–70) Clark, 1975 Cat: (9–77)
Golgi tendon organ (see above)				

Receptor		Adequate stimulus		Rhythm/spontaneous activity	Reference and conduction velocity (m/sec)
Paciniform ending (see Cutaneous mechanoreceptors, Pacinian corpuscle)					
Joint nociceptors	Aδ	Extreme bending	Threat or damage	—	Burgess and Clark, 1969b Cat: 12–33
	C	Unknown	—	—	Clark and Burgess, 1975 Cat: <30
Visceral mechanoreceptors					
Intestine		Distension, tension on mesentery or blood vessels (intestine)	Movement	May have respiratory, cardiovascular or gastrointestinal rhythm	Bessou and Perl, 1966 Cat: (2–21) Ranieri et al., 1973 Cat: (0.6–5) Clifton et al., 1976 Cat: Aδ or <2.5 Morrison, 1977 Cat: (0.6–30) Dog: (0.5–36)
Bladder		Distension or contraction	Tension	Maybe	Winter, 1971 Cat: (<2–>22) Clifton et al., 1976 Cat: Aδ
		Distension	Volume	Maybe	Clifton et al., 1976 Cat: <2.5
		Mesenteric Pacinian corpuscles	Vibration	May have cardiac rhythm	Ranieri et al., 1973 Cat: (61–70)
Visceral nociceptors		Intense mechanical, thermal, and chemical stimuli	Threat or damage	Little or none	Clifton et al., 1976 Cat: <2.5

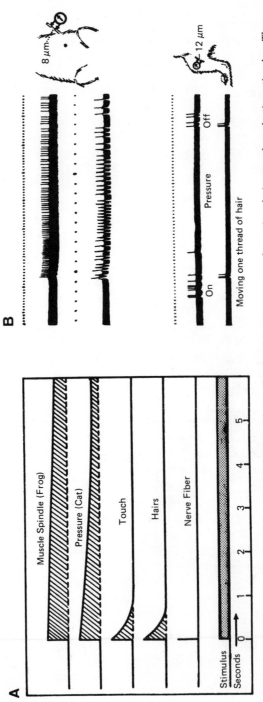

Fig. 2.1. A. The durations of the responses of slowly and rapidly adapting receptors are shown in relation to a long-lasting stimulus. The nerve fiber discharges just once at the start of the stimulus. (From Adrian, 1928). B. Illustration of the discharges of an afferent from a slowly adapting tactile receptor (above) and of an afferent from a rapidly adapting hair follicle receptor (below). Time marks 10 ms. (From Maruhashi *et al.*, 1952.)

cording to the most likely property of the stimulus for which they code (Burgess and Perl, 1973). For slowly adapting cutaneous mechanoreceptors, this may be the amount of indentation of the skin. The discharge rate of such receptors would then be a function of skin displacement (Fig. 2.2). Rapidly adapting receptors might signal the rate at which the skin is displaced (stimulus velocity) or some higher derivative of skin position (acceleration, jerk). Thus, the number of discharges that occur when such receptors are activated is a function of stimulus velocity, acceleration, or jerk (Fig. 2.3). Receptors signaling acceleration or jerk can be lumped together as transient detectors. Sometimes a given receptor will behave as if it signalled two properties of the stimulus. For instance, the slowly adapting, or "static," response of a displacement detector might be preceded by a velocity-sensitive "dynamic" response (Fig. 2.4C). Such a receptor would signal both velocity and displacement.

Cutaneous Displacement and Velocity Detectors. Two kinds of slowly adapting cutaneous mechanoreceptors have been described; both signal displacement and velocity. They are usually referred to as type I and type II slowly adapting mechanoreceptors, but each has synonyms.

Type I slowly adapting mechanoreceptors are associated with Merkel-cell complexes. Merkel cells are specialized cells in the epidermis adjacent to the basement membrane. Afferent nerve terminals contact the Merkel cells. The sense organs take the form of domelike structures in some animals (Fig. 2.4A), including the cat (also the rabbit, mouse, rat, and guinea pig), but domes are difficult to demarcate in the skin of primates (including man). These morphological features give rise to alternative names—Merkel cell ending, tactile dome, touch corpuscle. (For details about the structural features of type I receptors, see Merkel, 1875; Pinkus, 1964; Munger, 1965; Smith, 1968, 1970; Iggo and Muir, 1969; Straile, 1969; Jänig, 1971a,b.)

In the absence of a stimulus, type I endings are normally silent. However, they discharge following indentation of the skin directly over the ending with a low threshold (less than 15 μm). They are relatively insensitive to displacement of the skin immediately adjacent to the dome and to skin stretch. A step-displacement stimulus produces a dynamic response followed by a static response (Fig. 2.4C). The discharges during the static response occur at irregular intervals. A given afferent can supply as many as seven separate domes, although more commonly there are two or three branches. (For more information about type I endings, see Frankenhaeuser, 1949; Maruhashi *et al.*, 1952; Witt and Hensel, 1959; Hunt and McIntyre, 1960a; Tapper, 1965; Werner and Mountcastle, 1965; Burgess *et al.*, 1968; Perl, 1968; Iggo

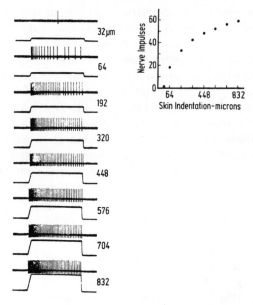

Fig. 2.2. Discharges of a slowly adapting cutaneous mechanoreceptor (type II) in response to a graded series of indentations of the skin are shown to the left. The graph at the right is an input–output curve relating the number of impulses to skin indentation in microns. (From Harrington and Merzenich, 1970.)

and Muir, 1969; Harrington and Merzenich, 1970; Hagbarth *et al.*, 1970; Horch *et al.*, 1974; Whitehorn *et al.*, 1974; see also Fig. 9.1.)

Type II slowly adapting mechanoreceptors have been identified with Ruffini endings (Fig. 2.4B) (Ruffini, 1894; Chambers *et al.*, 1972). These endings are located in the dermis. There is generally one low-threshold spot for each type II fiber. They may show a background discharge in the absence of an overt stimulus, and they respond to small displacements of the skin either directly over the receptors (threshold ≤15 μm) or as a result of stretch of the skin from a distance. The discharge has both dynamic and static responses to step displacements of skin, but the responses are smaller than is typical of the type I receptor (Fig. 2.4C). The discharges of type II endings are quite regular during the static response, in contrast to the type I receptor. (See Burgess *et al.*, 1968; Perl, 1968; Harrington and Merzenich, 1970; Hagbarth *et al.*, 1970; Chambers *et al.*, 1972; see also Figs. 9.1 and 9.2.)

Cutaneous Velocity Detectors.   There are at least five kinds of cutaneous sensory receptors that detect stimulus velocity. Four of these are found in hairy skin; these include G_2 hair-follicle receptors (and T hair-follicle receptors), D hair-follicle receptors, field receptors, and C mechanoreceptors. The velocity detector in glabrous skin is Meissner's corpuscle in primates (including man) and Krause's end-bulb in the cat.

Hair follicles of many mammals can be subdivided into three types—tylotrichs, guard hairs, and down hairs (Noback, 1957; Straile, 1960, 1961). Tylotrichs are the largest and least numerous of the hair types. Guard hairs are smaller than tylotrichs. Tylotrichs and guard hairs arise individually from follicles. Down hairs are the smallest type of hair; they are wavy; and they arise in groups from single follicles.

The afferent fibers supplying guard-hair follicles can be subdivided into two groups, based on their response properties. G_1 hair-

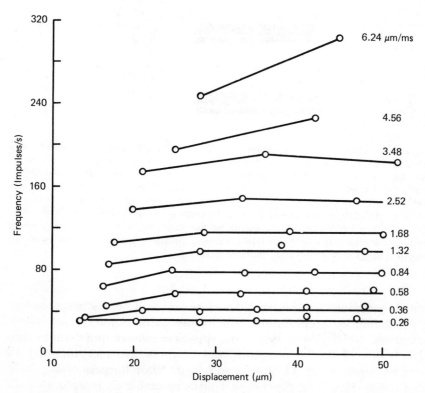

Fig. 2.3. Input–output curves for a rapidly adapting receptor (T hair follicle unit) that signals stimulus velocity. The stimuli were constant-velocity displacements of the hair. The graph shows the instantaneous frequency of the afferent at different amounts of displacement for a series of stimuli applied over a range of velocities. The family of curves indicates that the discharge rate is constant for a given stimulus velocity over much of the range and that the discharge rate is a function of stimulus velocity. (From A. G. Brown and Iggo, 1967.)

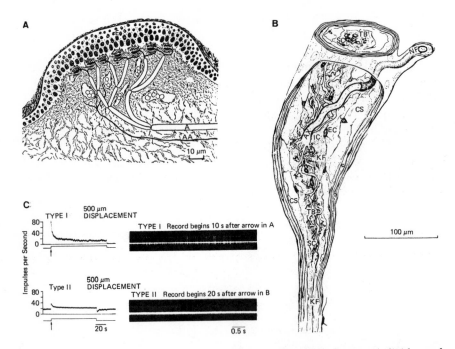

Fig. 2.4. A. Drawing of the structure of a type I ending. The afferent (A) divides and ends in relation to a series of Merkel cells in the base of the epidermis in a tactile dome. An adjacent unmyelinated axon (AA) is also shown. (From Iggo and Muir, 1969.) B. Drawing of a Ruffini, or type II, ending. (From M. R. Chambers *et al.*, 1972.) C. The responses of typical type I and II endings. The histograms at the left show the dynamic and static responses of the endings to step indentations of the skin. The characteristic discharge patterns during the static responses of the two types of endings are seen at the right. For type I endings, the discharges are irregular, while for type II endings they are regular. (From Burgess *et al.*, 1968.)

follicle receptors are transient detectors and will be discussed below. G_2 hair-follicle receptors are velocity detectors. Some T hair-follicle receptors, which supply tylotrichs, appear to behave in a manner similar to that of the G_2 receptors, and so these two receptors will be lumped together (A. G. Brown and Iggo, 1967; Burgess *et al.*, 1968; Perl, 1968). However, other type T units resemble G_1 receptors (A. G. Brown and Iggo, 1967).

G_2 (and T) hair follicle receptors respond to the velocity of hair movement (Fig. 2.5B); thresholds in the cat to ramp movements of individual hairs are 0.5–1.5 μm/ms; when the stimulus is applied to the skin, the threshold is less than 0.05 μm/ms. While the hair is moved gently, there is a steady discharge. However, no discharge occurs during a maintained stimulus. A given afferent supplies some ten or so guard hairs (Burgess *et al.*, 1968).

D hair follicle receptors also signal stimulus velocity (Fig. 2.5A), but their thresholds are lower than those of G_2 receptors (for hair movement, responses are first seen with ramp stimuli of 0.1–1.0 μm/ms). These receptors are extremely sensitive and can be activated by movement of either down hairs or of guard hairs. There is no discharge in the absence of an overt stimulus, but very small movements of the skin will activate them (A. G. Brown and Iggo, 1967; Burgess *et al.*, 1968; Perl, 1968; Merzenich and Harrington, 1969). They may appear to be slowly adapting when activated by a hand-held stimulator, perhaps because of repeated stimulation by physiological tremor.

Field receptors can be distinguished from hair-follicle receptors by the fact that they cannot be activated by movements of single hairs. They are excited by brushing large numbers of hairs, probably by mechanical stimulus spread to the underlying skin. Direct stimulation of the skin, along with hair movement, is the best stimulus. The morphology of the field-receptor sense organ is unknown. Field receptors signal stimulus velocity and have low thresholds to ramp stimuli (0.1–1.0 μm/ms). Some field receptors have a tendency to continue to discharge during a maintained discharge; several categories of field receptors (F_1, intermediate, F_2) can be distinguished on the basis of gradations between rapidly or slowly adapting responses (Burgess *et al.*, 1968; Perl, 1968; Burgess and Perl, 1973).

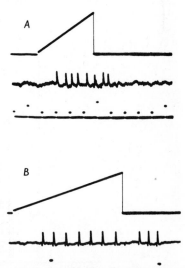

Fig. 2.5. Responses of hair follicle receptors to ramp displacements of single hairs. (A) The activity was produced in a type D hair-follicle receptor, (B) type T hair-follicle receptor. The responses that follow the termination of the stimulus were "off" responses. (From A. G. Brown and Iggo, 1967.)

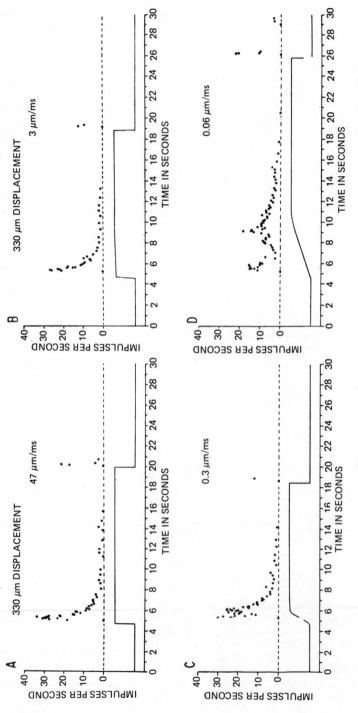

Fig. 2.6. Responses of a C mechanoreceptor to indentation of the skin at different velocities. (From Bessou *et al.*, 1971.)

C mechanoreceptors are sensitive mechanoreceptors that have un-myelinated afferent fibers. They respond to skin indentation, but they are especially sensitive to stimuli that move slowly across the receptive field. They signal chiefly velocity, although there is a tendency for their discharge to continue during a maintained stimulus (Fig. 2.6) (Iggo, 1960; Bessou et al., 1971). Following cessation of stimulation, there may be an after-discharge. (For additional detail, see Zotterman, 1939; Douglas and Ritchie, 1957; Iggo, 1960; Iriuchijima and Zotterman, 1960; Bessou and Perl, 1969; Bessou et al., 1971; Iggo and Korn-huber, 1977). C mechanoreceptors are not distributed universally. They are not found in the pad of the cat's foot (Bessou et al., 1971; Beck et al., 1974) nor in the glabrous skin of the monkey hand (Georgopoulos, 1976), and they have not yet been identified in recordings from human subjects (Van Hees and Gybels, 1972; Torebjörk, 1974).

In the glabrous skin, there appears to be just a single velocity-sensitive receptor. The morphology of this receptor varies, even within a single species (Malinovský, 1966). However, it appears that the receptor, which is often called a rapidly adapting, or RA, receptor, can be identified with Meissner's corpuscle (Fig. 2.7A) in the primate (including human) glabrous skin (see Figs. 9.8 and 9.9; Meissner, 1859; Cauna, 1956; Cauna and Ross, 1960; Munger, 1971; Quilliam, 1975) and with Krause's end-bulb in the cat foot and toe pads (Krause, 1859; Lynn, 1969; Jänig, 1971a,b; Iggo and Ogawa, 1977). Meissner's corpuscles and Krause's end-bulbs are likely to be variants of the same ending, and both may be morphological equivalents for glabrous skin to hair follicle endings (Malinovský, 1966; Munger, 1971). Golgi–Mazzoni corpuscles resemble Krause's end-bulbs and Meissner's corpuscles (Chouchkov, 1973); presumably they have comparable functional properties.

The glabrous-skin velocity detector or RA receptor is one of two kinds of rapidly adapting receptor that respond to stimuli applied to the glabrous skin; the other is the Pacinian corpuscle (PC receptor), which is a transient detector and is discussed below.

The RA receptor has a localized receptive field, and its threshold in the skin of the cat is low (often less than 10 μm of indentation; ramp thresholds average 2 μm/ms); there is no discharge during a maintained stimulus (Jänig et al., 1968a; Jänig, 1971b; Iggo and Ogawa, 1977). The RA receptors in primate glabrous skin have similar properties, although their thresholds seem to be higher than in the cat. They are activated best when repetitive stimuli at rates of 5–40 Hz are used (Fig. 2.7A) (for further detail, see Lindblom, 1965; Talbot et al., 1968; Knibestöl, 1973; K. O. Johnson, 1974).

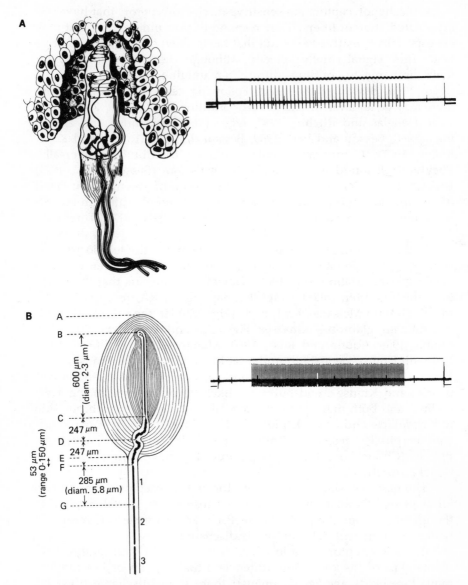

Fig. 2.7. A. Structure of a Meissner corpuscle (From Quilliam, 1975). Recording (right) is from an afferent supplying a rapidly adapting receptor in the glabrous skin of the monkey's finger. The stimulus was a sinusoidal indentation of the skin at 40 Hz, 18 μm. (From Talbot *et al.*, 1968.) B. Structure of a Pacinian corpuscle (From Quilliam and Sato, 1955). Recording (right) is from the afferent supplying a PC receptor. The stimulus was a sinusoidal indentation of the palmar surface of a monkey's hand at 150 Hz, 19 μm. (From Talbot *et al.*, 1968.)

Cutaneous Transient Detectors.   There are two types of cutaneous receptors that are designed to detect transients—G_1 hair-follicle receptors and Pacinian corpuscles. G_1 hair-follicle receptors are activated by rapid movements of guard hairs, especially the longest ones (the threshold-to-ramp stimuli exceed 80 μm/ms when single hairs are moved and are 5–20 μm/ms when the skin is stimulated (Burgess *et al.*, 1968).

Pacinian corpuscles are subcutaneous receptors that are very sensitive to mechanical transients resulting from cutaneous stimulation. The capsule of the Pacinian corpuscle (Fig. 2-7B) serves as a mechanical filter, allowing mechanical transients to affect the terminal but preventing lower-frequency mechanical events from doing so. (For details about the structure, distribution, and mechanical properties of Pacinian corpuscles, see Vater, 1741; Pacini, 1840; Quilliam and Sato, 1955; Pease and Quilliam, 1957; Cauna and Mannan, 1958; Hubbard, 1958; Loewenstein and Skalak, 1966; Malinovský, 1966; Lynn, 1969; see also Fig. 9.8.) Pacinian corpuscles adjacent to the interosseous membrane or beneath the pads of the cat's foot are extraordinarily sensitive. They can be activated by hair movement, as well as by stimuli applied to the skin; the threshold to indentation is often less than 1 μm (Hunt and McIntyre, 1960b; Hunt, 1961; Jänig *et al.*, 1968a; Lynn, 1969, 1971). Pacinian corpuscles are activated best by frequencies of vibration in the range of 60–300 Hz (Fig. 2.7B) (Talbot *et al.*, 1968), but they can follow 500 Hz or even higher frequencies (Hunt, 1961; Burgess *et al.*, 1968). Pacinian corpuscles do not appear to project by way of cutaneous nerves in the monkey, although they do in cats (Merzenich and Harrington, 1969). PC afferents have been recorded from in human subjects and have properties similar to those in cats and monkeys (Knibestöl, 1973).

Cutaneous Nociceptors.   Nociceptors respond to stimuli that threaten to damage or that actually damage tissue. Receptors that respond at threshold to moderate pressure are included in the nociceptive category, since they respond progressively more as stimulus intensity is increased, with the greatest response to damaging stimuli. Some nociceptors in the skin respond just to intense mechanical stimuli. There are two categories of mechanical nociceptor—Aδ and C, named according to the sizes of the afferent fibers supplying them. Other cutaneous nociceptors respond to various combinations of intense mechanical, thermal, and chemical stimuli. These receptors include Aδ heat nociceptors, Aδ and C cold nociceptors, and C polymodal nociceptors.

Aδ mechanical nociceptors (plus low-sensitivity and moderate-pressure mechanoreceptors) are excited best by mechanical stimuli

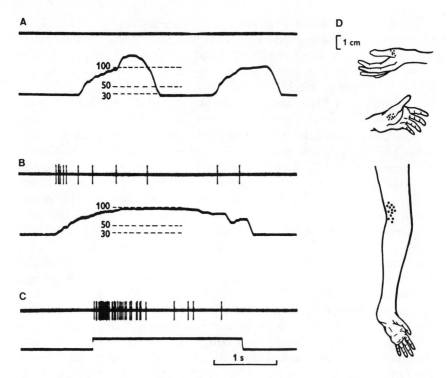

Fig. 2.8. A–C. The responses of an Aδ mechanical nociceptor in the glabrous skin of a monkey to pressure or to damaging stimuli. In A there was no response to pressure by a probe with a 2.2-mm tip diameter (numbers indicate force applied), whereas in B there was a response when pressure was applied by a needle tip. In C the stimulus was pinching with a serrated forceps.   D. Receptive fields of three different Aδ mechanical nociceptors in the skin of the monkey. The receptive fields consist of a set of punctate spots separated by insensitive zones. (From Perl, 1968.)

that damage the skin (Fig. 2.8) (Burgess and Perl, 1967; Perl, 1968). Thresholds for these receptors vary; some have thresholds that are clearly in the innocuous range. The receptive field of a single afferent consists of a set of small spots (Fig. 2.8C) distributed over an area of about 2 cm². There is no response to noxious heat or to intense cold, nor is there one to algesic chemicals (Burgess and Perl, 1967; Burgess et al., 1968; Perl, 1968; Beck et al., 1974; Georgopoulos, 1976). However, repeated applications of noxious heat stimuli may sensitize these receptors to heat (Fitzgerald and Lynn, 1977). The morphology of these as well as other nociceptors is unknown; it is presumed that the terminals of nociceptors are free endings and that the specificity of the responses of different types of nociceptor depends upon the particular membrane properties of each (and perhaps in part upon the investing tissues).

Mechanical nociceptors with unmyelinated afferent fibers have also been described. These C mechanical nociceptors have properties similar to those of the Aδ mechanical nociceptors, although the receptive fields are smaller (Iggo, 1960; Bessou and Perl, 1969; Beck et al., 1974; Georgopoulos, 1976). It is possible that some of these receptors are the same as the C cold nociceptors (see below), since adequate cold stimuli may not always have been used in characterizing them (Bessou and Perl, 1969).

Aδ heat nociceptors respond well both to noxious heat stimuli (greater than 45°C) and to intense mechanical stimuli. Thresholds can be in the innocuous range. Some of these receptors also respond to intense cold. (See Iggo and Ogawa, 1971; Beck et al., 1974; Georgopoulous, 1976, 1977.) Aδ fibers that can be activated by noxious mechanical, heat, and cold stimuli may be considered to be Aδ polymodal nociceptors, similar to the C polymodal nociceptors (see below); however, the sensitivity of such units to chemical agents needs to be assessed before a complete parallelism can be established (Georgopoulos, 1977).

Aδ and C cold nociceptors respond both to extreme cold and to intense mechanical stimuli (Iggo, 1959; Bessou and Perl, 1969; Georgopoulos, 1976, 1977).

C polymodal nociceptors are an abundant receptor type, especially in primates. They respond well to noxious mechanical, thermal, and chemical stimuli (Fig. 2.9) (Bessou and Perl, 1969). As for many other nociceptors, threshold stimuli may be in the innocuous range. The effective thermal stimuli are noxious heat (greater than 45°C) and sometimes intense cold. Effective chemical stimuli include topical application of acid or injections of algesic chemicals. (For more detail, see Iggo, 1959; Iriuchijima and Zotterman, 1960; Fjällbrant and Iggo, 1961; Bessou and Perl, 1969; Van Hees and Gybels, 1972; Beck and Handwerker, 1974; Beck et al., 1974; Torebjörk, 1974; Georgopoulos, 1976, 1977; Handwerker and Neher, 1976; Croze et al., 1976; see also Figs. 9.16 and 9.17.)

Cutaneous Thermoreceptors. Two kinds of receptors in the skin signal innocuous changes of temperature. These specific thermoreceptors include cold receptors and warm receptors. Thermoreceptors do not (or only poorly) respond to mechanical stimuli. As already mentioned, the discharges of several kinds of mechanoreceptors can be affected by innocuous temperature changes (Werner and Mountcastle, 1965; Iggo, 1969; Hahn, 1971; Duclaux and Kenshalo, 1972; Booth and Hahn, 1974), but there is no compelling evidence that such alterations

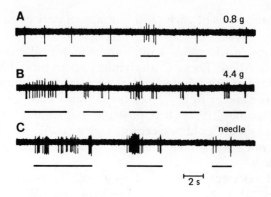

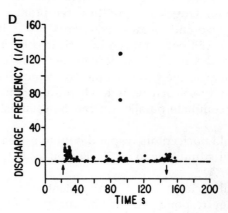

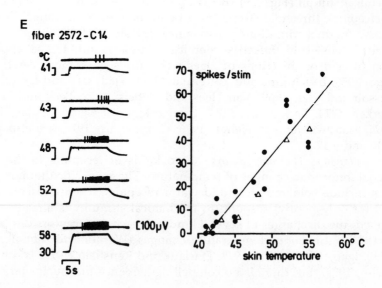

play a role in thermoreception (however, cf. Poulos and Lende, 1970b; Burton *et al.*, 1972).

The morphology of cold receptors has been found to differ from that of other free endings (Fig. 2.10) (Hensel, 1973a; Hensel *et al.*, 1974). The afferents from cold receptors may be myelinated or unmyelinated; they are chiefly myelinated in man (Fruhstorfer *et al.*, 1974).

Cold receptors are activated by changes in skin temperature as small as 0.1°C. They show a background discharge at normal skin temperature. With cooling, there is an increase in discharge rate, with both a dynamic and a static response (Fig. 2.11). The dynamic response signals the rate at which the temperature is changed, while the static response signals the temperature level. Static discharges are seen at temperatures from 5 to 43°C (Fig. 2.12). The maximum static discharge occurs between about 18–34°C. (For further information about cold receptors, see Hensel and Boman, 1960; Hensel *et al.*, 1960; Iriuchijima and Zotterman, 1960; Perl, 1968; Iggo, 1969; Hensel and Iggo, 1971; Darian-Smith *et al.*, 1973; Hellon *et al.*, 1975; Pierau *et al.*, 1975; Dykes, 1975; Kenshalo and Duclaux, 1977; see also Fig. 9.22.) It is of interest that the static discharge rate is the same for pairs of temperature readings above and below the optimum temperature. Cold receptors tend to have a bursting pattern of discharge in the lower range of temperatures (Fig. 2.11) (Dodt, 1952), and it has been suggested that this bursting may permit the central nervous system to distinguish between temperatures above and below the optimum (Iggo, 1969; Poulos, 1971; Dykes, 1975). The coding for static temperature by bursts in cold fibers may be more important for thermoregulation than for thermal perception (Dykes, 1975). Noxious heat may also evoke a discharge in cold receptors, the "paradoxical cold response" (Dodt and Zotterman, 1952b); this depends in part upon the core body temperature (Long, 1977).

The morphology of warm receptors is unknown, but they are presumed to be free endings. Warm receptors are a distinctly separate group from cold receptors. They are active at normal body tempera-

---

Fig. 2.9. In A are shown the responses of a C polymodal nociceptor to stimulation with a von Frey filament bending with a force of 0.8 g. A greater response is shown in B, when the stimulus was a 4.4 g von Frey filament. A needle that penetrated the skin was used for C. The discharge produced in a C polymodal nociceptor by the application of dilute acid to the skin is shown in D. (A-D are from Bessou and Perl, 1969.) In E are the responses of a C polymodal nociceptor to graded thermal stimuli. The relationship between discharges produced by each stimulus and skin temperature is shown by the graph at the right. (From Beck *et al.*, 1974.)

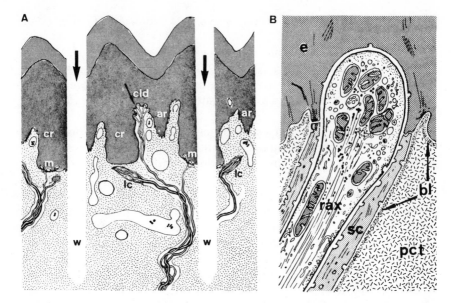

Fig. 2.10. Schematic representation of structure of a cold receptor (in cat's nose). A. The large arrows represent wire holes (w), which marked the location of the receptor. The cold receptor (cld; small arrow) is at the top of a dermal papilla. Other receptors are also present (Merkel cell, m; lamellated receptors, lc). The epidermal columnar ridge (cr) and adhesive ridge (ar) are indicated.   B. A magnified view of the cold receptor. The receptor axon (rax), Schwann cell (sc), epidermis (e), papillary connective tissue (pct), and basal lamina (bl) are labeled. (From Hensel et al., 1974.)

ture. Their discharge slows with cooling of the skin, and it accelerates with warming, reaching a maximum at temperatures of about 45°C (Fig. 2.12). However, warm receptors are silenced by noxious levels of heat (above 48°C). They have unmyelinated axons. (For additional detail, see Dodt and Zotterman, 1952a; Hensel et al., 1960; Iriuchijima and Zotterman, 1960; Martin and Manning, 1969, 1972; Iggo, 1969; Hensel and Iggo, 1971; Stolwijk and Wexler, 1971; Pierau et al., 1975; Hellon et al., 1975; Konietzny and Hensel, 1975; Handwerker and Neher, 1976; Duclaux and Kenshalo, 1978; see also Fig. 9.22.)

Muscle Receptors

Receptors in and around skeletal muscles include the stretch receptors (muscle spindles, Golgi tendon organs) and pressure–pain endings (Barker, 1962) with either myelinated or unmyelinated afferents. There are also Pacinian corpuscles in fascial planes; these respond like the ones found in subcutaneous tissue (see above).

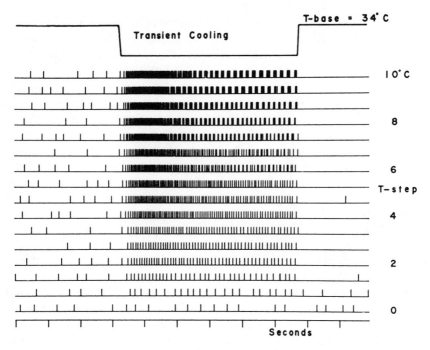

Fig. 2.11. Responses recorded from the afferent supplying a cold receptor following graded cooling pulses. (From Darian-Smith *et al.*, 1973.)

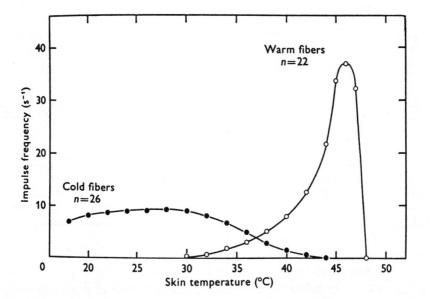

Fig. 2.12. Average static discharge rates for populations of cold and warm receptors. (From Hensel and Kenshalo, 1969.)

Stretch Receptors. The structure and function of the stretch receptors have been reviewed thoroughly by Matthews (1972). No attempt will be made here to provide an inclusive reference list for these important receptors. (For a bibliography of recent literature, see Eldred *et al.*, 1977.)

Muscle spindles have two types of sensory endings—primary and secondary. The primary ending of a muscle spindle is supplied by a large myelinated fiber classified as group Ia (Fig. 2.13). The ending is responsive both to the rate of stretch of the spindle (dynamic response) and to the new length (static response). The sensitivity of the dynamic response is set, in part, by the activity of dynamic fusimotor fibers (Bessou *et al.*, 1968). The secondary endings are supplied by afferent fibers of intermediate size, the group II fibers. Secondary endings show little dynamic responsiveness; instead, they have just a static response, which signals spindle length. Static responsiveness is controlled, in part, by static fusimotor fibers (Appelberg *et al.*, 1966).

Golgi tendon organs are located in the dense connective tissue of muscle tendons and aponeuroses. Their afferents are large myelinated fibers classified as group Ib. They respond at a high threshold to muscle stretch (Fig. 2.13B), but at a low threshold to the contraction of motor units ending on the tendon slip containing the receptor (Fig. 2.13D) (Houk and Henneman, 1967). Golgi tendon organs signal tension. There is only a small dynamic response to stretch (Fig. 2.13B).

Pressure–Pain Endings. There are numerous free endings in the fascia and in the adventitia of blood vessels of muscles. These form as much as 75% of the sensory innervation of skeletal muscle (Stacey, 1969). Some free endings are supplied by myelinated afferent fibers (group III), while others are supplied by unmyelinated (group IV) fibers. A few free endings are connected with afferents larger than group III (Paintal, 1960; Stacey, 1969).

Group III afferents can be excited by mechanical stimuli applied either directly to the muscle or indirectly through the tendon. However, there is no maintained discharge in response to prolonged stretch of the muscle. Threshold stimuli range from gentle pressure to frankly damaging pressure (Paintal, 1960; Bessou and Laporte, 1961). Group III afferents can also be activated by intraarterial injections of algesic chemicals (Mense, 1977; Kumazawa and Mizumura, 1977b; see also Hnik *et al.*, 1969) and by thermal stimuli applied to the muscle belly (Hertel *et al.*, 1976; Kumazawa and Mizumura, 1977b). Another effective stimulus is the injection of hypertonic sodium chloride solution into the muscle (Paintal, 1960).

Group IV muscle afferents are in general similar in their response properties to group III afferents, except that their thresholds to me-

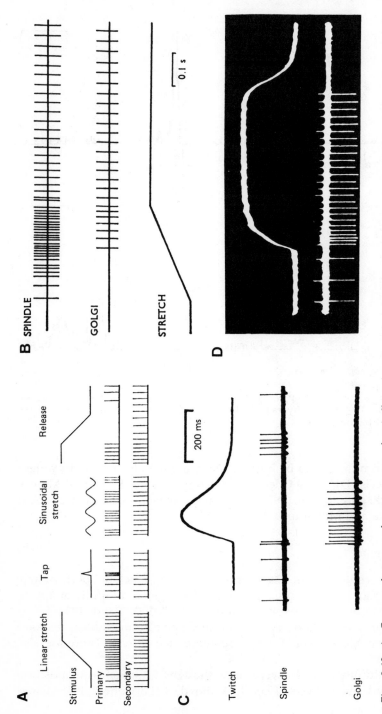

Fig. 2.13. A. Contrast between the responses of spindle primary and secondary endings to ramp stretch, tap, and sinusoidal stretch. B. Comparison of the responses of a muscle spindle primary ending and a Golgi tendon organ to a ramp stretch of skeletal muscle. C. Unloading of a muscle spindle afferent and the discharge of a Golgi tendon organ during a twitch contraction of the muscle. D. Activation of a Golgi tendon organ by stimulation of a single motor unit. (From Matthews, 1972.)

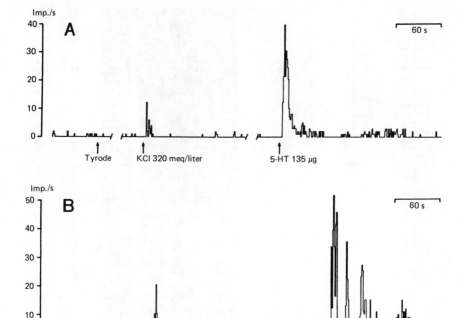

Fig. 2.14. Responses of a group IV muscle afferent to the intraarterial injection of algesic chemicals (5-HT = 5-hydroxytryptamine; Brad. = bradykinin; Hist. = histamine). (From Mense and Schmidt, 1974.)

chanical stimuli tend to be higher. Many are readily activated by algesic chemicals (Fig. 2.14) (Mense and Schmidt, 1974; Franz and Mense, 1975; Fock and Mense, 1976; Hiss and Mense, 1976; Mense, 1977; Kumazawa and Mizumura, 1977b).

Joint Receptors

The receptor types associated with joints include both slowly adapting (Golgi tendon organs, Ruffini endings) and rapidly adapting (paciniform) mechanoreceptors (Gardner, 1944; I. A. Boyd, 1954; Skoglund, 1956). The Golgi tendon organs and paciniform endings respond like comparable endings found elsewhere (see above). There are also nociceptors.

The Ruffini endings were once thought to signal joint position (I. A. Boyd and Roberts, 1953; I. A. Boyd, 1954; Cohen, 1955; Skoglund, 1956, 1973). However, it has been shown that these endings are seldom active at intermediate positions of the joint (at least for the cat knee joint), and so it is unlikely that they signal position (Fig. 2.15). Instead, they appear to signal the torque that develops as the joint is extended, flexed, or rotated to the extreme of its range (Burgess and Clark, 1969b; McCall et al., 1974; Clark and Burgess, 1975; Clark, 1975; Grigg, 1975; 1976; Grigg and Greenspan, 1977).

Joint nociceptors have not been studied in detail. However, many of the Aδ fibers supplying joints respond only when intense, often damaging stimuli are applied (Burgess and Clark, 1969b; F. J. Clark and Burgess, 1975; F. J. Clark, 1975).

Visceral Receptors

A variety of receptor types has been identified in viscera. Only those that enter the spinal cord will be considered here. These gain access to the cord either by way of the splanchnic nerves and sympathetic chain or by way of the pelvic parasympathetic nerves. Some enter the cord over the ventral roots. The receptor types include mechanoreceptors, nociceptors, and possibly thermoreceptors.

Visceral mechanoreceptors include Pacinian corpuscles located in the mesentery and in connective tissue around visceral organs (Sheehan, 1932). They behave like Pacinian corpuscles elsewhere, except that it has been noted that they sometimes discharge in phase with the heartbeat; it is not known if signals from these receptors are of consequence in cardiovascular regulation (Gammon and Bronk, 1935; Gernandt and Zotterman, 1946).

Other visceral mechanoreceptors have been found associated with the mesentery, the serosal surface of the gut or of other organs, and along blood vessels (Bessou and Perl, 1966; Ranieri et al., 1973; Paintal, 1957; Todd, 1964; Morrison, 1973, 1977; Floyd and Morrison, 1974; Floyd et al., 1976; Clifton et al., 1976). They appear to respond to movements or to distention of the viscera. However, the discharges do not signal intraluminal pressure or volume with precision, since the receptors are activated at a distance from the contractile region (Morrison, 1977). Another type of visceral mechanoreceptor seems to be inserted in series with smooth muscle and responds either to distention or to contraction of the muscle; such receptors are typical of the bladder (Iggo, 1955; Winter, 1971; cf. Floyd et al., 1976).

Visceral nociceptors have been described (Gernandt and Zotterman, 1946; Lim et al., 1962; Peterson and Brown, 1973; Kumazawa and Mizumura, 1977a). One type that has been found recently has multiple spotlike receptive fields in the mucosal lining of the rectal canal (Fig.

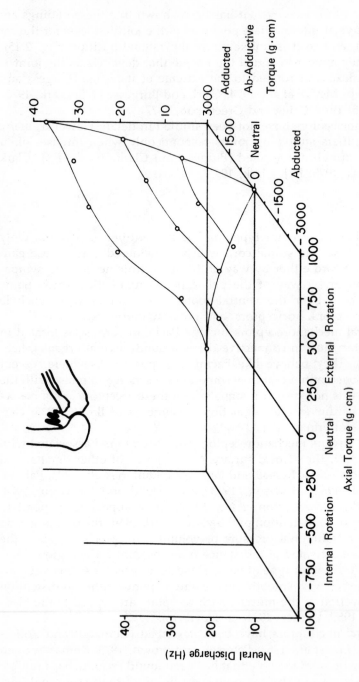

Fig. 2.15. Discharge rate of a slowly adapting joint afferent in response to axial and abductive torque applied to the knee joint. (From Grigg, 1975.)

2.16). This receptor has an unmyelinated axon and it responds to noxious mechanical, thermal, and chemical stimuli, thus resembling the C polymodal nociceptors of the skin (Clifton *et al.*, 1976).

Thermoreceptive responses have been recorded from afferent units supplying the abdominal wall (Riedel, 1976).

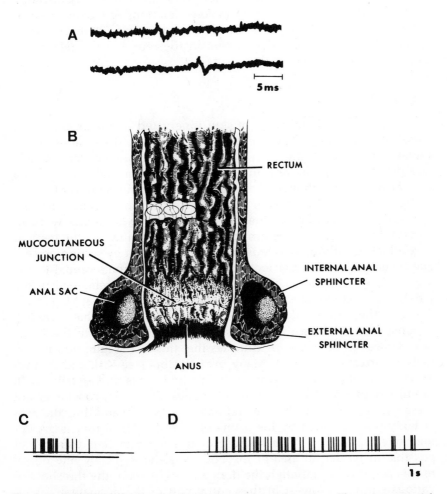

Fig. 2.16. Responses of a C mucosal receptor supplying the rectum. The action potential recorded from a ventral root filament with two sets of electrodes is shown in A. The conduction delay indicated that the afferent was unmyelinated. The receptive field consisted of several punctate zones on the rectal mucosa, as shown in B. The responses to pinch and to cold water are illustrated in C and D. (From Clifton *et al.*, 1976.)

THE DORSAL ROOT

The axons of each dorsal root are thought to be the sensory channels for one segment of the body wall. The axons in each root travel centrally to the spinal cord, where they are said to bifurcate into cranial and caudal branches, and collaterals of these branches pass to various parts of the spinal gray matter. Two facets of the organization of the dorsal roots are important in considerations of sensory mechanisms in the spinal cord: (1) the dermatomes and (2) the reported segregation of small and large fibers in the root and the relation of these fibers to the tract of Lissauer.

Dermatomes

A dermatome is that area of skin innervated by the axons of one dorsal root. The importance of the dermatomes in discussions of the spinal cord is that the spinal roots and dermatomes are widely regarded as among the best indicators of the segmental nature of the spinal cord. Although there were several earlier nineteenth century investigations as to the areas of skin supplied by dorsal roots, the first satisfactory delineation of the dermatomes came from the work of Sherrington (1893, 1898). Sherrington's strategy, known as the method of residual sensitivity, was to isolate one dorsal root by sectioning several (usually three) dorsal roots cranial and three roots caudal to the root under consideration. The area of sensation that remained in the otherwise anesthetic area that resulted was the dermatome. Maps were drawn of the different dermatomes, and it was assumed that each dermatome resulted from the sensory axons that remained in the intact root. However, recent work indicates that this last assumption is partially incorrect (see below). Many investigators (see Kirk and Denny-Brown, 1970, for references) used the method of residual sensitivity to produce dermatomal maps for many species. The major conclusions of these studies were: (1) that the dermatomes overlap and thus the area of body wall supplied by the axons of a single dorsal root is greater than one segment, (2) that because of this overlap, it is usually not possible to render an area of the body anesthetic if only one dorsal root is cut, (3) that although the dermatomes overlap, the threshold to various stimuli is lowest in the central part of the dermatomal field, and (4) that the dermatomes for the limbs do not extend to the midline of the body. A corollary of point 4 is that axial lines are found in the extremities. Axial lines result when dermatomes from discontinuous spinal levels abut. The axial lines are located at the dorsal and ventral midlines, and for the upper extremity the line occurs between segments C4 and T2 and for the lower extremity between segments L3 and S3. Other methods for determining dermatomes are: (1) the reflex method of vasodilatation, (2) the measurement of sensitive skin areas after herpes zoster infection, (3) the application of strychnine to spinal segments, (4) the measurements of dorsal root potentials, and (5) the locations of sensory levels after spinal cord section (see Kirk and Denny-Brown, 1970, for references). The results from these studies are in general agreement with the original conclusions of Sherrington, except for the observation that the method of reflex vasodilatation produced dermatomes somewhat smaller than those produced by the method of residual sensitivity.

Prior to the work of Denny-Brown *et al.* (1973), the major study with conclusions that differed significantly from the above was that of Keegan and Garrett (1948), who studied patients with dermatomal symptoms due to invertebral disk compression of spinal roots. Keegan and Garrett stated that all dermatomes extended to the midline dorsally, thus denying the presence of dorsal axial lines, and they also stated that the "primitive" dermatomes did not overlap. This work has been criticized on several grounds, however, and most people accept the formulations of Sherrington rather than those of Keegan and Garrett.

Another study, that of Denny-Brown *et al.* (1973), although not disagreeing with the results of Sherrington (1893, 1898), greatly extended his work to the extent that a profound reevaluation of ideas concerning the organization of the dermatomes will probably be necessary. Denny-Brown *et al.* (1973) sectioned the roots distal to the ganglion rather than proximal as all other investigators had done and showed that the size of each dermatome was enlarged. Strychnine also greatly enlarged the size of each dermatome, but cutting six roots on either side of an isolated root resulted in a smaller dermatome than by Sherrington's method of cutting three roots. These size differentials were traced to a mechanism involving the fibers in the lateral and medial parts of Lissauer's tract and were felt to be facilitation or inhibition of the first synapse in the dermatomal pathway by primary afferent fibers from different segments (Denny-Brown *et al.*, 1973). Another implication of the study by Denny-Brown *et al.* (1973) is that axons in any particular dorsal root spread over at least five segments of the body, or to say it another way, any point on the body is innervated by axons from at least five different dorsal roots. The maximal size of any particular dermatome seems to come when (1) the neighboring dorsal roots are sectioned distal to the ganglia, (2) when strychnine is given to the animal, or (3) when the lateral part of Lissauer's tract is cut. Thus, a dermatome is not a simple sensory pattern that is

the result of the anatomic distribution of the sensory axons of a particular dorsal root. Instead, the size of the dermatome and probably also
the quality of the sensation is determined by an interaction of primary
sensory fibers from various segments with neurons whose axons are in
Lissauer's tract (Denny-Brown *et al.*, 1973). Furthermore, although the
dorsal roots appear to be segmental structures, the segmental nature of
the dermatomes is blurred by a great deal of overlap and what appears
to be a very important interaction of primary afferents from different
segments. It is obvious that much further work needs to be done, but
the studies of Denny-Brown and colleagues indicate the danger in taking too simplistic a view of the segmental nature of the spinal cord,
and they reemphasize the necessity of understanding the organization
and synaptic interconnections of the primary afferent fibers if we are
to understand what it means to say that the spinal cord is a segmental
structure.

*In summary, the dermatomes have been demonstrated by many tech-
niques, including the method of residual sensitivity of Sherrington, and
published maps of them are available. Each dermatome has been assumed to
represent the distribution of primary afferent axons from one dorsal root,
but recent work has shown this assumption to be incorrect. Various manip-
ulations, such as cutting the medial or lateral parts of the tract of Lissauer
or administering strychnine, greatly change the size of the dermatome, as
measured clinically, and this probably implies that the size of the dermatome, and possibly the quality of sensation, is determined in part by a
synaptic interaction of primary afferent fibers.*

The Large and Small Fiber Divisions of the Dorsal Roots

One of the early observations on the gross anatomy of the spinal
cord is that each dorsal root breaks up into a group of small rootlets or
fascicles, which in turn attach to the spinal cord. In 1886, Lissauer
noted that the axons in the proximal parts of each rootlet were not ran-
domly distributed in regard to size, but that the small myelinated
axons congregated on the lateral side of the rootlet as it entered the
cord, leaving the larger axons in central and medial parts of the rootlet.
Lissauer further noted that the small lateral fibers passed to the apex of
the posterior horn, thus forming the pathway that bears his name,
whereas the larger fibers passed centrally to travel in the dorsal columns. The importance of these findings was emphasized when Ranson and his collaborators published a series of studies on Lissauer's
tract that are of fundamental importance in present understanding of
spinal cord organization.

Ranson (1914) confirmed Lissauer's findings but noted that un-myelinated fibers, which are much more numerous than the smallest myelinated fibers, also are segregated in the lateral parts of each root-let. Ranson further stated that smallest myelinated and unmyelinated axons entered only the medial parts of the tract of Lissauer and that the remaining axons in the medial part of the tract and all the axons in the lateral part of the tract were endogenous (had their cell bodies in the spinal cord). Ranson suggested that impulses indicating "pain" were carried by unmyelinated fibers. On this basis, Ranson sub-divided the axons of the dorsal root into two systems, a medial large-fiber dorsal-column system, primarily concerned with fine touch, and a lateral small-fiber system involved with the tract of Lissauer and substantia gelatinosa that was primarily concerned with pain. He regarded touch as "epicritic" sensation and pain as "protopathic" sen-sation (see Chapter 1), but he realized in later years that these con-cepts were oversimplifications. Ranson and Billingsley (1916) stated that cutting the lateral side of the dorsal root, where the small myelinated and unmyelinated fibers were located, abolished several types of be-havior and reflexes that were associated with pain. By contrast, cutting the medial part of the root had no such effect. This formulation was undoubtedly the forerunner of the lemniscal and extralemniscal categories of central nervous system sensory transmission (see Chap-ter 1).

The notion that there is a segregation of large and small fibers in the dorsal roots has been confirmed in a general way by many inves-tigators (Ingvar, 1927; O'Leary et al., 1932; Szentágothai, 1964; Sindou, et al., 1974; Kerr, 1975a). It has also been denied or at least modified by several others. Among those who disagreed with Ranson's formu-lation are Earle (1952), who stated that the fine fibers were mixed with other fibers in the root and the subdivisions medial and lateral apply primarily to Lissauer's tract rather than to the fibers in the roots, and Wall (1962), who felt that Ranson had confused the fine fibers in the dorsal roots with dorsal deflections of fibers in Lissauer's tract.

The most detailed examination of the fine fiber–coarse fiber sub-division of the dorsal root has been done by Snyder (1977), who exam-ined serial sections of the dorsal root–spinal cord junction in light and electron microscopes. He found that there was almost no segregation of fine and coarse fibers in the cat, but there was some in the rhesus monkey. Unfortunately, however, it would probably be almost impos-sible to interrupt the fine fibers surgically and also leave the coarse fibers intact, even in the monkey. Thus, although the formulation of Ranson is confirmed by many, others deny it, and the most detailed study indicates that, although there is some segregation of coarse and fine fibers in the monkey, it would probably be impossible to section either type of fiber without damaging the other.

If it is accepted that it is probably impossible to destroy the fine fibers selectively by cutting the lateral edge of the entering dorsal rootlet, then Ranson's physiological results, which indicated that a cat so treated did not respond to painful stimuli, must be explained. Wall (1962) suggested that Ranson's results were probably due to infarction of the dorsal horn rather than to cutting of the fine fibers in the dorsal roots. Sindou et al. (1974) agreed with Wall (1962) and attributed the lessening of spastic symptoms that follow dorsal rhizotomy to this vascular damage that occurs when dorsal roots are cut. Thus, the view that Ranson's physiological results depend primarily on vascular damage rather than sectioning a specific nerve fiber bundle would probably be accepted at the present time.

In summary, early investigators, particularly Ranson, stated that fine fibers congregated on the lateral side of each entering dorsal rootlet. The fine fibers were regarded as passing to the tract of Lissauer, the coarse fibers to the posterior white columns. This finding has been confirmed in a general way by some investigators and denied by others, but it seems clear that the fine fiber-coarse fiber separation is not such that the fine fibers can be selectively lesioned. Accordingly the results of Ranson and his colleagues who correlated absence of responses to painful stimuli with selective damage to the fine fiber primary afferent system are no longer accepted. Instead, the physiological results are thought to be due to an infarction of part of the dorsal horn due to interference with the spinal blood vessels that enter the spinal cord along the dorsal roots.

THE VENTRAL ROOT

The ventral root is usually regarded as part of the motor system and so would not normally be considered in discussions on sensory mechanisms of the spinal cord. In recent years, however, it has become clear that there are large numbers of sensory fibers in certain ventral roots. This particular group of fibers has obvious relevance to considerations of spinal sensory mechanisms and will be considered below.

It has been known since the time of Sherrington that there are a few myelinated fibers that survive on the distal side and degenerate on the proximal side of a ventral rhizotomy (Sherrington, 1894; Windle, 1931). These fibers were called "recurrent fibers" by Sherrington. Physiological recordings from fine filaments of ventral roots show that there are myelinated sensory fibers in the ventral root (Dimsdale and Kemp, 1966; Kato and Hirata, 1968; Ryall and Piercey, 1970; Kato and Tanji, 1971; Clifton *et al.*, 1976; Coggeshall and Ito, 1977). If the reasonable assumption is made that the sensory fibers, as determined physiologically, are the recurrent fibers of Sherrington, then it seems clear that there are a few myelinated sensory fibers in the ventral root. If only the myelinated sensory fibers are considered, however, then the numbers are so few that they probably do not require a revision in the law of separation of function of the spinal roots, and they are probably not very significant in terms of the sensory mechanisms of the spinal cord.

With the advent of the electron microscope to biology, the unmyelinated fibers could be studied properly. When a number of cat ventral roots were examined with the electron microscope, a large number of unmyelinated fibers were seen (Coggeshall *et al.*, 1974). Many of these fibers came from dorsal root ganglion cells and, like the myelinated recurrent fibers of Sherrington, degenerated proximal and survived distal to a ventral rhizotomy (Coggeshall *et al.*, 1974; Applebaum *et al.*, 1976; Emery *et al.*, 1977). Physiological recordings from fine filaments of ventral roots revealed unmyelinated sensory fibers (Clifton *et al.*, 1976; Coggeshall and Ito, 1977). On the assumption that the unmyelinated ventral root sensory fibers are the unmyelinated recurrent fibers, then 15–30% of the axons in six cat ventral roots are sensory.

It is an important question as to whether the unmyelinated sensory ventral root axons enter the spinal cord directly through the ventral root or whether they curve back to enter the spinal cord through the dorsal root. The latter possibility has been suggested to explain the phenomenon of recurrent sensibility (Magendie, 1822; Bernard, 1858; Frykholm, 1951; Frykholm *et al.*, 1953). There is other evidence, however, that at least some of these fibers enter the spinal cord directly through the ventral root (Maynard *et al.*, 1977; Yamamoto *et al.*, 1977). Thus, this particular issue is not completely resolved yet.

As yet, no special spinal sensory mechanisms have been demonstrated for the ventral root afferents. Since their large numbers have been appreciated only recently, however, such functions may yet be demonstrated. It should be understood that these fibers may necessitate a revision in the law of separation of function of the spinal roots.

In summary, certain ventral roots are now known to have large numbers of sensory fibers. It seems clear that some of them enter the spinal cord directly via the ventral root but it is by no means certain that all or even the majority do. To the extent that the ventral root afferents enter the

spinal cord directly through the ventral roots, the law of separation of
function of the spinal roots would not hold and it would be impossible to
deafferent by dorsal rhizotomy alone.

DORSAL ROOT GANGLION

Morphology

The cell bodies of primary afferent fibers to the spinal cord are
located in dorsal root ganglia, although there is a possibility that some
sensory neurons are located in the visceral plexuses. Several types of
neurons have been described in dorsal root ganglia (Fig. 2.17). Most of
the cells are of the simple unipolar or pseudounipolar type (Dogiel,
1896; Ranson, 1912). The term "pseudounipolar" is based on the em-
bryologic origin of these cells from bipolar cells whose processes fuse
(Ramon y Cajal, 1909). Unipolar cells can be subdivided into large and
small classes. The somata of the large cells have diameters of 60–120
μm; the axon may be highly convoluted, forming a "glomerulus" between the cell body and the point of bifurcation (Dogiel, 1896; Ramon
y Cajal, 1909; Ranson, 1912). The somata of the small cells have diameters of 14–30 μm; their axons are thin and travel directly toward the
central region of the ganglion where they bifurcate (Dogiel, 1896;
Ramon y Cajal, 1909; Ranson, 1912). The large ganglion cells give rise
to large myelinated fibers, and the small ganglion cells are connected
with small myelinated or unmyelinated axons (Ranson, 1912). From
the axonal bifurcation, the two processes travel in opposite directions.
The central process enters the dorsal root to project into the spinal
cord; the peripheral process enters the spinal nerve to project distally
through a somatic or automatic nerve to supply sensory receptors. The
central process is generally smaller than the peripheral process
(Dogiel, 1896; Ranson, 1912). Sometimes the central process enters the
cord through a ventral root and there is evidence for trifurcating axons
(Dogiel, 1896), two of which project centrally through both the dorsal
root and the ventral root and the other peripherally.

There are a number of other cell types in the dorsal root ganglion
(Dogiel, 1896; Ramon y Cajal, 1909; Ranson, 1912). These include cells
whose axons give off collaterals that terminate within the capsule of
the cell of origin or in other parts of the ganglion. Another type of cell
gives off several branches that reassemble to form a single axon. These
varieties of dorsal root ganglion cells account for only about 3% of the
total number in the dorsal root ganglia of the dog (Ranson, 1912).
Some of the cells have a fenestrated appearance. A final type of dorsal

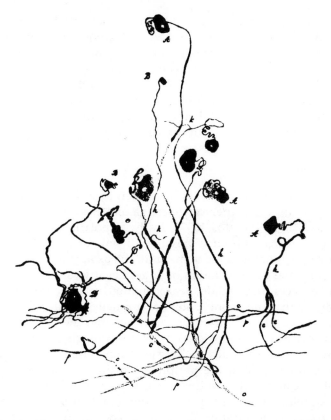

Fig. 2.17. A and B are large and small unipolar dorsal root ganglion cells. D is a multipolar ganglion cell. The division of the axons (h) of the ganglion cells into peripheral (p) and central (c) processes is shown for several neurons. Note the trifurcation of the axon of cell A at the right. (From Dogiel, 1896.)

root ganglion cell has multiple dendritic-like processes that terminate near the cell body (Dogiel, 1896; Ranson, 1912). There is no evidence that any of these cell types function differently from the more commonplace unipolar neurons.

Of the total population of dorsal root ganglion cells, some 60–70% are of the small unipolar type (Ranson, 1912). This is in keeping with the preponderance of unmyelinated fibers over myelinated fibers in the dorsal root.

In addition to neurons within the dorsal root ganglion proper, there are similar ganglion cells located in an aberrant position along the ventral root (Schäfer, 1881; Sherrington, 1894; Windle, 1931; Webber and Wemett, 1966; Willis *et al.*, 1967; Kato and Hirata, 1968; Stacey, 1969; Yamamoto *et al.*, 1977). It has been suggested that these cells are responsible for the ventral root afferent projections, but they are not abundant enough to account for all of the afferent fibers now known to enter the cord over the ventral root.

There have been reports of autonomic fibers that terminate in the dorsal root ganglion (Dogiel, 1896; Owman and Santini, 1966). Some of them appear to end in relation to the dorsal root ganglion cells (Owman and Santini, 1966), but their function is unknown.

Electrophysiology

Resting and action potentials have been recorded from dorsal root ganglion cells by a number of investigators (Svaetichin, 1951, 1958; Sato and Austin, 1961; Ito, 1957). By hyperpolarizing the cell body through a microelectrode, it is possible to slow or block the invasion of the spike potential into the soma from the axon (Ito, 1957). This observation plus the demonstration of large, negative spike potentials in extracellular recordings made near ganglion cells (Svaetichin, 1951, 1958) indicate that the action potential normally invades the ganglion cell body. However, no activity reflects back into the axon under normal circumstances. It is not clear what function the action potential has in the ganglion cell body, since the action potential is presumably transmitted directly from the peripheral to the central process at the point of bifurcation of the unipolar process.

Neurochemical studies of dorsal root ganglion cells indicate that there is a high concentration of glutamic acid in them (Duggan and Johnston, 1970; J. L. Johnson and Aprison, 1970). Furthermore, there are receptors for γ-aminobutyric acid on the surface membrane of dorsal root ganglion cells, and so they are useful as a model for studies on the mechanism of synaptic action of this candidate transmitter (De-Groat *et al.*, 1972). However, it is not certain that the action of GABA is identical on the cell body membrane and, for example, 'at axoaxonal synapses. Immunohistochemical studies suggest that small dorsal root ganglion cells contain either substance P or somatostatin, two other candidate transmitters (Hökfelt *et al.*, 1976).

In summary, there are two main categories of dorsal root ganglion cells—large and small unipolar cells. These cells give rise to large myelinated axons and small myelinated and unmyelinated axons, respectively. The central process of a dorsal root ganglion cell enters the spinal cord over the dorsal root or, in some cases, the ventral root, while the peripheral process supplies sensory receptors. Other types of dorsal root ganglion cells have been described, but it is not likely that they have different functions. Nor is the function known of the autonomic fibers that terminate in the ganglion. The action potential in primary afferents invades the cell bodies of dorsal root ganglion cells. The functional significance of this is not known. Neurochemical studies of dorsal root ganglion cells suggest several candidate transmitters, including glutamic acid, substance P and somatostatin.

CONCLUSIONS

1. Peripheral cutaneous, joint and visceral nerves may contain $A\alpha\beta$ and $A\delta$ myelinated afferent fibers and C or unmyelinated afferent fibers. Muscle nerves contain afferent fibers belonging to groups I, II, III, and IV; type IV are unmyelinated.

2. The conduction velocities of myelinated fibers can be predicted by multiplying the axonal diameter in microns by 6 (for large myelinated fibers) or by 4.5 (for small myelinated fibers). Unmyelinated fibers conduct at rates below 2.5 m/s.

3. Electrical stimulation of peripheral nerves can only rarely be shown to activate a population of afferents from a single receptor type. Generally, natural forms of stimulation must be used to determine the responsiveness of central neurons to particular classes of sensory receptors.

4. Cutaneous sensory receptors include mechanoreceptors, nociceptors and thermoreceptors.

5. Cutaneous mechanoreceptors can be classified as slowly or rapidly adapting. Alternatively, they can be subdivided according to the information they signal—position, velocity, or transients.

6. Two slowly adapting cutaneous mechanoreceptors are called type I and type II. Each signals both position and velocity. Type I receptors are associated with Merkel-cell complexes, often in tactile domes, while type II receptors are associated with Ruffini endings.

7. Cutaneous velocity detectors in hairy skin include G_2 (and T) hair-follicle receptors, D hair-follicle receptors, field receptors, and C mechanoreceptors. The velocity detector in glabrous skin is the Meissner's corpuscle in primates and Krause's end-bulb in cats. Velocity detectors of different types are tuned to different best frequencies.

8. Cutaneous transient detectors include the G_1 hair-follicle receptors and, in subcutaneous tissue, the Pacinian corpuscle.

9. Several types of cutaneous nociceptor respond to various kinds of intense stimuli—mechanical, thermal, or chemical. The nociceptors include $A\delta$ mechanical, C mechanical, $A\delta$ heat, $A\delta$ and C cold, and C polymodal nociceptors.

10. The specific thermoreceptors of the skin include cold and warm receptors.

11. Skeletal muscle contains stretch receptors and pressure–pain endings. One type of stretch receptor, the muscle spindle, has two different sensory endings, primary and secondary. The primary ending signals position and velocity and the secondary ending position. The other stretch receptor is the Golgi tendon organ, which signals tension. Pressure–pain endings are apparently free endings supplied by small myelinated and unmyelinated (group III and IV, respectively) fibers.

12. Joint receptors include Ruffini endings, which appear to signal torque. Other joint receptors include nociceptors.

13. Visceral receptors can detect mechanical or noxious stimuli. Some respond to distention or movement of viscera, others to distention or contraction, and still others to threatening or damaging stimuli.

14. Dermatomes, as measured clinically, seem to reflect not only the distribution of dorsal root fibers to a particular area of the body wall, but also a physiological interaction of dorsal root fibers with one another after they enter the spinal cord.

15. Because of the physiological interactions of dorsal root fibers, the normal dermatome is much smaller in area than the distribution of peripheral axons from one dorsal root to the body wall.

16. The small fiber–large fiber subdivision of the dorsal root does not seem to hold in the cat, at least in the sense that the small fibers can be selectively destroyed at the dorsal root entrance to the spinal cord.

17. Physiological data that seem to indicate that an animal can be made insensitive to pain without affecting other sensory modalities by cutting fine fibers in the dorsal root selectively are now ascribed to vascular damage of the dorsal horn.

18. Large numbers of sensory axons are found in certain ventral roots.

19. To the extent that sensory axons enter the spinal cord directly through the ventral roots, they negate the law of separation of function of the spinal roots.

20. There are several types of dorsal root ganglion cells. Most are unipolar, but some have collaterals or are multipolar. The axon bifurcates into a peripheral process and a central process. Large dorsal root ganglion cells give rise to large myelinated fibers; small cells give rise to small myelinated and unmyelinated fibers.

21. The nerve impulse in a primary afferent fiber invades the cell

body of the dorsal root ganglion cell. The functional significance of this is not known.

22. Dorsal root ganglion cells are useful for neurochemical and neuropharmacological studies of synaptic transmitters and presynaptic receptors.

3 Structure of the Dorsal Horn

This chapter will take as its primary mission the description of the structure of the dorsal horn, in particular laminae I–VI of Rexed (Fig. 3.1). The format will be to describe each of the laminae in turn, with interludes for issues that are not strictly related to the structure of a particular lamina. This format can be justified because almost all recent studies on the anatomy and physiology of the dorsal horn have used the laminae as landmarks, and it will be one of the purposes of this chapter to show to what extent the laminae are meaningful, not just in terms of being landmarks, but in terms of the fundamental organization of the spinal cord. Three relatively arbitrary cut-off points were chosen to keep the length of this chapter within reasonable bounds. First, only the dorsal six laminae are considered. Second, although the primary afferent input to each of the laminae is considered, the equally important descending input is not. Third, the considerations of dorsal horn structures are primarily restricted to studies on chick, rat, cat, monkey, and man.

To review briefly, ever since the spinal cord has been studied grossly, it has been known that two materials of different texture, the white matter and the gray matter, make up the spinal cord. In early times, the white matter was characterized as having a glistening appearance and the gray matter appeared pinkish because of the relative absence of myelinated fibers and the presence of large numbers of capillaries filled with blood. However, when the spinal cord was exposed to formalin, which was the most frequently used early fixative, the hemoglobin turned gray, and so the term "white" was used to characterize myelinated fiber tracts and the term "gray" was used to characterize neuropil or unmyelinated fiber systems.

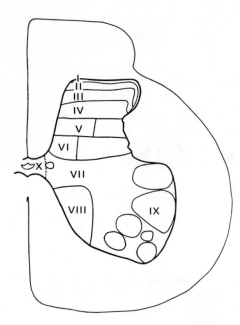

Fig. 3.1. A schematic indicating the location of Rexed's laminae from segment L7 of the cat spinal cord. In this study we will consider laminae I–VI, which make up the dorsal horn. (From Rexed, 1952.)

After the recognition of the white and gray matter, the first landmark to be described in the gray matter of the dorsal horn was the substantia gelatinosa (gelatinous substance) of Rolando (1824, quoted from Ramon y Cajal, 1909). Rolando noted that there was an area near the apex of the dorsal horn that had a distinctly more gelatinous and less fibrous texture than the rest of the gray matter, and to this day, the substantia gelatinosa is an important landmark in the spinal cord.

The next step in the organization of the gray matter of the spinal cord was to subdivide it into nuclei, which reflected neuronal groupings as seen in cytoarchitectonic (Nissl) stains, and these studies are summarized by Rexed (1952, 1954) in his excellent historical reviews. Early cytoarchitectonic studies were in agreement that the superficial part of the dorsal horn consisted of two layers or laminae: (1) the marginal cell layer and (2) the substantia gelatinosa. The studies were not in agreement, however, as to the organization of the dorsal horn deep to the substantia gelatinosa, and it is Rexed's contribution to point out that the entire dorsal horn seems to consist of recognizable concentric laminae.

Finally, it should be pointed out that cytoarchitectonic studies have limited usefulness because only the nucleus and cytoplasm of the cells is seen. An analysis of the structure of the spinal gray matter is essentially an analysis of a complex field of neuropil, and to understand a neuropil, it is much more important to understand dendritic arborizations and axonal connections than it is to be able to describe the shape of the nucleus and cell body. Thus, the most important early studies on the structure of the gray matter of the spinal cord are those by Lenhossek (1895) and especially by Ramon y Cajal (1909), who described the dendritic and axonal arborizations of various neurons in the dorsal horn as well as the afferent input to these neurons, as revealed by the method of Golgi and its variants. These last two studies still have an important impact on present-day analyses of the structure of the spinal cord.

LAMINA I

Rexed (1952) defined lamina I of the spinal cord as "a thin veil of gray substance, forming the dorsal-most part of the spinal gray matter" (Fig. 3.1). Bundles of myelinated axons penetrate this lamina, giving it a spongy or reticular appearance and sometimes making the boundary between lamina I and the overlying white matter indistinct. Although the superficial border of lamina I is often indistinct, its lower border is sharp, because there is an abrupt change from the relatively scattered neurons of lamina I, whose cell bodies have a primarily horizontal arrangement, to the densely packed, radially arranged, small neurons of lamina II (Rexed, 1952, 1954). The cell bodies of the neurons of lamina I vary in size. The largest were noted long ago by Clarke (1859), and they have been seen and described by almost all investigators since that time (see Rexed, 1952, p. 428). Waldeyer (1888) referred to the large lamina I neurons as marginal cells (*marginale Zellen* or *marginale Hinterzellen*), which is the name that is now in general use for these cells, and this layer of spinal cord is usually referred to as the marginal zone of Waldeyer.

Most investigators concerned with the anatomy or physiology of lamina I cells deal primarily with the large cells, presumably because they are prominent and easily studied. For this reason, we will also be concerned primarily with the marginal cells, but the caution of Rexed (1952) should be remembered. Rexed noted that there were many neurons in lamina I and that in terms of numbers, the large marginal cells are only a small fraction of the total. Thus, although most discussions about lamina I concentrate on the large marginal cells, the remaining neurons will also have to be studied if the function of lamina I as a unit is to be understood.

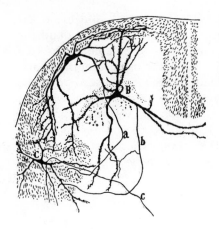

Fig. 3.2. A schematic diagram of a Golgi-stained section of spinal cord. Cell A is a large marginal cell. Note that the majority of the dendrites of cell A pass tangentially over the surface of the dorsal horn, but some pass ventrally into the gray matter of the dorsal horn. The axon (a) of cell A arises from a ventral dendrite and disappears in the lateral funiculus. Cell B is a large cell in the center of the dorsal horn. The dendrites pass medially, laterally, and dorsally, and the axon of this cell (b) also passes to the lateral funiculus. Cell C is located in the white matter and does not belong to the dorsal horn. (From Ramon y Cajal, 1909.)

Cell Bodies and Dendritic Organization

The marginal cell bodies are large and flattened between the overlying white matter and the underlying lamina II (Figs. 3.2 and 3.3) (Waldeyer, 1888; Rexed, 1952; Scheibel and Scheibel, 1968). The flattening of the cell bodies of the marginal cells reflects the dendritic organization of these neurons. The dendrites of the marginal cells (e.g., Lenhossek, 1895; Ramon y Cajal, 1909; Scheibel and Scheibel, 1968) travel in the plane between the white matter and the outer cells of lamina II (Figs. 3.2 and 3.3). The dendrites are long, but they do not branch frequently, and dendrites from neighboring marginal cells overlap. The dendrites usually remain in the relatively narrow space between the tract of Lissauer and lamina II, but occasionally dendritic branches dip down into the underlying lamina II (Figs. 3.2 and 3.3) (Ramon y Cajal, 1909; Scheibel and Scheibel, 1968). At this point the dentrites are suddenly studded with thorns, and for this reason, the Scheibels speculate that the dendrites of marginal cells are more densely covered with presynaptic terminals when they are in deeper laminae than when they are in lamina I. The shape of the dendritic fields is discoid in that they extend for long distances in the mediolateral and craniocaudal axes, but they are flattened and occupy relatively little space in the dorsoventral axis (Fig. 3.4).

Axonal Projections

Two destinations for the axons of the marginal cells have been proposed. One commonly accepted view is that these cells project to the thalamus, and their axons make up part of the spinothalamic tract.

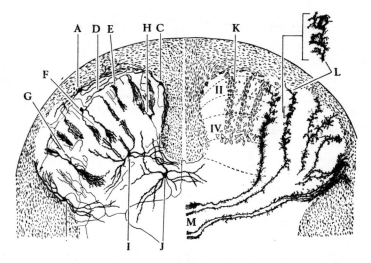

Fig. 3.3. A schematic diagram of the organization of the dorsal horn. Cells A and C are marginal (lamina I) cells of Waldeyer. D is a transitional cell that has characteristics of both marginal cells and cells of the substantia gelatinosa. Cell I is a lamina IV cell, and cell J belongs to the intermediate nucleus of Ramon y Cajal. On the right-hand side of this diagram are the cell bodies of neurons and glial processes in the dorsal horn. (From Scheibel and Scheibel, 1968.)

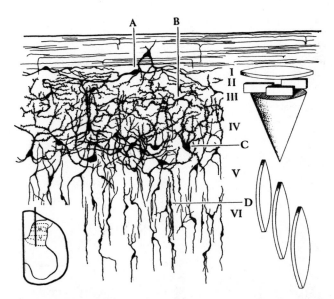

Fig. 3.4. Shapes of the dendritic patterns of the cells in laminae I–VI. The geometric patterns of the dendritic fields are shown in the right-hand side of the picture. (From Scheibel and Scheibel, 1968.)

The evidence for this is discussed in Chapter 8, and it seems clear that many of the large marginal cells of Lissauer project to the thalamus via a pathway in the contralateral white matter of the spinal cord.

The other idea about the projected destination of the axons of the marginal cells is that they "form propriospinal links along the inner surface of the dorsal and dorsolateral white matter" (Scheibel and Scheibel, 1968). Szentágothai (1964) mentions that the axons of the marginal cells usually send their axons into Lissauer's tract or the lateral fasciculus proprius, rather than into the region of spinal white matter where the spinothalamic tract is found. Bok (1928) regarded these cells as association neurons, and both Ramon y Cajal (1909) and Lenhossek (1895) illustrated marginal cells with axons passing to the ipsilateral or contralateral lateral fasciculus proprius. Finally, Burton and Loewy (1976) showed that some of the marginal cells were labeled when horseradish peroxidase was injected into the dorsal horn two to eight segments caudal to the labeled cells. These observations make it highly likely that some of the marginal neurons project to other segments of the spinal cord via propriospinal pathways.

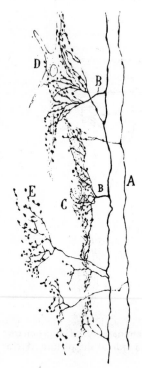

Fig. 3.5. Collaterals (B) from fibers, both myelinated and unmyelinated (A), that form synaptic boutons on proximal dendrites and cell bodies (C and D) of marginal cells. (From Ramon y Cajal, 1909.)

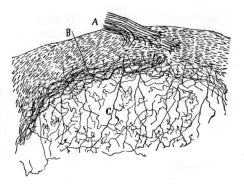

Fig. 3.6. A view of the fine fibers that permeate dorsal parts of the dorsal horn. A indicates fibers of the dorsal root, B the fine fibers of the marginal plexus, and C fine fibers that penetrate the substance of the substantia gelatinosa. (From Ramon y Cajal, 1909.)

Primary Afferent Input into Lamina I

Ramon y Cajal (1909) noted that there was a plexus of fine fibers that surrounded and came into synaptic contact with the large neurons in the marginal layer (Figs. 3.5 and 3.6). Ramon y Cajal called this plexus the marginal plexus and noted that the fibers making up the plexus arose as collaterals from axons in or near the tract of Lissauer. Most of the studies using the Golgi method that dealt with the axons and neurons of lamina I confirmed Ramon y Cajal's description of the marginal plexus (Szentágothai, 1964; Scheibel and Scheibel, 1968; Beal and Fox, 1976). Cajal felt that many of these fibers were primary afferent axons because they arose as collaterals from axons in the tract of Lissauer, which he felt consisted of fine primary afferent fibers. More recent evidence has shown, however, that the tract of Lissauer consists primarily of propriospinal fibers (Szentágothai, 1964).

As a brief digression, the reason that Ramon y Cajal (1909) had some difficulty determining whether the marginal plexus consisted of propriospinal or primary afferent fibers is a difficulty inherent in the study of single sections of Golgi-impregnated spinal cord. To determine whether a fiber is a primary afferent fiber by this technique, it would be necessary to trace the fiber into the dorsal root; and to determine if the fiber is a propriospinal fiber, it would be necessary to follow it to a neuron in the spinal cord. This is not usually done in Golgi-impregnated spinal cord. The fibers arise as collaterals from axons in the white matter of the spinal cord, and then they take a relatively tortuous path in the gray matter of the spinal cord. Accordingly, if single sections of spinal cord are studied, which is usually the case, the fiber almost always leaves the plane of section before it gets to a location that would definitively label its origin. Thus, when a user of the Golgi technique identifies an axon in the dorsal horn as propriospinal or primary afferent in nature, it usually means that he or she could trace the axon to some part of the white matter of the spinal cord and that that part has been previously identified as containing primarily propriospinal fibers or primarily sensory fibers. Since a constantly recurring question in the study of the fiber connections of the spinal cord is whether a fiber is propriospinal or whether it belongs to some other category, the student should review what is known about the propriospinal pathways in the spinal cord. An excellent place to begin is with the review by Nathan and Smith (1959).

Organization of the Neuropil

Ralston (1968a) examined the neuropil of lamina I in the electron microscope and noted that the majority of axons are "in a horizontal array, parallel to the surface of the cord" (Ralston, 1968a), as opposed to the primary longitudinal or radial orientation of the axons in lamina II. Ralston also noted the presence of "complex synaptic arrays" in lamina I. These structures consist of a widened central unmyelinated axon that synapses with a number of dendrites, both large and small, and upon which are ending small axonal terminals (Ralston, 1968a). According to Ralston (1968a), these structures are morphologically the same as the glomeruli in laminae II and III. A more extended discussion of the glomeruli is given in the section of this chapter concerned with the neuropil of lamina II.

Kerr (1970a), who studied lamina I in cervical spinal cord as well as in the equivalent area in the spinal trigeminal nucleus, did not completely agree with these observations. Kerr (1970a) pointed out that "the richness of end knobs in the marginal zone far exceeds that in any other part of the primary nucleus (trigeminal or spinal)." The marginal layer is characterized by clusters of terminals, "in which a small number of terminals are in synaptic contact with a dendrite of medium or large size, while the remainder establish some synaptic contacts with each other and with occasional fine dendrites which may pass through or near the cluster" (Kerr, 1970a). Kerr specifically states that these complexes are more irregularly arranged than the glomeruli of the substantia gelatinosa (see the section on the neuropil of lamina II). These clusters, according to Kerr, make lamina I easy to recognize.

Ralston (1968b) studied the fine structure of lamina I after the dorsal root was cut. He noted that there were very few degenerating fiber terminals in lamina I after dorsal root section and those that were found were on small dendrites (Fig. 3.7). If these findings are accepted, it would imply that the bulk of the fibers making up the tangential plexus are not of primary afferent origin, because it is clear that many of the terminals of axons in the tangential plexus are on the

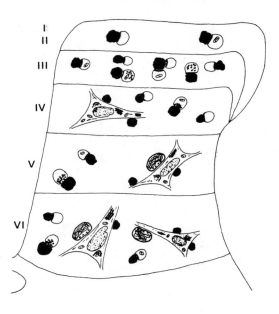

Fig. 3.7. A diagram of the location of degenerating primary afferent fibers in laminae I–VI. Degenerating axonal terminals are pictured in solid black. (From Ralston, 1968b.)

cell bodies and proximal dendrites of lamina I neurons (Ramon y Cajal, 1909). The difficulty with this analysis is that Heimer and Wall (1968) and others (Petras, 1968; Réthelyi and Szentágothai, 1969) noted that degenerating terminals in laminae I and II were numerous if the appropriate time for degeneration was allowed. This issue will be considered in more detail when lamina II is considered, because the controversy was more intense for that area of the spinal cord, but it does raise the possibility that not all the degenerating primary afferent terminals in lamina I were seen by Ralston. Kerr (1970b, 1975a) also examined the marginal zone after the dorsal root was cut. In agreement with Heimer and Wall (1968), he noted that there were degenerating axons in the marginal plexus and degenerating terminals in the marginal zone. But in accord with the findings of Ralston (1968b), the degenerating terminals were not found on cell bodies of the marginal neurons, rather they were found on small dendrites in this layer. Although direct proof was lacking, Kerr felt that the small dendrites originated from the large marginal cells in this lamina. If this is correct, the primary afferent terminals in lamina I end on the distal ends of the dendrites of the large marginal cells.

Kerr (1970b, 1975a,c) also analyzed the location of the terminals that arise from the propriospinal fibers. Kerr did this by comparing the degeneration patterns after dorsal rhizotomy with the degenera-

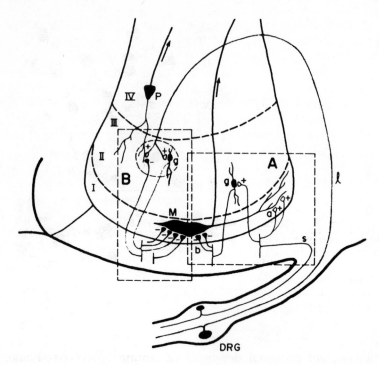

Fig. 3.8. A schematic diagram of Kerr's ideas about the synaptic connections to the marginal neurons (M). Note that fine primary afferent fibers (s) end on distal dendrites of the marginal cell (M). Note that the synapses on the cell body of the marginal cell (M) arise from small cells in laminae II and III. Kerr speculates that the synapses on the distal dendrites are excitatory (+) and those on the cell body are inhibitory (−). (From Kerr, 1975a.)

tion patterns that follow sections of the tract of Lissauer. The justification for this procedure is that, although early investigators stated that the axons in the tract of Lissauer were the fine primary afferents from the dorsal root (Lissauer, 1885; Ranson, 1914), more recent work has shown that the large majority of fibers in this tract are propriospinal. When the tract of Lissauer was sectioned, most of the degenerating terminals were found on the cell bodies and the proximal dendrites of the neurons in the marginal layer (Kerr, 1975a). Kerr then speculated that the marginal cells receive their primary afferent input on their distal dendrites and their propriospinal input on the soma and proximal dendrites (Fig. 3.8). Kerr (1970a) further speculated that the primary afferent input was excitatory and the propriospinal input was inhibitory (Fig. 3.8). These interesting ideas will have to be checked by further work.

A recent study, which is at the present time available only in abstract form, offers promise for further resolution of the axonal connections in lamina I (Light and Perl, 1977). These investigators marked individually identified high-threshold afferents, which conducted at 7–40 m/s, and followed them into lamina I. Kumazawa and Perl (1978) further suggest that fine myelinated afferents terminate almost exclusively in lamina I. It yet remains to examine these marked fibers in the electron microscope, but these findings indicate that there is an important primary afferent input into lamina I.

The input into the marginal layer of Waldeyer seems to be primarily from fine fibers. The coarse collateral primary afferent input that is so prominent in slightly deeper layers of the dorsal horn (see the following section of this chapter), particularly in lamina III, does not enter lamina I (Ramon y Cajal, 1909; Kerr, 1975a).

Duncan and Morales (1973a,b) emphasize an intriguing aspect of neuropil organization in the upper part of the dorsal horn in cat and dog. Kerr (1970a) noted that many of the terminals in the upper part of the dorsal horn contain dense core vesicles. Duncan and Morales pointed out that the dense-core-vesicle-containing axons are extremely numerous along the medial and lateral edges of the dorsal horn, more specifically the medial and lateral edges of laminae I, II, and III. The vesicles are round, with diameters ranging between 750 and 1500Å. The cores almost fill the vesicles and range in density from barely discernible to very electron dense (Duncan and Morales, 1973a,b). The chemical contents of the vesicles are not known.

Function of Lamina I Neurons

A major breakthrough in our understanding of the function of the marginal cells came from the observations of Christensen and Perl (1970). These investigators noted that the marginal cells respond to peripheral stimulation in one of three ways; the first group of cells were responsive only to mechanical nociceptive information, which was brought to them by slowly conducting (small) myelinated axons. The second group was responsive to both mechanical and thermal nociceptive stimuli, the former apparently being carried by small myelinated fibers, the latter by unmyelinated axons. Finally, there was a third group of cells that responded to innocuous temperature changes as well as mechanical and thermal nociceptive stimuli. Thus, it appears that these cells are part of a pain pathway, and further consideration of these cells will be taken up in the chapter dealing with the cells of origin of the spinothalamic tract.

In summary, the neurons of lamina I can be recognized by their pre-dominantly horizontal orientation. The dendrites of these cells are relatively long and unbranched and most of them travel tangentially over the surface of the dorsal horn. A few dendrites, however, penetrate more deeply into the substance of the dorsal horn. The axonal projections of the cells seem to be primarily to the thalamus or to other areas of the spinal cord. The major-ity of afferent fibers to this layer are fine, and they arise as collaterals from the tract of Lissauer. The plexus they form is named the marginal plexus. Cajal was of the opinion that the majority of these were primary afferents but present opinion is that the majority are propriospinal. The neuropil contains axodendritic, axosomatic, and axoaxonic synapses. In addition there are relatively complex synapses that resemble the glomeruli of la-minae II and III. Primary afferent terminals appear to be primarily on fine dendrites. Propriospinal terminals appear to be primarily on the cell body and proximal dendrites.

THE SUBSTANTIA GELATINOSA AND ITS RELATIONSHIP TO LAMINAE II AND III

If this discussion were to proceed with a morphological analysis of lamina II followed by a similar analysis of lamina III, a fundamental debate that permeates recent structural and functional studies on the dorsal horn would be obscured. The main concern in the debate is whether or not lamina II of Rexed is the same as the substantia gela-tinosa of earlier authors or whether both lamina II and lamina III rep-resent the substantia gelatinosa. This debate is not a simple search for historical identity; rather it hinges on whether or not the region of the spinal cord between the superficial marginal cells of Lissauer and the deeper large projection neurons of lamina IV can legitimately be sub-divided into two separate layers or whether, as far as we can tell at present, this is a single region with one overall structural plan. To focus this issue, it should be understood that early investigators usually subdivided the dorsal horn into the marginal cell layer, the substantia gelatinosa, and the rest of the dorsal horn. As pointed out previously, it was Rexed's (1952) contribution to point out that the whole dorsal horn, not just its superficial part, could be divided into concentric laminae. Without denying the importance of Rexed's overall conception, however, there has been some question as to his justification for subdividing the area between the marginal cell layer (lamina I) and the superficial part of the base of the dorsal horn (lam-ina IV) into two laminae (laminae II and III) and then equating the substantia gelatinosa only with lamina II.

In Rexed's original formulation, lamina II was made up of many small, closely packed neurons, most of which were arranged radially, in contrast to the prevailing horizontal arrangement of the lamina I cells. The cells of lamina III are then demarcated from the cells of lamina II by being slightly larger and farther apart than the cells in the inner layer of lamina II. In addition, there are some columns in lamina III that are due to the ascending dendrites from the large cells in lamina IV. These are not impressive differences, and in 1964, Szentágothai pointed out that cells from both layers had essentially the same dendritic patterns and the same axonal projections. Thus, he regarded the two laminae as a functional unit and equated both to the substantia gelationsa of earlier workers. Wall (1967) agreed with this formulation.

One finding that would have clearly distinguished lamina II from lamina III was reported by Ralston (1965, 1968b) and Sterling and Kuypers (1967). These investigators noted that dorsal rhizotomy resulted in a great deal of primary afferent degeneration in lamina III but relatively little or almost none in lamina II. This finding aroused much interest, because it implies that lamina II had almost no primary afferent input and thus could clearly be distinguished in an important way from lamina III. By contrast, however, Escolar (1948), Sprague and Ha (1964), and Szentágothai (1964) noted degenerating terminals throughout the substantia gelatinosa, by which they meant both lamina II and III. This difficulty was resolved by Heimer and Wall (1968), who showed that degenerating primary afferent terminals could be found throughout lamina I–III, but that the degenerating terminals appear and disappear rapidly in laminae I and II, whereas those in lamina III appeared and disappeared at a much more leisurely pace. Thus, there is a difference in the time it takes primary afferent terminals to degenerate, but all the superficial spinal laminae seem to have sizable numbers of primary afferent terminals (for percentages of degenerating spinal afferents in laminae I–IV) (see Ralston, 1977).

Although a suggested major difference between laminae II and III, namely that there was no primary afferent input to lamina II, cannot be accepted, there are other differences in addition to the cytoarchitectonic patterns noted by Rexed. First, there is the above-mentioned difference in degeneration time of the primary afferent terminals in lamina II as opposed to lamina III. Recently it has been suggested that these differences might reflect the different degeneration times for small as opposed to large afferent fibers (LaMotte, 1977; Réthelyi, 1977). If this were the case, it would indicate a fundamental difference in terms of axonal input into laminae II and III. Ralston also mentions that myelinated axons are far more numerous in lamina III than in lamina II. Several investigators have noted that complicated synaptic glomeruli are found in laminae II and III, and Ralston (1971) and Kerr (1975a) noted that they are more numerous in lamina III. These various differences, even though their functional implications are not clear, allow the experienced morphologist to distinguish between the laminae. Nevertheless, the dendritic fields and axonal projections of the neurons in the two laminae have many points of similarity and so the argument of Szentágothai (1964) and Wall (1967) that the two laminae are, in certain respects, a functional and structural unit still has force. Furthermore, since the dendritic fields and axonal projections are similar, it is probable that major differences between the laminae will probably be in terms of different modalities of afferent input. Major progress in this regard has recently been reported (A. G. Brown, 1977; A. G. Brown et al., 1977c; Light and Perl, 1977; Kumazawa and Perl, 1978). For these reasons, the laminae will be considered separately, but the similarities will be pointed out as we progress.

In summary, there has been some discussion as to whether just lamina II or both laminae II and III represent the substantia gelatinosa of earlier investigators. The two laminae can be distinguished in cytoarchitectonic stains, but there are many common features of dendritic and axonal organization of the neurons in the two layers. An early suggestion was that lamina II neurons received little primary afferent input in contrast to lamina III neurons, but this view is not generally accepted at present. Evidence is accumulating, however, to indicate that different types of primary afferent fibers end in each lamina.

LAMINA II

Lamina II is equated by Rexed (1952, 1954) to the substantia gelationosa. As was pointed out in the introduction to this chapter, the substantia gelatinosa is found just ventral to the marginal cell layer of Waldeyer (1888). This layer can be recognized because the cells are small and closely packed and they have a slight radial orientation with respect to the surface of the cord in cytoarchitectonic stains. There is an absence of myelinated fibers in this lamina. According to Rexed (1952), the neurons in lamina II (the substantia gelatinosa) can be distinguished from the neurons of lamina I (the marginal cell layer) by the predominantly radial orientation of the lamina II cells as opposed to the horizontal orientation of most lamina I neurons, and they can be distinguished from the neurons of lamina III because the neurons of lamina II are slightly smaller and closer together than those in lamina III.

Cell Bodies and Dendritic Organization

Most early investigators noted only one cell type in the substantia gelatinosa, but Ramon y Cajal (1909) described two cell types: (1) the "cellules centralis," or central cells, which were the typical and by far the most common cells in the substantia gelatinosa, and (2) the "cellules limitrophes," or border cells, which were larger and were found in the superficial region of the substantia gelatinosa. These two cell types will be described separately.

Central Cells ("Cellules Centralis")

Dendritic Organization. The name "central cell" is a slight misnomer, because these cells are found throughout the substantia gelatinosa and not just in central areas. The central cells are small and relatively close to one another. In cytoarchitectonic (Nissl) stains, only a thin rim of cytoplasm can be seen around the relatively small nucleus. Various investigators noted that these cells seem to have a radial orientation, in contrast to the horizontal lamination of the cells in lamina I (Rexed, 1952), and this is due to the fact that the major dendrites of most of these neurons emerge from the apical and basal portions of the cell (Szentágothai, 1964).

The early descriptions of the dendritic arborizations of the central cells of the substantia gelatinosa are given by Lenhossek (1895) and Ramon y Cajal (1909). Ramon y Cajal's description is the more complete, and he mentions that the central cells are the smallest in the spinal cord. He notes, however, that in spite of the small cell body, the cells have large numbers of fine dendrites and each dendrite is extensively branched (Figs. 3.9 and 3.10). The dendrites of each central cell ramify in and among the lobules of the substantia gelatinosa, the lobules being defined by the flame-shaped axonal arborizations of the coarse afferent collaterals (see below and Fig. 3.9). According to Ramon y Cajal, it is these extraordinarily complex dendritic ramifications that give the substantia gelatinosa its finely granular or plexiform appearance when the cord is stained with carmine or hematoxylin.

Later descriptions of the dendrites of the cells of the substantia gelatinosa are in general agreement. Szentágothai (1964) emphasizes the radial orientation of the dendrites and points out that this seems to be due to the fact that the main-stem dendrites usually emerge from

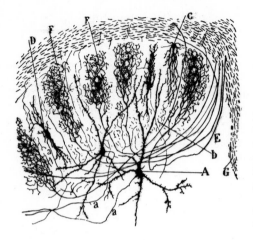

Fig. 3.9. Ramon y Cajal's picture of the coarse primary afferent collaterals (E) that end in bushy arborizations (F) in the substantia gelatinosa. Cell D is a central cell of the substantia gelatinosa. Cell C is a "limitrophe" cell. Cell A is a large cell in the central part of the dorsal horn. (From Ramon y Cajal, 1909.)

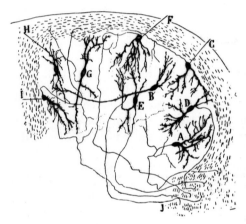

Fig. 3.10. Various cell types found in the substance of Rolando. Cells C and F are probably "limitrophe" cells, but Ramon y Cajal refers to them as "cellules limitantes." The varying dendritic organization of the remaining neurons fits fairly well with the idea that the majority of cells of the substantia gelatinosa have radial dendritic fields, but some clearly do not. (From Ramon y Cajal, 1909.)

the dorsal and ventral poles of the cell and then they break up into the rich dendritic plexus described by Lenhossek and Ramon y Cajal. This can be seen to some extent in Figs. 3.9 and 3.10, but it is clear that the dendritic shapes are often not radially arranged (cf. Figs. 3.11, 3.12, and 3.13). Nevertheless, enough have radial dendrites so that there is a slight radial orientation to the cells of this layer in Nissl stains. Scheibel and Scheibel (1968) note the presence of numerous spines on the dendrites, many of the spines being 10 μm long.

Various investigators such as Ramon y Cajal (1909), Pearson (1952), and Sterling and Kuypers (1967) mention that the dendritic spread of the cells is widest in a longitudinal direction. However, Scheibel and Scheibel (1968) show this most dramatically (Fig. 3.4).

They consider both laminae II and III to be the substantia ¦
They state that a typical cell in the substantia gelatinosa ha¦
tic field that extends 15–20 μm in the mediolateral plane, 50–200 μ..¦
the dorsoventral plane, and 200–500 μm in the craniocaudal plane
(Scheibel and Scheibel, 1968). Thus, Scheibel and Scheibel regard
these dendritic domains as thin rectangular sheets (Fig. 3.4). These
findings lead to the typical depiction of central cells as having relatively thin, radially oriented dendritic fields (Figs. 3.3 and 3.4).

Mannen (1975), Sugiura (1975), and Mannen and Sugiura (1976),
although they do not directly disagree with the size of the dendritic
domains as measured by Scheibel and Scheibel (1968), point out that a
limitation of previous Golgi analyses is that some of the processes of

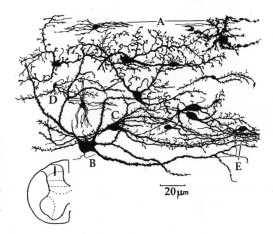

Fig. 3.11. A composite sagittal
section of Golgi-impregnated
spinal cord. The purpose of this
picture is to show the longitudinal extent of the dendrites of
cells in laminae I–IV. (From
Scheibel and Scheibel, 1968.)

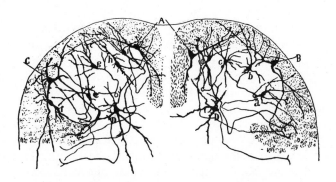

Fig. 3.12. A composite picture showing the dendritic patterns and axonal projections of
cells in the dorsal horn. Cells A, B, and C are marginal cells. Cells b, c, d, g, h, and i are
central cells of the substantia gelatinosa. Cell D is in the center of the dorsal horn. (From
Ramon y Cajal, 1909.)

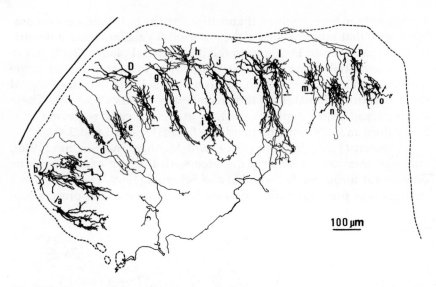

Fig. 3.13. Diagram of the cells of lamina II. These cells were reconstructed from serial sections of Golgi-stained spinal cord. Most of the cells are regarded as variants with characteristics of both central or inner cells and "limitrophe," or outer cells of the substantia gelatinosa. (From Suguira, 1975.)

cells in laminae II or III almost always pass out of a section of spinal cord no matter how thick the section is. Thus, these authors developed a method for following the dendrites and axons of neurons in laminae II and III through as many as fourteen 100-μm-thick serial celloidin sections of kitten spinal cord. The study by Suguira (1975) is primarily concerned with neurons in lamina II (Fig. 3.13). The central cells, or as Suguira calls them, the inner neurons, do not have dendritic fields that are particualrly flattened. The dendritic domains are 80–100 μm mediolaterally, 150–230 μm dorsoventrally, and 200–250 μm craniocaudally. In support of these findings, Ramon y Cajal illustrates some central neurons in the substantia gelatinosa with relatively wide dendritic fields (Fig. 3.12), but others clearly have a distinctly radial dendritic organization (Fig. 3.12). Thus, the dendritic fields of most lamina II cells seem to be wider than Scheibel and Scheibel (1968) report, but they are still somewhat flattened in a mediolateral plane. The determination of the width of the dendritic fields might seem to be an esoteric matter, but it has some importance when one considers the flame-shaped arbors (Fig. 3.9) (Scheibel and Scheibel, 1968) that are the terminations of the recurrent collaterals from large primary afferent fibers (see below). Both Scheibel and Scheibel (1968) and Réthelyi and Szentágothai (1973) emphasize that the cells of the gelatinosa are small and numerous and that their dendritic fields, although extensive in the dorsoventral and rostrocaudal dimension, are thin (flattened in the mediolateral dimension). Thus, they feel that there are a large number of gelatinosa neurons embedded in the thick swirl of axonal branchings that come from one primary afferent fiber, and presumably, therefore, one afferent fiber makes extensive synaptic contact on a particular group of neurons of the substantia gelatinosa. By the same reasoning, although Scheibel and Scheibel (1968) and Réthelyi and Szentágothai (1973) do not mention this, the gelatinosa cells that are between the flame-shaped arbors would receive no input from the arbors. Since recent evidence indicates that the flame-shaped arbors arise from axons whose distal ends are associated with hair follicles (A. G. Brown, 1977; A. G. Brown et al., 1977c), this might imply that there is a strong input from bending hairs to one fraction of the central neurons of the gelatinosa and little or no such input to another large group of central gelatinosa neurons. The fact that the dendritic fields of some central cells may be wider than indicated by the Scheibels (cf. Ramon y Cajal, 1909; Sugiura, 1975) may blur this picture somewhat, but this idea should be tested. To do so, it will probably be necessary to record from central neurons as large primary afferents are stimulated. It might be noted that the first successful recordings from the central neurons have recently been obtained (Yaksh et al., 1977; Hentall, 1977; Cervero et al., 1977b). As a final point in the above argument, it should be noted that Scheibel and Scheibel (1968) and Réthelyi and Szentágothai (1973) regard the substantia gelatinosa as consisting of both lamina II and lamina III. Brown et al. (1977c), however, state that the flame-shaped arbors are restricted to lamina III. If this finding is confirmed, then the reasoning in the preceding paragraph would apply only to cells of lamina III.

In summary, the central cells of the substantia gelatinosa are small, but their dendritic ramifications are fairly extensive. The dendrites most frequently emerge from the apical and basal poles of the cell, thus giving an overall appearance of radially oriented cells in this area in cytoarchitectonic stains. The dendrites of the lamina II cells remain, by and large, within lamina II, and several investigators make the point that the central cells have flattened dendritic fields, thus being relatively extensive in a dorsoventral and craniocaudal direction but relatively restricted in the mediolateral direction.

Axonal Projections

Central cells can be split into two categories on the basis of their axonal projections: (1) those neurons that send their axons into the tract of Lissauer or into the posterior or lateral propriospinal pathways surrounding the apex of the dorsal part of the dorsal horn and (2) those cells whose axons do not leave the gray matter of the dorsal part of the dorsal horn (Ramon y Cajal, 1909; Nathan and Smith, 1959; Szentágothai, 1964; Scheibel and Scheibel, 1968). Ramon y Cajal would regard cells in category 1 as funicular cells and those in category 2 as short-axoned cells. These two types of cells will be considered separately.

Axonal Projections of Funicular Cells

Lenhossek (1895) noted that the axons of the cells of the substantia gelatinosa, after a complex and tortuous path across the dorsal horn, enter the tract of Lissauer or lateral proprious bundle. Ramon y Cajal (1909) was also struck by the complex path of the axons of these cells within the dorsal horn (Figs. 3.9, 3.10, and 3.12). He was able to trace them only in embyronic chicks, and he confirmed Lenhossek's observation that they pass into the tract of Lissauer or the lateral proprius bundle (*"fasceau de la corne posterieure"*); in addition, Ramon y Cajal noted some axons passing into the dorsal proprius bundle. Szentágothai (1964) confirmed these observations but also noted that some of the axons of the medial cells in the substantia gelatinosa went into the posterior commissure to be distributed in laminae II and III of the opposite side of the spinal cord. Sugiura (1975) noted that the axons of central cells, which he called inner cells, could not be contained in single sections of spinal cord, even if they were 150 μm thick, and so he traced the axons through serial celloidin sections. The extraordinary complexity of the axonal path taken by these cells is well illustrated in his pictures (Fig. 3.13), but in general his conclusions do not differ from those of earlier investigators.

One problem in the analysis of Golgi-impregnated funicular central cells of the substantia gelatinosa is that it is almost impossible to follow the axons of these cells to their terminations. The difficulty is that even in well-impregnated material, the axons take a right-angle bend and then travel with a large number of similar-sized fibers in the white matter. The nearest to being able to trace an axon of a central funicular cell to its termination is cell E of Sugiura (1975). The axon could be followed from the cell body to the tract of Lissauer, and then longitudinally for 1200 μm in the tract of Lissauer. The axon then left the tract, reentered lamina II, and ended. Sugiura (1975) does not say, however, whether it truly ended or just could no longer be followed. The finding that the axon reentered lamina II and there seemed to end fits well with the conclusion of Szentágothai (1964) that the substantia is a closed system (see below).

A clever experiment was done by Szentágothai (1964) to get evidence as to the axonal terminations of the central cells of the substantia gelatinosa. Szentágothai isolated a slab of dorsal horn by (1) cutting a dorsal root, (2) undercutting the denervated dorsal horn, and (3) crushing the spinal cord at the anterior and posterior borders of the denervated segment (Fig. 3.14). The pial vessels were left intact by not cutting through the pia meter, and the result was "a dorsal sector of the spinal cord with all neural connections cut, but supplied with blood by the known arcuate vessels connecting the ventral and dorsal longitudinal tracts" (Szentágothai, 1964). These isolated dorsal horns were allowed to survive for 2 months, and then the animals were sacrificed and the isolated dorsal horn was studied in light and electron microscopes. In this preparation, all afferent and long propriospinal fibers would be severed, and the axons that are left must be intrinsic to this part of the spinal cord. Szentágothai stated that the fibers of lateral fasciculus proprius and the lateral part of Lissauer's tract are intact, thus indicating that they are still attached to their cell bodies. Furthermore, although there is considerable degeneration in the medial part of the tract of Lissauer, a finding that Szentágothai ascribes to

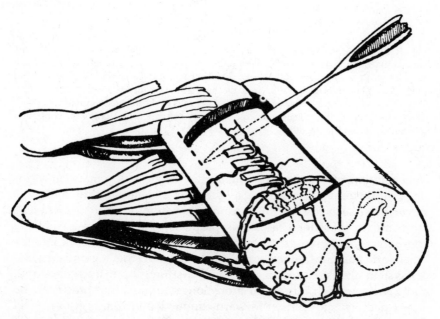

Fig. 3.14. A diagram of the operation used by Szentágothai to provide an isolated segment of dorsal horn. Note that the blood vessels into the isolated segment are still intact. (From Szentágothai, 1964.)

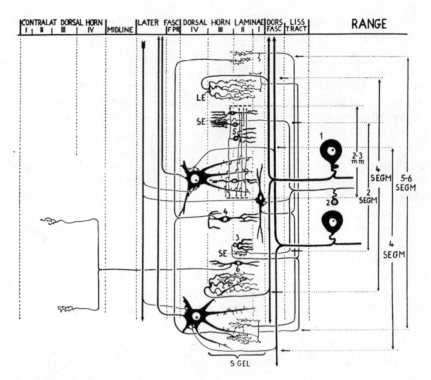

Fig. 3.15. A "highly schematized diagram showing neuronal connections of the SG (substantia gelatinosa) in an imaginary longitudinal section plane that runs through all relevant structures" (Szentágothai, 1964). Note that the large lamina IV neurons send their prominent dorsal dendrites into the substantia gelatinosa (laminae II and III). There the dendrites are contacted by axons of the cells of the substantia gelatinosa (5, 6). Thus, according to this scheme, the large lamina IV cells are the output of the substantia gelatinosa. (From Szentágothai, 1964.)

degeneration of primary afferents, many fibers still remain and thus are propriospinal. Therefore, "as the cells of laminae II and III have never been seen to send their axons anywhere other than Lissauer's tract and to the lateral fasciculus proprius, and in addition both of these tracts only give rise to collaterals, which again turn back into the substantia gelatinosa, the conclusion is that . . . this region is a cellular system almost closed in itself with a strong input from the dorsal roots and very rich interconnections longitudinally, but practically no direct pathways for further forward conduction" (Szentágothai, 1964). It might be remembered that some axons of the gelatinosa cells pass to the dorsal fasciculus proprius or dorsal bundle of the posterior commissure (Szentágothai, 1964), but in general, Szentágothai's reasoning is well taken and is a cornerstone of present-day understanding of the wiring diagram of the substantia gelatinosa (Fig. 3.15).

Axonal Projections of Short-Axoned Cells

As mentioned in the preceding section, Ramon y Cajal (1909) noted that some of the central cells of the substantia gelatinosa had axons that never left the substantia gelatinosa. These would be short-axoned cells in his terminology. Again this may be slightly misleading, because the axons of some of these cells, even though they do not enter the white matter, are quite long. Nevertheless, the axons are shorter than those of the funicular central neurons of the gelatinosa. It should be emphasized that as far as present knowledge goes, the dendritic arborizations and afferent connections of the two types of central neurons, short-axoned and funicular, do not differ. It is only their axonal projections that vary.

Several studies that followed that of Ramon y Cajal confirmed that there were cells in the substantia gelatinosa whose processes did not

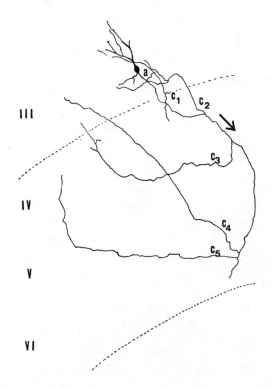

Fig. 3.16. Matsushita's depiction of the axonal tree of a lamina III cell. Note that some branches from junction C2 ramify back into the general region of the cell body. Also note that the axonal tree of this cell passes to laminae IV and V and is not restricted to lamina III. (From Matsushita, 1969.)

leave the gray matter of the dorsal horn (Szentágothai, 1964; Scheibel and Scheibel, 1968; Sugiura, 1975). Szentágothai (1964) felt that these intrinsic or short-axoned cells give rise to the "intrinsic longitudinal axon system of the substantia gelatinosa," and it should be understood that the substantia gelatinosa consists of both laminae II and III for Szentágothai. This plexus should not be confused with the longitudinal axon system of primary afferent origin that permeates laminae III and IV (Sterling and Kuypers, 1967) or laminae III, IV, and the upper part of V (Réthelyi and Szentágothai, 1973). The evidence for Szentágothai's conclusion was that the longitudinal axon system was intact in relatively short isolated segments of the dorsal horn (this procedure is described in the previous section).

Thus, since the intrinsic longitudinal axon system of the substantia gelatinosa survived the dorsal horn isolation procedures, Szentágothai (1964) felt that the axons came from cells in the substantia gelatinosa, "largely from the smaller neurons in lamina II." Furthermore, by relating the length of the isolated segments of spinal cord to the presence or absence of fibers in the intrinsic longitudinal plexus and the propriospinal pathways of the white matter, Szentágothai (1964) was able to estimate that the axons from gelatinosa cells that entered Lissauer's tract or the lateral fasciculus proprius (the funicular central cells of the gelatinosa) traveled longer distances (up to six segments) than the axons of the short-axoned central cells (maximum of 2–3 mm). Scheibel and Scheibel (1968) confirmed the descriptions of Ramon y Cajal (1909) and Szentágothai (1964), and they brought up the question as to whether the short-axoned cells in the substantia gelatinosa are Golgi type II cells, which is an important consideration in physiological reasoning about the arrangement of neurons in the spinal cord.

Although there is no universally accepted definition of the term "short-axoned cell," it would generally be accepted that a typical short-axoned or Golgi type II cell had an axon that (1) is short, (2) is confined to the region of gray matter where the parent cell is located, and (3) arborizes in the region of the dendritic field of the parent cell (Scheibel and Scheibel, 1966). Early debate on this matter seems to have begun with Ramon y Cajal (1909), who noted that Golgi, Kolliker, Lenhossek, and Van Gehuchten described the presence of numerous short-axoned cells in the spinal cord. Ramon y Cajal (1909) himself, however, vehemently denied the presence of any short-axoned cell in the spinal cord except for a few which he saw in the substantia gelatinosa. This view is generally accepted *for the dorsal horn* (Matsushita, 1969), and interest has therefore focused on the short-axoned cells of the substantia gelatinosa.

Scheibel and Scheibel (1968) state that "some of the axons (of central neurons in the substantia gelatinosa) appear to beak up in the immediate vicinity of the cell, producing a dense, spatially limited neuropil field, which can only be characterized as typical of Golgi type II cells. In these cases, when no axonal branches can be followed into white matter, it is a reasonable presumption that these elements may be true short-axoned cells" (Scheibel and Scheibel, 1968). Thus, Scheibel and Scheibel (1968) believe that some of the short-axoned cells in the substantia gelatinosa are true short-axoned, or Golgi type II, cells.

Matsushita (1969), however, is not as certain about the presence of short-axoned, or Golgi type II, cells, because he notes that although there are many dorsal-horn neurons that give axonal collaterals that ramify in the vicinity of the parent cell, the main process of the axon usually travels on for a considerable distance (Fig. 3.16). Mannen (1975), Sugiura (1975), and Mannen and Sugiura (1976) agree and reinforce the message of Matsushita. These investigators followed the processes of neurons impregnated by the Golgi method through serial sections, and they noted that the axonal and dendritic trees of neurons in the various laminae are much more extensive than is usually depicted (Figs. 3.13, 3.16, 3.27, and 3.30). By this method, however, they confirm that there are many neurons whose axons never leave the gray matter of the spinal cord. Interestingly enough, some of these cells are outside the substantia gelatinosa, being located in laminae VII, VIII, and X (Mannen, 1975). However, none of the cells identified by these

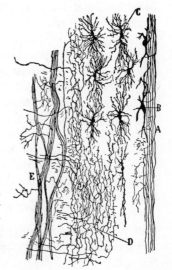

Fig. 3.17. Ramon y Cajal's picture of a horizontal section through the dorsal horn. The cell labeled B is identified as a "limitrophe" cell in Fig. 150 (Ramon y Cajal, 1909) and a marginal cell in Fig. 128 (Ramon y Cajal, 1909). The longitudinal plexus of the dorsal horn is represented by the letter D. (From Ramon y Cajal, 1909.)

investigators would be short-axoned cells in the sense that the axonal ramifications exist only in the region of the cell body. In all cases, at least one axonal branch traveled a considerable distance away from the cell body and the total distance traveled in the gray matter often exceeded 5 mm. These investigators also noted, as did Matsushita (1969) before them, that many neurons, regardless of whether they had a process entering the white matter or not, had a system of recurrent collaterals that ramify in the region of the parent cell body, and recent studies of physiologically identified neurons that are injected with a morphologically visualizable substance confirm this finding (Snow *et al.*, 1976; Czarkowska *et al.*, 1976).

Thus, it seems clear that there are in the spinal cord many neurons whose axons never leave the spinal gray matter. These cells are reported to be limited to the substantia gelatinosa, but recent evidence indicates that they are found in other areas of the spinal cord as well. These cells, even though their axons are restricted to gray matter, send at least one axonal process a long distance away from the cell body. Thus, these cells should probably not be regarded as short-axoned cells, even though they fulfill two major criteria for Golgi type II cells, namely that their axons are restricted to the gray matter in which the parent cell body is found and that they have axonal collaterals that ramify in the region of the parent cell body. It also seems to be true that many cells in the spinal cord, including some that send axons into the white matter, have axonal collaterals that ramify extensively in the region of the parent cell body. These recurrent collaterals may be responsible for the activity recorded by physiological techniques that led to the postulation of the presence of Golgi type II cells in various areas of the spinal cord.

In summary, the central cells of the substantia gelatinosa can be split into two groups on the basis of their axonal projections: (1) funicular cells and (2) short-axoned cells. The axons of the funicular cells project either to the tract of Lissauer or to the other parts of the white matter around the top of the dorsal horn, particularly the dorsolateral fasciculus proprius. The axons of short-axoned cells stay within the gray matter of the substantia gelatinosa. The axons of both the funicular cells and short-axoned cells are thought to end within the substantia gelatinosa and do not project to other areas. On this basis, the substantia gelatinosa is regarded as a closed system.

The short-axoned cells deserve further comment because they are thought to represent Golgi type II neurons in the spinal cord. Golgi type II neurons should have short axons, axons restricted to the gray matter of the

*parent cell body, and axonal arborizations that are restricted to the region
of the dendritic arborizations of the parent cell. There seem to be no cells in
the spinal cord, including the short-axoned cells of laminae II and III, that
fulfill all of these criteria. There are many cells, however, that have axonal
collaterals that arborize in the region of the dendrites and cell body of the
same cell, even though other parts of the axonal tree travel on for a long
distance. These recurrent collaterals probably are responsible for the physiological activity ascribed to Golgi type II cells.*

Border Cells ("Cellules Limitrophes")

The *"cellules limitrophes,"* or border cells, are large cells in the dorsal part of the substantia gelatinosa that Ramon y Cajal believed were
distinct from the equally large marginal cells of Waldeyer (Ramon y
Cajal, 1909). These cells have, according to Ramon y Cajal, ovoid or
piriform or semilunar-shaped cell bodies, and the dendrites extend
ventrally or laterally as well as horizontally, in contrast to the dendrites of either the marginal cells of Waldeyer (in lamina I) or the central cells of the substantia gelatinosa (in lamina II) (Fig. 3.10). It is possible, however, that Ramon y Cajal himself was not completely certain
about the separation of the marginal cells and the border, or *"limitrophe,"* cells. In his famous text, for example, Ramon y Cajal (1909)
reproduces the same figure twice [Figs. 128 and 150, Ramon y Cajal
(1909), Vol. I, p. 346 and 413] (Fig. 3.17 in this chapter). In Fig. 128,
cell B is an example of the *"cellules marginales de la substance de Rolando"* and in Fig. 150 the same cell is an example of the *"cellules limitrophes de la substance de Rolando."* This may be an error by Dr. Azou-
lay, who translated Ramon y Cajal's work from Spanish to French, but
if so, it is unfortunate, because the adjective *"marginale"* is usually
used by Ramon y Cajal to describe the cells of Waldeyer in the
marginal layer. At any rate, it does raise the question as to whether
there are two large cell types in the outer part of the dorsal horn—(1)
the marginal cells whose dendrites run tangentially over the surface of
the dorsal horn, except where they dip ventrally into deeper layers of
the dorsal horn, and (2) the *"cellules limitrophes"* (border cells,
marginal cells of the substance of Rolando), whose dendrites pass
anteriorly and laterally as well as tangentially in the upper part of
the dorsal horn—or whether there is just one large cell type whose
dendritic organization is somewhat variable. The axonal projections
of the border cells are much the same as for the marginal cells
of Waldeyer.

The Question as to the Separation of "Cellules Limitrophes" and Marginal Cells

The distinction between the *"cellules marginales"* and *"cellules limitrophes"* was used by Rexed to justify his splitting of lamina II into two parts, "a thin outer and a broad inner zone" (Rexed, 1952). Rexed (1952) states that "it is easy to see that it [lamina II] consists of a dorsal or *outer zone* and a ventral or *inner* zone. . . . The cells are more tightly packed and perhaps also in general a little smaller in the outer zone which therefore, stands out as a thin dark dorsal border of the second layer" (Rexed, 1952, p. 429). Since the *"cellules limitropes"* are large and relatively solitary, however, it is difficult to see how they could account for the dorsal layer of lamina II, whose cells are characterized as being small and closely packed (Rexed, 1952).

Sugiura (1975) also described one *"cellule limitrophe"* or outer neuron. This neuron was somewhat larger than the inner neurons (which are the central cells of Ramon y Cajal). The axon of this cell was bifurcate with one branch ending in lamina I and the other traveling into the neuropil of the substantia gelatinosa and dorsally "along the dorsal border of the substantia gelatinosa in the medial and lateral directions in the transverse plane" (Sugiura, 1975). These latter dendrites are thus passing tangentially along the surface of the dorsal horn in the same general pattern as marginal cell dendrites. Sugiura (1975) further describes two cells that are intermediate in dendritic organization between the inner and outer cells and thirteen cells that are variants of these forms. These numbers are not particularly strong support for the notion that there are two distinct cell types in the dorsal part of the substantia gelatinosa.

Presumably because of the similarity of *"cellules limitrophes"* to marginal cells, many investigators of neurons in the marginal layer and dorsal parts of the substantia gelatinosa do not mention the *"cellules limitrophes."* Scheibel and Scheibel (1968) are among these, but in Fig. I of their paper (Fig. 3.3) they mention that cell D is a "transitional cell sharing characteristics of both marginal and gelatinosal cells" (Scheibel and Scheibel, 1968). At the present time, until more definitive differences between the two cell types can be demonstrated, this is probably the best way to describe the *"cellules limitrophes,"* rather than making them a separate cell type as Ramon y Cajal did.

In summary, Ramon y Cajal stated that there were two cell types in the substantia gelantinosa, central cells and "cellules limitrophes." The limitrophe cells are large cells on the outer border of the substantia gelatinosa whose dendrites pass longitudinally over the dorsal horn as well as radially into the substance of the gelatinosa. The axons of these cells are not, so far as is known, distinctive, and the dendritic patterns resemble a combination of marginal-cell and central-cell dendritic organization. Thus, it would probably be better to regard these cells as neurons having characteristics of both marginal and central cells and avoid calling them a separate cell type until more is known about their function and specific afferent and efferent connections.

The Primary Afferent Input into Lamina II

The primary afferent input into the spinal cord is said to consist of collaterals that arise from anterior or posterior divisions of dorsal root afferent fibers (Ramon y Cajal, 1909; Réthelyi and Szentágothai, 1973). More recent work, however, indicates that some of the coarse afferents (see below) are not collaterals of anterior or posterior branches of primary afferent axons; rather they seem to rise from fibers that come directly from the dorsal root (A. G. Brown *et al.*, 1977c). Since this last finding is very new and thus needs confirmation and since classical descriptions state that primary afferent fibers that synapse in the gray matter are collaterals, we will continue to describe the primary afferent input in this way, even though it appears that it may not be a correct way to describe all the primary afferent fibers into the spinal cord.

The classical account of the primary afferent innervation of the substantia gelatinosa goes back to the work of Ramon y Cajal (1909). Ramon y Cajal noted that there were two groups of collaterals that enter the substantia gelatinosa from the white matter of the spinal cord: (1) the coarse collaterals that arise in white matter in the posterior columns at the dorsomedial edge of the substantia gelatinosa (Fig. 3.9) and (2) the fine collaterals that arise in the tract of Lissauer or the nearby white matter (Fig. 3.6). The coarse afferents have been regarded by all investigators as primary afferents; the fine afferents are not so easily characterized, but the usual opinion is that these fibers are a mixture of primary afferents and propriospinal fibers (Szentágothai, 1964).

Coarse Primary Afferent Collaterals

The coarse afferents to the spinal cord were first described by Ramon y Cajal (1909). He showed large-caliber collaterals entering the dorsomedial part of the dorsal horn from the adjacent white matter (Fig. 3.9). These collaterals curve laterally through the medial part of the dorsal horn and enter the substantia gelatinosa from below. When they reach the substantia gelatinosa, each coarse collateral breaks up into a characteristic flame-shaped arborization as illustrated in Ramon

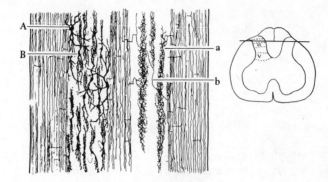

Fig. 3.18. Another horizontal section through the dorsal horn. Compare with Fig. 3.17. Cell A is a marginal cell of Waldeyer and cell B is a typical neuron of the substantia gelatinosa. Fiber b is a coarse collateral that breaks up into its terminal arborization field a. Note that the coarse primary afferent collateral arborization system extends much farther in a longitudinal than in a mediolateral direction. Thus, since this arborization has depth, it forms a sheet extending in the longitudinal plane of the substantia gelatinosa. (From Scheibel and Scheibel, 1968.)

y Cajal's well-known drawing (Fig. 3.9). Although Ramon y Cajal could not follow the coarse collaterals to axons in the dorsal root, he clearly felt that they were terminals of primary afferent fibers. This speculation has been proven correct by the degeneration studies of Szentágothai (1964) and the single primary afferent fiber injection results of A. G. Brown (1977).

From Figure 3.9 it can be seen that the arborization of each coarse collateral occupies a relatively restricted area of the substantia gelatinosa. However, within that restricted area, the fine processes from one coarse collateral are very numerous, and between the arbors, there are no fibers from the coarse primary afferent collaterals. Szentágothai (1964) mentioned that there were six to ten coarse-fiber arborizations in a given cross-sectional area of cat spinal cord, and he called each coarse-collateral arborization a "lobule." Scheibel and Scheibel (1968) added several important findings to this picture. First, they emphasized that the flame-shaped arborizations are cross-sectional views of long sheets of a large-axonal arborization (Fig. 3.18). The dimensions given by Scheibel and Scheibel for the arborization of a single coarse collateral in the lumbosacral area of spinal cord in kittens are 20 μm in a mediolateral direction and 150–500 μm in a craniocaudal direction. The depth of these fields is not given by Scheibel and Scheibel, but from their diagrams, the arbors can be seen to span laminae II and III, a distance of approximately 200–400 μm. Thus, the flame-shaped arborizations are in reality cross-sections of sheets of an extensive axonal plexus that have large dorsoventral and craniocaudal extents but are thin in the mediolateral direction (Fig. 3.18)).

The Scheibels (1968) also point out that the flame-shaped arborizations are discrete only in the cervical and lumbosacral enlargements. In the rest of the spinal cord, the coarse afferents break up into a more diffuse plexus and the lobules are not apparent (Fig. 3.19). In a previous section of this chapter, it was pointed out that Szentágothai (1964) and Scheibel and Scheibel (1968) stated that the fact that each coarse collateral breaks up into a discrete flame-shaped arbor means that those gelatinosal cells that are enmeshed in the arbor receive extensive synaptic contacts from one coarse afferent and that the gelatinosal cells that are between the arbors receive almost no such contacts. It now turns out that this is a characteristic only of the cervical and lumbosacral enlargements and not of the rest of the spinal cord, where the gelatinosa cells apparently receive a relatively uniform innervation from coarse collaterals. This presumably implies that there is a major difference in the segmental organization of the coarse collaterals in the spinal cord.

In 1976, Beal and Fox carefully repeated the experiments of Ramon y Cajal (1909), Szentágothai (1964), and Scheibel and Scheibel (1968). They noted that the main stem of the coarse collateral, just before it broke up into its axonal arbor, was 4.2 μm in diameter and on this basis was almost certainly myelinated. These investigators called the terminations of the coarse collaterals the "confined ansiform axonal complexes," and they indicated that some of the central terminals of the glomeruli of laminae I–III almost certainly arise from the coarse collaterals. We will return to this point when we consider the organization of the neuropil in lamina II.

By contrast to all the above authors, LaMotte (1977) felt that the main projection of the coarse collaterals is not to laminae I, II, or III but rather to laminae IV, V, and VI. This conclusion is based on the

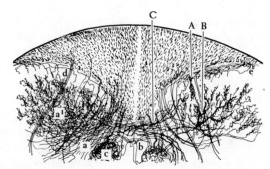

Fig. 3.19. A Golgi section demonstrating that the coarse primary afferent aborization does not form discrete lobules in the substantia gelatinosa of segments of the spinal cord outside of the cervical and lumbosacral enlargements. Axonal field a' is such a terminal field. Compare with Fig. 3.9. (From Scheibel and Scheibel, 1968.)

finding that when she cut the posterior white column, which she stated would damage only the coarse or large collaterals, the degeneration, as seen by the Nauta and Fink–Heimer methods for degenerating axons and terminals, was largely confined to laminae IV–VI. It is difficult to reconcile these findings with the large number of papers showing the arborization of the coarse collaterals in the substantia gelatinosa or at least in lamina III, and LaMotte mentions that species differences or the fact that her work was not done at lumbosacral areas of the spinal cord might explain her results. Another possibility is that it may be very difficult to selectively cut only coarse afferent fibers by cutting laterally in the posterior white column. Whatever the explanation, the study by LaMotte (1977) is the one suggestion that the coarse primary afferent collaterals have little input into laminae II and III, particularly lamina III.

One point might be made about the laminar distribution of the coarse collaterals into the dorsal part of the dorsal horn. From the studies by Ramon y Cajal (1909), Szentágothai (1964), Scheibel and Scheibel (1968), and Beal and Fox (1976), it seems clear that the flame-shaped arborizations that arise from the coarse collaterals do not enter lamina I, the marginal cell layer of Waldeyer. It is interesting, however, that all the above-quoted authors either wrote before the small cell part of the dorsal horn was split into laminae II and III (Ramon y Cajal, 1909), or they studied laminae II and III as a unit (Szentágothai, 1964; Scheibel and Scheibel, 1968; Beal and Fox, 1976). Thus, the possibility that the coarse collaterals might be restricted primarily to lamina III was not discussed by the investigators. However, in recent years, there has been a considerable debate as to the number of primary afferent terminals in lamina II. The issue is not completely settled as yet, but one fact seems to be that the most of the primary afferent terminals in lamina II degenerate much more rapidly than those in lamina III. It has been suggested that this difference in degeneration time might be a reflection of the size of the parent axon (LaMotte, 1977; Réthelyi, 1977). If this is the case, the rapid primary afferent degeneration in lamina II might reflect fine-fiber input and the slow primary afferent degeneration in lamina III might reflect coarse-fiber input. In this regard, A. G. Brown (1977) and A. G. Brown et al. (1977c) report arborizations of individually identified coarse primary afferent collaterals are found primarily in laminae III and IV and are not seen in lamina II. This might be due to a difficulty in filling the finer processes of a coarse collateral with horseradish peroxidase, but it is probably due to a restriction of the flame-shaped arbors to lamina III and below. Thus, there are strong suggestions that the primary afferent input into lamina III is from coarse collaterals. One way to provide further evidence would be to destroy the fine or coarse afferents selectively.

Recently, a powerful combined physiological and anatomic technique has given insight into the termination and function of both the coarse and fine collaterals. Large primary afferent collaterals were impaled with a microelectrode filled with a concentrated solution of horseradish peroxidase (A. G. Brown, 1977; A. G. Brown *et al.*, 1977c). The electrical characteristics of the electrode were good enough so that the receptive field of the afferent fiber could be determined. Then the axon was filled with peroxidase, which can be visualized after appropriate treatment (Fig. 3.20). By this method A. G. Brown (1977) and

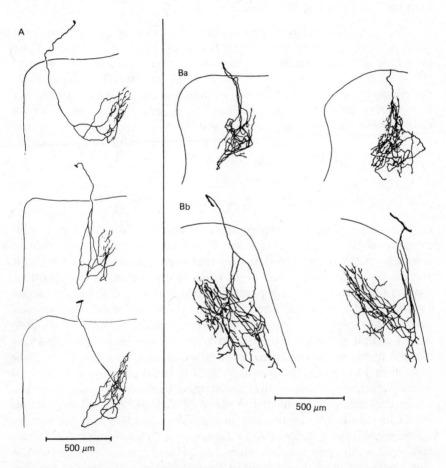

Fig. 3.20. A depiction of single, individually identified, hair afferents that have been filled with a visible marker and then reconstructed in serial sections. (From A. G. Brown, 1977.)

A. G. Brown *et al.* (1977c) demonstrated that the coarse collaterals arise from axons that innervate hair follicles. Furthermore, A. G. Brown *et al.* (1977c) found that the rostrocaudal and mediolateral extent of the axonal fields of the coarse collaterals were greater than Scheibel and Scheibel (1968) had indicated. A. G. Brown *et al.* (1977c) found that the axonal arborizations could extend for distances up to 1700 μm in the rostrocaudal direction and 150–400 μm in the mediolateral direction. Because of possible limitations on the spread of the enzyme, Brown felt that these were minimum estimates of the distances. Using the same technique, Light and Perl (1977) noted that finer myelinated fibers, which could be classified as mechanical nociceptors, ended in laminae I and the upper part of II.

In summary, the coarse primary afferent collaterals arise from large axons in the lateral part of the dorsal funiculus. They pass ventrally along the medial side of the dorsal horn, then curve into the gray matter and enter the substantia gelatinosa, where they break up into the characteristic flame-shaped arborizations that are relatively restricted mediolaterally but have a very long craniocaudal extent. Early studies suggested that the flame-shaped collaterals spanned the substantia gelatinosa (lamina II and III), but more recent suggestions are that they are restricted to lamina III. They are apparently the terminals of hair fibers.

Fine Primary Afferent Collaterals

The other major group of fibers that come into synaptic relationship with the cells in lamina II are fine collaterals that can be traced to axons in the white matter that surrounds the dorsal horn. It should be understood that most early studies used the method of Golgi to demonstrate these processes (see Ramon y Cajal, 1909; Szentágothai, 1964; Scheibel and Scheibel, 1968). As stated before, the method of Golgi is an extremely powerful method, but a major difficulty is that although the axons in lamina II can be followed back to the white matter of the spinal cord, they cannot be followed to their cells of origin or into the dorsal root. This is because the axons blend with the other fine axons that are stained in the white matter or because the axons pass out of the plane of section. A similar situation exists for the coarse fibers, but degeneration studies and the single-axon injection technique of A. G. Brown (1977) clearly indicate that the coarse fibers are primary afferents. The evidence is not so clear for the fine fibers. At the present time, it seems certain that some of the fine fibers in the tract of Lissauer are primary afferents, but the majority seem to be propriospinal.

Ramon y Cajal (1909) noted that fine fibers that formed synaptic contacts with neurons in the substantia gelatinosa came from three places: (1) the tract of Lissauer; (2) the dorsal part of the dorsal proprius bundle, and (3) the dorsal part of the lateral proprius bundle. Thus, in general, the fine axons in the substantia gelatinosa are collaterals whose parent axons are in the white matter that surrounds the top of the dorsal horn. Because of earlier work that indicated that many of the fibers in the tract of Lissauer were small primary sensory axons, Ramon y Cajal regarded most of these fine processes coming from the tract of Lissauer as collaterals of primary sensory axons. It seems clear, however, that he was not as certain about this as he was about the coarse collaterals. The fibers coming from medial and lateral sides of the dorsal horn, Ramon y Cajal felt, were predominately propriospinal. Ramon y Cajal did not note any peculiarities about the arborizations of these fine fibers except that the fibers tended to break into their terminal arborizations in areas of the substantia gelatinosa near their entrances.

Studies following Ramon y Cajal (1909) were generally confirmatory. Pearson (1952), for example, noted that fine axons entered the substantia gelatinosa from the tract of Lissauer and nearby white matter. He stated that some of the fine primary afferent axons circled the substantia gelatinosa and entered it from below and the others just passed directly into the substantia gelatinosa and there ended. He assumed that all these fibers were primary afferents. He regarded the coarse fibers as passing through the substantia gelatinosa to end on cells in the nucleus proprius.

In 1964, Szentágothai made a major contribution to our understanding of the organization of the substantia gelatinosa. Szentágothai regarded the substantia gelatinosa as representing both laminae II and III of Rexed, and he noted five types of afferent fibers into the gelatinosa. The first were the coarse collaterals already described by Ramon y Cajal (and many others) that looped through the dorsal horn to enter the substantia gelatinosa from the ventral surface (Fig. 3.9). The second group of fibers emerge from the tract of Lissauer and coarse ventrally, some taking part in the marginal plexus already described by Ramon y Cajal and the rest entering the substantia gelatinosa. These are the fine fibers of Ramon y Cajal. Each of these fine fibers arborizes into a "columnar area about half the depth of the substantia gelatinosa in length and around 10–20 μm breadth" (Szentágothai, 1964). These arborizations of the fine and coarse axon collaterals overlapped so that a "plexus of high density results" (Szentágothai, 1964). Another group of fibers come from the dorsal most part of the lateral fasciculus proprius. According to Szentágothai,

these fibers curve around the ventrolateral edge of the substantia gelatinosa and then enter the substantia gelatinosa from below. In size
they appear to be intermediate between the large coarse collaterals and
the fine fibers that come from the tract of Lissauer. Their axonal fields
resemble the flame-shaped arborizations from the coarse collaterals,
except that they are smaller and arise from axons on the lateral side of
laminae II and III rather than from axons on the medial side, which is
where the coarse collaterals enter. Szentágothai also notes fibers coming through the dorsal part of the posterior commissure to end in medial parts of the substantia gelatinosa. Finally, he noted fibers coming
into the substantia gelatinosa from below, and he thought they originated from an axonal plexus in the center of the dorsal horn. Szentágothai was somewhat hesitant as to whether they were ending in the
substantia gelatinosa or just passing through. He raised the possibility
that these last axons came from the pyramidal tract and emphasized the
importance of working out in greater detail the connections of the substantia gelatinosa with fibers that enter from deeper regions of the spinal cord.

In this same paper, Szentágothai (1964) described the experiment
where he maintained an isolated segment of dorsal horn (Fig. 3.14)
with an intact blood supply for approximately 2 months. After this
time, the isolated dorsal horn was studied histologically, and most of
the axons in the tract of Lissauer were intact and the axons in the dorsal lateral fasciculus proprius remained "completely intact (Szentágothai, 1964). Furthermore, the commissural fibers were also
regarded by Szentágothai as coming from the substantia gelatinosa of
the opposite side. Thus, Szentágothai regarded the majority of fine
axons ending in the substantia gelatinosa as intrinsic (i.e., coming
from substantia gelatinosa neurons). The fine primary afferent collaterals, he felt, were restricted to two bundles, one on the medial side
and one on the lateral side of the entering dorsal root. It is clear, however, that Szentágothai regards these as in the minority as compared
to the intrinsic or propriospinal fibers.

Scheibel and Scheibel (1968) restudied the dorsal horn with Golgi
techniques. They emphasized that the flame-shaped arborizations that
arose from the coarse collaterals were cross-sections of long sheets of a
large axonal arborizations (see the section on coarse primary afferent
collaterals, above). Scheibel and Scheibel (1968) then noted two systems of fine fibers. The first system consists of small fibers that
"emerge from the region of Lissauer's tract," and these fibers form
capping plexuses over the apical (superficial) region of the flame-
shaped arborizations (Fig. 3.21). The second system of fine fibers can
be traced to the most ventral portion of the dorsomedial white matter

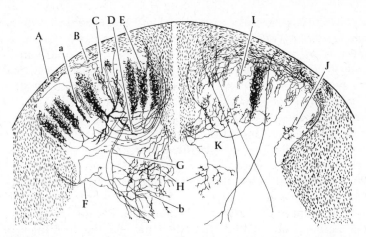

Fig. 3.21. The apical and basal fine-fiber plexuses in the substantia gelatinosa. The apical capping plexus is indicated at C. The fibers at K are forming the basal infiltrations of the flame-shaped afferents. Other prominent structures are a substantia gelatinosa neuron (a), a flame-shaped arborization (E), and fine fibers in Lissauer's tract (A). (From Scheibel and Scheibel, 1968.)

(Fig. 3.21), a region of the dorsal white column often referred to as the cornu-commissural tract or zone of Marie (Nathan and Smith, 1959). These fibers form rather simple terminal arborization patterns with clusters of terminal boutons. Some of these boutons end on dendrites of cells in lamina IV, but most of the processes follow the large afferents into the substantia gelatinosa, where they form a plexus around the bases of the flame-shaped arborizations (Fig. 3.21). Scheibel and Scheibel (1968) regarded the apical plexus fibers as being primarily propriospinal, whereas the fibers forming the basal plexuses they regarded as being a mixture of primary afferents and propriospinal fibers.

Scheibel and Scheibel (1968) suggest that the apical and basal capping plexuses might be the explanation for the primary afferent depolarization (Wall, 1962) that results in the presynaptic inhibition that is found in the dorsal horn. They also suggest that these fibers might provide the presynaptic boutons in the axoaxonic contacts that are numerous in this region of the spinal cord.

In a recent study, Beal and Fox (1976) carefully repeated previous Golgi studies. They extended Ramon y Cajal's work by noting that there are two types of fine collaterals in the substance of Rolando. The first type is found throughout laminae II and III, and these are fibers with fine terminal branches bearing small *"bouton en passant"* endings. These resemble the identifiable collaterals of the central neurons of the substantia gelatinosa and so Beal and Fox regard the fibers with *"bouton en passant"* endings as the propriospinal axons that arise from the neurons in the substantia gelatinosa. The other fibers are found primarily in the lamina II, and end in *"boutons terminaux"*. Beal and Fox believe they are fine descending collaterals from primary afferents. In a somewhat similar analysis, Réthelyi (1977) described "small diameter fibers, apparently of dorsal root origin which fan out from a narrow region corresponding to the dorsal root entry zone to spread medially and ventrally in the superficial dorsal horn." They are most apparent in sagittal sections. They give off longitudinal side branches and the branches give rise to large end bulbs, which are usually preceded by two to three equally large *"en passant"* enlargements. These areas of termination are restricted to lamina II. Because these fibers are so fine, Réthelyi speculated that they may be the terminals of unmyelinated afferents. He then suggests that only unmyelinated afferents terminate in lamina II, whereas the myelinated afferents (the coarse primary afferent collaterals of Ramon y Cajal) are restricted to lamina III.

LaMotte (1977) attempted to determine the distribution of the coarse and fine afferents to the dorsal horn. She sectioned the dorsal root or injected a dorsal root ganglion with radioactive amino acids, and these procedures label (either by degeneration or by transport of radioactive material) both the large and small afferents that make up the dorsal root. She compared this with the degeneration data obtained from a section of the tract of Lissauer, the latter procedure being designed to sever both the fine primary afferents and propriospinal fibers in this pathway. One of LaMotte's major conclusions was that the fine afferents terminate in laminae I, II, and III, whereas the coarse afferents, which are collaterals from dorsal column axons, terminate in laminae IV, V, and VI. The reason for these conclusions was that a Lissauer's-tract lesion caused maximum degeneration in laminae I–III and the dorsal-column lesion caused maximum degeneration in laminae IV–VI. It is difficult to accept part of this conclusion, however, since other investigators that studied the afferents to lamina III or the substantia gelatinosa by the Golgi method noted the flame-shaped arborizations that come from collaterals of large axons in the dorsal column (Ramon y Cajal, 1909; Pearson, 1952; Szentágothai, 1964; Scheibel and Scheibel, 1968; Beal and Fox, 1976). Furthermore, Brown (1977) injected large primary afferents with rapid conduction velocities, and terminal arborizations were demonstrated in laminae III and IV. Thus, it seems likely that coarse primary afferent collaterals synapse in lamina III. The second conclusion, namely that the fine afferents synapse in laminae I, II, and III might be correct, but the speculation by Réthelyi (1977) that unmyelinated fibers are restricted to lamina II and large myelinated fibers to lamina III should be remembered.

La Motte (1977) then subdivided the fine afferents into two populations based on differences in degeneration times. The more rapidly degenerating fibers distribute primarily to laminae II and III and the slowly degenerating fibers to lamina I and the outer part of lamina II. This subdivision of the fine-fiber systems fits well with the demonstration by Kumazawa and Perl (1978) that slowly conducting myelinated fibers end in lamina I and the unmyelinated fibers in lamina II.

A last point might be made here. It appears obvious from the above discussion that many earlier investigators felt that there was a fine-fiber input into the substantia gelatinosa. More recently, however, there have been suggestions that there was little degeneration in lamina II, as opposed to lamina III, when the dorsal root was cut (Ralston, 1965, 1968b, 1971; Sterling and Kuypers, 1967; Shriver et al., 1968). This result was disputed (Sprague and Ha, 1964; Szentágothai, 1964; Heimer and Wall, 1968; Petras, 1968; Réthelyi and Szentágothai, 1969). This dispute is now thought to be related to differences in degeneration times for coarse and fine afferents (Heimer and Wall, 1968; LaMotte, 1977), but the issue is probably not completely settled yet. Of interest in this regard is the general paucity of degenerating terminals in the upper four spinal laminae after dorsal rhizotomy (see Ralston, 1977), a relatively surprising finding for an area of spinal cord that is thought to have such an important primary sensory input.

In summary, the fine fiber input to the gelatinosa is complex and there are differences in the various descriptions of these fibers. Ramon y Cajal noted that the fine fibers of the gelatinosa arise as collaterals from fibers in the tract of Lissauer and the nearby fasciculi proprii. Szentágothai confirmed the location of these fibers and also mentioned that other fibers enter from the posterior commissure, from the lateral white matter, and from deeper parts of the spinal gray matter. Scheibel and Scheibel noted fine fibers that emerged from the region of Lissauer's tract and formed capping plexuses over the tops of the flame-shaped arborizations and a basal plexus that emerged from the cornu-commissural tract. The relation of these various plexuses to each other is not completely clear. Ramon y Cajal felt that the majority of fibers in this plexus were probably primary afferents, but later opinion is that the large majority of the fine fibers in this area are propriospinal. Recent suggestions have been that fine fibers are restricted to lamina II and coarse fibers to lamina III.

Organization of the Neuropil

When the neuropil of the dorsal horn is examined in the electron microscope, one of the interesting findings is that it is very difficult to distinguish laminae I, II, and III by variations in synaptic architecture. There are slight differences, of course, but the overall pattern seems remarkably similar. The most prominent structures in the neuropil in lamina II are the glomeruli, and so these will be considered first and then the "nonglomerular" neuropil will be described.

Glomeruli

The neuropil of lamina II is characterized by the synaptic arrangements called "complex synaptic arrays" by Ralston (1965, 1968a, 1971); "glomeruli" by Kerr (1966, 1970a, 1975a,c), Coimbra *et al.* (1974), Knyihár and Gerebtzoff (1973), and Knyihár *et al.* (1974); and "large synaptic complexes" by Réthelyi and Szentágothai (1969). These glomeruli, as we will call them, make up approximately 5% of the synapses in laminae I–III (Ralson, 1971). It is clear that, despite the different names, the same structure is being examined but the descriptions vary somewhat (Figs. 3.22–25). Since most authors regard the glomerulus as a key structure in the synaptic organization of the neuropil of the dorsal horn, it is important to understand the various ideas about the organization of this structure.

All investigators agree that the central element or terminal of the glomerulus consists of an enlarged axonal bouton (Figs. 3.22–25). The bouton contains predominately round, clear vesicles whose dimensions range (depending on which study is consulted) from 300 to 700 Å. Mitochondria and a few dense-core vesicles are also seen. Most investigators report that these boutons are relatively electron dense, so that they appear to be dark in electron micrographs. Knyihár and Gerebtzoff (1973) note that there seems to be a population of neurofilaments that increases the density of the terminal, but most investigators state that the axoplasm itself has an inherent electron density. The central terminals are boutons *"en passage"* (Ralston, 1971; Knyihár and Gerebtzoff, 1973). Ralston stated that the axons that give rise to the central element are unmyelinated, but Knyihár and Gerebtzoff (1973) mention that the preterminal fibers are sometimes covered by a thin myelin sheath.

The central terminal in the glomerulus is in synaptic contact with a group of neuronal processes, and it is in the arrangement of these processes and the question of other synapses on the processes and

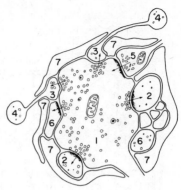

Fig. 3.22. Kerr's schematic diagram of the glomerulus of the substantia gelatinosa. The labeled components are: (1) the central bouton; (2) dendrites, probably from lamina IV neurons; (3 and 4) a spine head from a substantia gelatinosa neuron dendrite; (5) a presynaptic bouton filled with flattened vesicles, (6) an unknown dendrite, and (7) a glial lamella. (From Kerr, 1975a.)

onto the central element where descriptions differ. Ralston (1965, 1968a, 1971) and Kerr (1966, 1970a, 1975a,c) present a view of the organization of the glomerulus that is simpler than other schemes (Fig. 3.22). These investigators state that most of the processes upon which the central element terminates are dendrites. The number of dendrites are not mentioned but the numbers illustrated are three to eight. Most of the dendrites are regarded by both Ralston and Kerr as probably coming from large cells in laminae IV and V (dendrites labeled 2 in Fig. 3.22). Kerr (1975a,c) adds two complicating factors: first, an occasional dendrite that contains vesicles, and he regards these as spines from dendrites that arise from the central neurons of the substantia gelatinosa (3 in Fig. 3.22); second, dendrites of unknown origin (6 in Fig. 3.22). The other feature of the glomeruli is that there are axonal terminals on the central element (5 in Fig. 3.22). This last junction is thus an axoaxonic synapse. The vesicles in the smaller axonal terminal may be round (Ralston, 1971), but usually they are flattened or pleomorphic (Ralston, 1971; Kerr, 1975a,c).

Kerr (1975a) speculated on the function of the glomeruli in the following way. The central terminal he regards as arising from a primary afferent. This point will be discussed later, but most investigators today agree. Impulses in the primary afferents would then depolarize the dendrites of the large neurons in lamina IV as well as the dendrites of the central cells of the substantia gelatinosa. The lamina IV cells probably send axons into the spinothalamic tract, and the substantia gelatinosa cells probably discharge back into the substantia gelatinosa to produce inhibition. This finding, Kerr suggests, might explain why spinothalamic cells fire briefly when their receptive field is activated

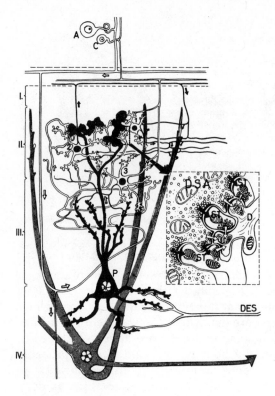

Fig. 3.23. Réthelyi and Szentágothai's schematic diagram of the golmerulus of the substantia gelatinosa. In the large diagram, 1, 2, and 3 are neurons of the substantia gelatinosa, and P is a large pyramidal neuron at the junction of laminae III and IV. In the inset, DSA is a terminal of neuron P, ST is a small-axon terminal, and D is the dendrite of a substantia gelatinosa neuron. (From Réthelyi and Szentágothai, 1973.)

and then are quickly inhibited. Kerr emphasizes that further data may well modify this scheme, but it seems to be a simple and straightforward beginning.

The scheme proposed by Réthelyi and Szentágothai (1969, 1973) is more complex (Fig. 3.17). They felt that the central axon terminal arises not from primary afferents as is now believed by several investigators (see below), but from a large pyramidal cell between laminae III and IV (P in Fig. 3.23). Réthelyi (1977), however, indicates that this is probably not correct. The central element then synapses on two types of fibers, the first of which are large dendrites, which Réthelyi and Szentágothai (1969, 1973) believe arise from central neurons of the substantia gelatinosa (D in Fig. 3.23). The second is a group of processes (ST in Fig. 3.23, inset) that contain small, round, clear vesicles and cytoplasmic densities that are interpreted as indicating that they are presynaptic to the dendritic (D) profiles. Thus, the ST processes appear to be incoming axons, and they are postsynaptic to DSA and presynaptic to D in Fig. 3.23 (inset). By contrast, in Fig. 3.22, the incoming axon is presynaptic to the central terminal (5 in Fig. 3.22). In

Réthelyi and Szentágothai's scheme, both the central element (DSA) and the axons (ST) synapse on the dendrites (D) of substantia gelatinosa cells. In addition, the central element (DSA) synapses on the incoming axon (ST).

The description by Coimbra *et al.* (1974) is intermediate between the above two descriptions. A picture based on their paper has been drawn to facilitate comparison (Fig. 3.24). These investigators state that the central terminal, which is relatively electron dense, ends on four to eight processes. Some of the processes "appear to be ordinary dendrites with pale cytoplasm, few mitochondria, and some agranular reticulum" (D in Fig. 3.24). These are postsynaptic to the central process or knob as they refer to it. The other processes contain vesicles and can be divided into two types. The first, called V_1, contains agranular vesicles that vary widely in number and size (the diameter ranged between 35 and 110μ m) and are irregularily scattered in the terminal (V_1 in Fig. 3.24). These processes also contain occasional large dense-core vesicles, smooth-walled cisternae and a single mitochondrion and are postsynaptic to the central process. The second, called V_2, contains numerous flattened vesicles. It appears to be presynaptic to the central knob (V_2 in Fig. 3.24). Occasionally, both V_1 and V_2 endings appear to be presynaptic to the small dendrites. Coimbra *et al.* (1974) state that the type V_1 terminals "were like adjacent dendritic profiles, postsynaptic to the central knobs, and usually contained few irregularly distributed vesicles sometimes hardly distinguishable from cross-sectioned smooth-walled cisternal profiles occuring in dendrites. . . . Furthermore, a few contained ribosomes . . . though this was an exceptional observation. Hence it is our impression that these terminals may be vesicle-containing dendrites . . . whose presynaptic contacts are rarely located in the immediate vicinity of the glomeruli."

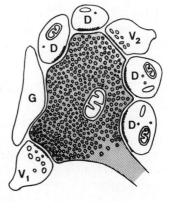

Fig. 3.24. A diagram of the structures of the glomerulus of the substantia gelatinosa according to the study of Coimbra *et al.* (1974). The central bouton is darkened. The processes D are "ordinary dendrites," V_1 is a terminal that contains clear vesicles of widely varying sizes, and V_2 is a terminal with round and flattened vesicles. G is a glial process.

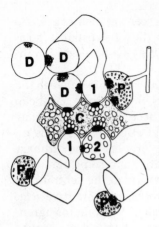

Fig. 3.25. Gobel's schematic diagram of the glomerulus of the substantia gelatinosa. C is the central bouton. 1 and 2 are dendritic spines that the central process (C) contacts. Type II spines also seem to synapse on type I spines. D are dendritic shafts that are contacted by the central element C, and these shafts also seem to form synaptic contacts with other shafts and with type I spines. The vesicles in the D endings are flattened. The P endings contain flattened vesicles and contact dendritic shafts, type I spines, and the central process. (From Gobel, 1974.)

Knyihár and Gerebtzoff (1973) and Knyihár *et al.* (1974) state that almost all the synapses in the glomerulus are axoaxonal, with the central bouton being presynaptic to the surrounding axons.

Finally, the construct of Gobel (1974, 1976) is most complicated of all (Fig. 3.25). It may be that some of the differences between Gobel's picture and those described above are due to the fact that Gobel examined the substantia gelatinosa of the spinal nucleus of the trigminal nerve. Nevertheless, the similarities between the substantia gelatinosa of the spinal nucleus of V and the substantia gelatinosa for the spinal nerves make it worthwhile to consider Gobel's formulation. As in all the other studies, the central element is dark and appears to be presynaptic to a number of other processes. Gobel then describes three types of processes to which the central terminal is presynaptic: (1) dendritic shafts (D in Fig. 3.25), (2) type I dendritic spines containing no synaptic vesicles (1 in Fig. 3.25), and (3) type II dendritic spines containing synaptic vesicles (2 in Fig. 3.25). In addition, there are P-type axonal endings, which are presynaptic to the central bouton. Gobel states that the central process and P endings have an inherent electron density. On the basis of morphological evidence, Gobel concludes that the type 2 dendritic spine is presynaptic to the type I dendritic spine, and that the dendritic shafts are presynaptic to one another and also to the type I dendritic spines. Furthermore, the P-type axonal endings contact not only the central ending but also the type I spines. The P endings and the endings on the dendritic shafts (D) are regarded as inhibitory. The central terminal (C) and type II (2) spine synapses are regarded as excitatory. If all this circuitry can be confirmed, then this would be an extremely complicated synaptic apparatus.

In a later publication, Gobel (1976) expanded his previous study and concentrated on the presumed synapses that the type 2 dendrites make on the central ending. If Gobel's assumptions are correct, then this would be a dendroaxonic synapse. Gobel speculated that the type 2 dendrite might be excitatory to both the central process (C in Fig. 3.25) and the type 1 dendrite (1 in Fig. 3.25), and the P ending might be inhibitory to both the central process and the type 1 dendrite. Much work will be needed to confirm or deny these suggestions.

The "Nonglomerular" Synapses in the Neuropil

Although the glomeruli are the most prominent and intensely studied elements in the neuropil of lamina II, they occupy a small amount of space and make up only about 5% of the synapses in this area (Ralston, 1971). The rest of the neuropil of lamina II is characterized by bundles of unmeylinated axons traveling either parallel to the surface of the cord or radially (Ralson, 1965, 1968a; Kerr, 1966). There is also an absence of myelinated axons in this area, except for the radially oriented, myelinated, coarse primary afferents in medial parts of this lamina. The commonest synaptic arrangement is axodendritic. There seems to be nothing particularly remarkable about these synapses. In the majority of cases, the vesicles in the axonal terminal are round, approximately 500 Å in diameter, and they are clustered against the presynaptic membrane. The cytoplasmic thickenings are characteristic of the typical asymmetrical type of synaptic bouton (Gray and Guillery, 1966). Some of the presynaptic terminals in these synapses, however, contain flattened or pleomorphic vesicles and, in this case, the cytoplasmic thickenings are symmetrical. Axoaxonal synapses are also seen in this lamina. Often the axon that is presynaptic to the terminal knob contains flattened or pleomorphic vesicles (Kerr, 1970b). There are a few synapses that contain densecore vesicles (Kerr, 1970a; Duncan and Morales, 1973a,b). Axosomatic contacts in lamina II are very rare, although Kerr (1970a) mentions that an occasional cell has them.

Primary Afferent Degeneration as Seen with the Electron Microscope

The Glomeruli. The glomeruli that characterize lamina II consist of a large, dark central bouton surrounded by several processes (Figs. 3.22–3.25). Although it seems clear that the processes around the central bouton do not all have the same origin, they will be referred to as the "outer processes" of the glomeruli for purposes of this discussion.
The Central Bouton. The characteristics of the central bouton are:

(1) that it forms synapses on most of the outer fibers of the glomeruli, (2) that the axoplasm of this process is relatively electron dense, and (3) that the acid phosphatase content of this terminal is relatively high (Knyihár and Gerebtzoff, 1973; Coimbra et al., 1974). When the dorsal root is cut, most investigators agree that some of the central boutons degenerate (Kerr, 1970b; Gobel, 1974; Knyihár et al., 1974; Coimbra et al., 1974). Thus, the weight of present evidence seems to indicate that the central bouton is of primary afferent origin.

It is interesting that some recent light microscopic studies on the organization of the primary afferents identify the coarse, flame-shaped collaterals as the source of the central boutons (Beal and Fox, 1976; Réthelyi, 1977). If this is the case, then the coarse collaterals would presumably travel to lamina II, since the glomeruli are in both laminae II and III.

One other point to note is that not all central boutons degenerate when the dorsal root is cut. Knyihár, et al. (1974) specifically state that only half of the central boutons are damaged by dorsal rhizotomy. It will be most interesting if further work indicates that there are two types of glomeruli, those that have central processes derived from primary afferents and those that have central processes derived from some other axon system.

The Outer Processes.   Most investigators either state that the outer processes are intact or do not mention any degeneration in the outer processes when the dorsal root is cut (Ralston, 1965, 1968b, 1971; Kerr, 1970b, 1975a; Gobel, 1974; Knyihár et al., 1974; Coimbra et al., 1974). Thus, although there is one study that is in disagreement (Réthelyi and Szentágothai, 1969), the weight of evidence seems to be that the outer processes of the glomeruli are not affected by dorsal rhizotomy and thus are probably not primary afferent fibers.

Kerr (1975a) notes in passing that sections of Lissauer's tract also have little affect on the outer processes of the glomeruli. Since Lissauer's tract is made up primarily of propriospinal fibers, Kerr thought that the outer processes are also not of propriospinal origin.

The "Nonglomerular" Synapses in the Neuropil of Lamina II

There has been some disagreement as to how many and which types of synapses are affected when the dorsal root is cut. Ralston (1965, 1968b, 1971) felt that very few synapses degenerated in lamina II after dorsal rhizotomy. Those processes that did degenerate were presynaptic to dendrites (Fig. 3.7). Thus, the degenerating synapses are a very small portion of the axodendritic synapses that are found in this lamina. Rarely there was a degenerating axoaxonal synapse, and in these "the degenerating synapse of dorsal root origin was invariably presynaptic in axoaxonal complexes" (Ralston, 1968b).

Several investigators using light microscopy disagreed with the conclusion of Ralston as to the number of synapses that degenerate after dorsal rhizotomy (Heimer and Wall, 1968; Réthelyi and Szentágothai, 1969), but there have not been many follow-up studies at the fine-structure level. Heimer and Wall (1968) did confirm their light microscopic findings in the electron microscope by noting many degenerating terminals in lamina II 1–3 days following dorsal rhizotomy. Kerr (1970b) also noted numerous degenerating terminals in his material, but he did not distinguish between laminae II and III, calling this whole region the substantia gelatinosa. Ralston (1977) notes that there are very few degenerating terminals in any of the upper spinal laminae in comparison to the total number of synapses in this area, but he also notes in his later study that the percentages of degerating terminals are approximately the same in laminae II and III. Thus, early ideas that there was little degeneration in lamina II as compared to lamina III are probably not correct. It does seem clear, however, that the synapses in the two laminae degenerate at different times, and there is a relative paucity of degenerating synapses in both laminae when the dorsal root is cut.

In summary, the most prominent structures in the neuropil of lamina II are the glomeruli. Each glomerulus consists of a central relatively dark axonal terminal and a group of peripheral processes, most of which are in synaptic contact with the central terminal. There is general but not complete agreement that the central terminal is an "en passant" ending of a primary afferent collateral. There is relatively little agreement about the peripheral processes. Axodendritic, axoaxonic, dendrodendritic, and dendroaxonic synapses are proposed by various investigators. The various individual schemes have been described in the text and diagrammed in Figs. 3.22–3.25.

The nonglomerular neuropil in lamina II consists of axodendritic and a few axoaxonal synapses. There are reported to be few axosomatic contracts in this area. When the dorsal roots are cut, a few axonal terminals on dendrites die, and the presynaptic fiber in a few axoaxonic contacts degenerates. A surprisingly small percentage of synapses show degeneration of either the pre- or postsynaptic element when the dorsal root is cut.

LAMINA III

Lamina III is a broad band across the dorsal horn (Fig. 3.1). This lamina borders on the white matter medially, but laterally it is covered by the ventral bend of laminae I and II (Fig. 3.1). The nerve cells are less closely packed than in lamina II, and thus, lamina III has a lighter appearance in cytoarchitectonic stains. The cells are spindle shaped and are oriented vertically to the surface of the lamina. The cells have little cytoplasm and there is only a small amount of Nissl substance. Thus, these cells resemble those of lamina II, but they are somewhat larger.

Cell Bodies and Dendrites

There are relatively few studies on the dendritic pattern of lamina III cells as opposed to lamina II cells. Ramon y Cajal (1909) and Pearson (1952) wrote before the laminae were understood, and Szentágothai (1964) and Scheibel and Scheibel (1968) regarded the substantia gelatinosa as both laminae II and III. In all these studies, therefore, the dendritic patterns of the laminae II and III cells were not distinguished, except that the cells in deeper parts of the substantia gelatinosa, which is probably lamina III, tend to be larger and their dendrites extend somewhat further. To our knowledge the only study that determined the dendritic pattern of cells specifically in lamina III was that of Mannen and Sugiura (1976). These investigators elucidated the dendritic pattern of three lamina III cells in serial sections. The dendritic patterns are relatively complex. One cell, for example, has dendrites extending through laminae I–IV, with one prominent dendrite extending almost to the outer surface of the dorsal horn (Fig. 3.26). The dendrites of the other two cells do not extend so far, being seen predominantly in lamine I–III, but they are still extraordinarily widespread. Thus, these dendritic patterns are more complex than the small dendritic arborizations seen in previous sketches of these cells (Fig. 3.3, 3.4, 3.11, 3.15, 3.16), but they probably fit the overall dendritic pattern of these cells that was described by previous authors.

Axonal Projections

As with the dendritic patterns, few studies have been done distinguishing the axonal projections of lamina III cells from the axonal projections of lamina II cells. Ramon y Cajal (1909), Szentágothai (1964), and Scheibel and Scheibel (1968) felt that the axons of the cells of the substantia gelatinosa either passed into the tract of Lissauer or into nearby white matter or never left the substance of the gelatinosa. On the basis of the work of Szentágothai (1964), both of these fiber types would be regarded as propriosphinal in that they return to the substantia gelatinosa after they leave the white matter, or they never

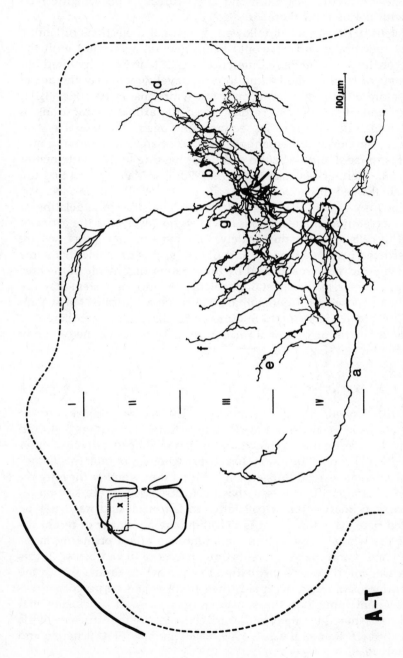

Fig. 3.26. Reconstruction of the dendritic and axonal arborizations of a lamina III cell. Serial sections were used. Note that both the dendritic field and axonal arborizations are more complex than the depictions by earlier investigators of these same cells. (From Mannen and Sugiura, 1976.)

leave the substantia gelatinosa and enter directly into synaptic relations with the neurons there.

Matsushita (1969, 1970) followed the axonal projections of lamina III cells specifically and he would be in general agreement with the above conclusions. The only difference is that Matsushita pointed out that axons of some of the lamina III cells travel widely over the dorsal horn before ending or passing into the white matter (see Fig. 3.16). Mannen and Sugiura (1976) reconstructed the axonal ramifications of three laminae III cells in serial sections, and again, the axonal system was very complex and the pattern was that of an axon ramifying outside of laminae II and III before ending or passing to the white matter (Fig. 3.26). Neither Matsushita (1969, 1970) nor Mannen and Sugiura (1976) challenged the notion that axons of lamina III cells formed part of an intrinsic system that was restricted to the substantia gelatinosa, defined as laminae II and III. It is obvious, however, that the axons of lamina III cells spread rather widely, and some of their processes are not restricted just to laminae II and III. Thus, it is probable that some of the synaptic junctions formed by these axons are outside of the area classically known as the substantia gelatinosa, and the system may not be quite as closed as Szentágothai's (1964) data indicate. Matsushita (1969, 1970) and Mannen and Sugiura (1976) also noted that there was often an arborization of axonal collaterals in the region of the cell body of the parent cell (Fig. 3.16).

Primary Afferent Input

Coarse Primary Afferent Collaterals.   The coarse primary afferent collaterals have been described (Ramon y Cajal, 1909) (Fig. 3.9), and almost all investigators agree that the flame-shaped afferents enter lamina III. The only question has been whether or not the flame-shaped afferents extend dorsally into lamina II or whether they are restricted to lamina III. The issue has been discussed in the section on the coarse primary afferent collaterals to lamina II and need not be repeated here. The only point is that there are a number of recent investigators who suggest that fine afferents are found primarily in laminae I and II and coarse afferents only in lamina III and below. If this is the case, and if Rexed's inclination to equate only lamina II with the substantia gelatinosa is accepted, then there would be no coarse primary afferent input into the substantia gelatinosa, a conclusion that would be disputed by many earlier investigators of the structure of the spinal cord (cf. Ramon y Cajal, 1909; Szentágothai, 1964; Scheibel and Scheibel, 1968).

There have been a large number of studies using methods of degeneration to determine if there is a topographic distribution of dorsal root afferents in the spinal cord (see Shriver et al., 1968). A concise summary of the somatotopic termination of primary afferent collaterals is given in a review of Réthelyi and Szentágothai (1973).

One topographic projection pattern was proposed by Szentágothai and Kiss (1949), who stated that large-caliber dorsal root afferents from dorsal cutaneous regions synapse laterally and those from ventral cutaneous regions synapse medially in the dorsal horn. Another type of somatotopic arrangement was suggested by Imai and Kusama (1969). These investigators state that if a cervical dorsal root is cut, ascending fibers tend to end in medial parts of the nucleus proprius (laminae III and IV) and descending fibers tend to end laterally in the nucleus proprius. The conclusions of Shriver et al. (1968) and Carpenter et al. (1968), however, are that these terminations are not so precisely distributed, and roots from different segments have somewhat different termination patterns. Still another type of somatotopic distribution of primary afferents is suggested by Sterling and Kuypers (1967) and LaMotte (1977). Sterling and Kuypers (1967) point out that the caudal dorsal roots of the brachial plexus project to medial parts of laminae III and IV, whereas cranial roots of the brachial plexus project laterally. LaMotte (1977) is in general agreement with these results. Again, Shriver et al. (1968) and Carpenter et al. (1968) urge caution in accepting precise somatotopic distribution patterns of primary afferents into laminae III and IV.

Finally, work is just beginning that will lead to more precise somatotopic maps than are presently available. This work involves the use of techniques that allow the receptive fields to be determined for individual axons and then the axonal ramifications are located by morphological examination (A. G. Brown et al., 1977c).

Fine Primary Afferent Collaterals.   Again early investigators either did not know of the laminar distributions of Rexed or they regarded the substantia gelationosa as consisting of both laminae II and III. Thus, the discussion of the fine afferents for lamina II will also suffice for those of lamina III, except for the suggestions that indicate a difference between the primary afferent innervation of the two areas.

Probably the first suggestion that there is a difference in primary afferent innervation between laminae II and III were the observations by Ralston (1965; 1968b; 1971), Sterling and Kuypers (1967), and Shriver et al. (1968) that dorsal rhizotomy produced little degeneration in lamina II and extensive degeneration in lamina III. These observations have been summarized earlier and need not be repeated here. Perhaps the only point to note is that the conflict over the question as to whether there are or are not large numbers of degenerating primary afferents in lamina II as opposed to lamina III may be resolved by the finding that fine afferents end in lamina II and coarse afferents in lamina III (Réthelyi, 1977; Kumazawa and Perl, 1978). Beal and Fox (1976) made a careful analysis of Golgi-impregnated material and would concur that fine primary afferent endings are found predominantly in lamina II and coarse primary afferent endings in lamina III. However, it should be remembered that in all the analyses of Golgi-impregnated material, it is impossible to be certain which fibers are primary afferents and which ones come from other sources. Further support of this notion that the fine primary afferents end in lamina II and the coarse primary afferents in lamina III come from combined anatomico-physiological studies. Injection of coarse primary afferents, as determined by conduction velocity, showed the flame-shaped arborizations ending only in lamina III (A. G. Brown, 1977; A. G. Brown et al., 1977c), whereas injection of fine primary afferents showed labeled axons in lamina I and the upper part of lamina II (Light and Perl, 1977).

There are, however, two studies that are at variance with the idea that fine afferents end in lamina II and coarse afferents in lamina III. Scheibel and Scheibel (1968) claim to demonstrate that fine fibers form apical (in lamina II) and basal (in lamina III) plexuses along the flame-shaped primary afferent arborizations. Interestingly enough, Scheibel and Scheibel (1968) feel that the basal plexus consists at least partially of fine primary afferent collaterals, whereas the apical plexus they regarded of propriospinal origin. Thus, the basal plexus would consist of fine primary afferent fibers that ended in lamina III. In another study, LaMotte (1977) stated that the fine fibers innervated laminae I–III and the coarse fibers laminae IV–VI.

Organization of the Neuropil

Several investigators have been struck by the similarity at the fine-structure level of the neuropil of laminae II and III. In both laminae, the most prominent feature of synaptic organization is the glomerulus, the commonest type of synapse is axodendritic, axosomatic synapses are rare, and axoaxonic synapses are seen. These features have been discussed in the section concerned with the neuropil of lamina II.

Although the similarities predominate, there are slight differences between laminae II and III. Kerr (1975a), for example, noted that there are more glomeruli per unit area in lamina III than there are in lamina

II. In addition, Ralston (1977) noted certain quantitative differences, namely that the dense-core vesicle containing synapses are more numerous in lamina II and that the presynaptic endings with flattened vesicles are much more numerous in lamina III.

In summary, lamina III can be differentiated from lamina II cytoarchitectonically because the cells in lamina III are slightly larger and farther apart that those in laminae II. The dendritic patterns of the lamina III cells resemble those of lamina II cells, but they are larger and more complex. The axonal projections of the lamina III cells are thought to be back into the substantia gelatinosa, in a manner similar to the lamina II cell axonal projections. The axons of some lamina III cells, however, travel through deeper laminae before they reenter the gelatinosa. Thus, these axons are not completely restricted to lamina II and III and this may have bearing on how closed the substantia gelationosa is. The descriptions of the primary afferent input to this lamina are the same as for lamina II, but there are recent suggestions that the coarse collaterals are restricted to lamina III and the fine collaterals to lamina II. The neuropil of lamina III is indistinguishable from that of lamina II, except that there seems to be slightly greater concentration of glomeruli and of flattened vesicle endings in lamina III as compared to lamina II.

LAMINAE IV–VI

Laminae IV, V, and VI represent the bulk of the dorsal horn deep to the substantia gelatinosa. Many different cyoarchitectonic subdivisions of the dorsal horn have been proposed for this part of the spinal cord, but with the exception of the Rexed laminae, none has been accepted. These previous organizational patterns have been summarized by Rexed in his excellent historical reviews (Rexed, 1952; 1954) and will not be considered further here. A major contributory factor to the general acceptance of these laminae was the study of Wall (1967), who noted that the receptive fields of dorsal horn neurons changed in a predictable way from lamina to lamina.

LAMINA IV

This is a relatively thick layer that extends straight across the dorsal horn. Its medial border is the white matter of the dorsal column and its lateral border is the ventral bend of laminae I–III (Fig. 3.1). The nerve cells in this layer are of various sizes, ranging from small ones of approximately 8 by 11 μm to the largest which are 35 by 45 μm. According to Rexed (1952), the largest cells are relatively infrequent, but they are so prominent that there is a general impression that this is a layer with large cells. Rexed himself was struck, however, by the heterogenity of cell sizes rather than the large cells as being most characteristic of this layer. In cytoarchitectonic terms, lamina IV can be distinguished from lamina III by the heterogeneity of the neuronal size and the presence of some very large cells as compared to more homogeneous, smaller cells that characterize lamina III. Lamina IV can be distinguished from lamina V because the neurons of lamina V are even more heterogenous than those of lamina IV and there are many myelinated axons in lamina V, particularly in its lateral half.

Cell Bodies and Dendritic Architecture

It is difficult to be certain of the exact laminar location of the cells that Ramon y Cajal illustrated in the basal part of the dorsal horn, but his cell A in Fig. 2.9 seems to be in the region of lamina IV. This cell has long, spine-studded dendrites that pass dorsally, laterally, and ventrally and an axon that passes to the lateral white matter. This is a general picture that would probably be valid for many of the large neurons in laminae IV and V.

Szentágothai (1964) emphasized particularly the dorsal dendrites of the large cells in lamina IV (and lamina V) (Figs. 3.9, 3.10, 3.12, 3.15). The reason for this is that the dorsal dendrites penetrate the substantia gelatinosa, thus allowing axons from the central cells of the gelatinosa to contact the dendrites. It should be remembered that Szentágothai (1964) provided evidence to show that the substantia gelatinosa is a system of cells with primary afferent input and rich synaptic interconnections but no obvious pathways for direct forward conduction. The importance of the large cells in laminae IV and V with dorsal dendrites that penetrate the gelatinosa is that they represent the output of this enigmatic region. This formulation has become a cornerstone of thought about the synaptic connectivity of the dorsal horn, and it has been pictured in a series of important wiring diagrams (Fig. 3.15).

The diagram of Szentágothai (Fig. 3.15) comes from his major 1964 paper in which he provided evidence showing that cells of the substantia gelatinosa (laminae II and III) formed a closed system whose axons arborized only in the substantia gelatinosa. The primary afferent input into this area, he thought, came primarily from the coarse collaterals, which curve around the medial edge of the substantia gelatinosa and enter from below, and the fine collaterals, which enter from the tract of Lissauer or nearby white matter and penetrate from above. Note that in the diagram there are three places where the coarse-fiber collaterals end. First, some collaterals end directly on the cell bodies of lamina IV cells. Second, coarse collaterals form the flame-shaped arbors that contact the dendrites of lamina IV cells. Third, the flame-shaped arbors also contact dendrites of substantia gelatinosa neurons. The fine collaterals are depicted as ending on dendrites of substantia gelatinosa neurons, but they may also end on the dendrites of lamina IV neurons. The large lamina IV cells are shown sending their axons to the lateral white matter, and presumably these axons will end in the lateral cervical nucleus or possibly in the thalamus. The axons of small neurons of the substantia gelatinosa either travel through the gelatinosa and then end or pass to one of the several sub-divisions of the white matter (dorsolateral fasciculus proprius, Lissauer's tract, lateral fasiculus proprius, posterior commissure), but these latter axons always return to the substantia gelatinosa of the same or the opposite side. The axons of the substantia gelatinosa neurons eventually end either on the dendrites of other cells of the substantia gelatinosa or on dendrites of the lamina IV cells. The large lamina IV cells, with their dorsally directed dendrites, are termed "antenna-type neurons" by Réthelyi and Szentágothai (1973). They are the only output of the substantia gelatinosa because no other neurons have axons that lead away from the substantia gelatinosa. The above construction is usually accepted today, at least in its overall details. The two key elements of this formulation are (1) that axons of the neurons of the substantia gelatinosa synapse within the gelatinosa and (2) that the output of this system is the antenna-type neurons in la-minae IV and V.

Scheibel and Scheibel (1968) repeated the analysis of the dorsal horn by the method of Golgi and its variants. They stated that lamina IV consisted of a relatively small number of moderate-to-large cells (20–40 μm) whose dendrites radiate medially, laterally, ventrally, and dorsally from the soma. They point out that these dendritic fields are cone-shaped, with the apex of the cone directed ventrally (Fig. 3.4). This is because the ventral dendrite is usually single, the longitudinal dendrites do not extend far from the cell body, and the dorsal dendrites ramify extensively.

Scheibel and Scheibel make a point that, from the point of view of presynaptic connections, the dendrites of lamina IV cells can be divided into three categories: (1) medial, (2) lateral, and (3) dorsal. The inputs to these three types of dendrites are different (see below).

Réthelyi and Szentágothai (1973), in a major article summarizing current knowledge about the distribution of primary afferent fibers in the spinal cord, point out that "it is difficult to translate into modern architectonic terms (lamination of Rexed, 1954) the classical expressions head (or center) of the dorsal horn (nucleus proprius cornus posterioris). The difficulty is caused mainly because the cytoarchitectonic borders do not match with those of dendroarchitectonics and neuropil architectonics." These authors then point out that laminae III, IV, and the upper part of V are dominated by a longitudinal axonal plexus that had previously been described by Sterling and Kuypers (1967). This plexus should not be confused with the intrinsic longitudinal axon plexus of laminae II and III that Szentágothai described in 1964. Within this area, Réthelyi and Szentágothai (1973) described three types of neurons on the basis of their dendritic projections: (1) antenna-type neurons, smaller in lamina III and larger in laminae IV and V, whose dendrites project dorsally into the substantia gelatinosa (these are the output neurons for the substantia gelatinosa); (2) central cells with longitudinally oriented dendrites; and (3) cells, primarily in lamina V, with transverse dendrites. Réthelyi and Szentágothai (1973) mention, however, that many cells in these laminae have all three types of dendrites.

Réthelyi and Szentágothai (1973) state that the main ascending relay cells in this part of the dorsal horn are the cells of the spinocervical tract. The large antenna-type neurons, located particularly in lamina IV, are regarded as the cells of origin of the spinocervical tract (Réthelyi and Szentágothai, 1973). The other cells in these layers are regarded as "propriospinal or even short local interneurons" (Réthelyi and Szentágothai, 1973).

The notion that the cells or origin of the spinocervical tract are antenna-type neurons has been tested by intracellular injection of horseradish peroxidase into identified spinocervical neurons (A.G. Brown et al., 1977b). These investigators report that "in our sample of twenty-two identified SCT cells only four had dendritic trees which could be loosely defined, according to the figures of Réthelyi and Szentágothai (1973), as antenna type. A further five cells had semicircular dendritic trees and, therefore, resembled "antenna type" neurons in that they lacked well developed ventral dendrites. Thus, although physiologically identified spinocervical-tract cells are located primarily in laminae IV and V, the dendritic arborization pattern is not usually that of an antenna-type neuron.

The other projection system whose cells of origin are found in lamina IV is the spinothalamic system. As reviewed in Chapter 8, there are large numbers of neurons that give rise to fibers of the spinothalamic tract in lamina IV and V, at least in the monkey. Unfortunately, nothing is yet known about the dendritic patterns of these particular neurons as compared with the dendritic patterns of the other neurons in this lamina.

Recently Proshansky and Egger (1977) noted that neurons in laminae IV, V, and VI could be distinguished on the basis of differences in dendritic spread. These investigators point out that most neurons in lamina IV have dense, bushy dendritic fields, much like the spinocervical-tract cell illustrated in Fig. 8.3. By contrast, lamina V has some cells with bushy dendrites and other cells with radiating dendritic fields, and lamina VI consists primarily of cells with radiating dendritic fields. Radiating dendritic fields means that the dendrites are relatively straight and have few branches. The dendritic spread, according to Proshansky and Egger (1977), is least for the lamina IV cells, intermediate for lamina V cells, and greatest for lamina VI cells. These investigators suggest that there may be a correlation between the increasing size of the receptive fields from lamina to lamina as measured physiologically (Wall, 1967) and the width of the dendritic spread as measured anatomically. A possible difficulty with the Proshansky and Egger (1977) classification of dendritic patterns comes from a consideration of the results of Mannen (1975). Mannen (1975) pointed out that many processes of Golgi-stained neurons are lost if the cells are not examined in serial sections. For example, the cell body of Mannen's cell P is located at the boundary of laminae IV and V (Fig. 3.27). The dorsal dendrites spread through laminae I–V of the ipsilateral side and some enter laminae III–IV of the opposite side of the spinal cord (Fig. 3.27). The ventral dendrites of this cell are extensive and reach down into lamina VII. The side-to-side spread of these dendrites is greater than any of those noted by Proshansky and Egger (1977), and the shape of a dendritic field does not resemble a cone, which is the shape suggested by Scheibel and Scheibel (1968). Mannen only studied one lamina IV cell by his serial section technique, which is not enough for statistical significance, but the results of this technique on cells from many laminae in the spinal cord (Mannen, 1975; Mannen and Sugiura, 1976) seem to imply that previous studies on Golgi-stained neurons are deficient because so many axonal and dendritic processes are lost unless serial sections are done.

Axonal Projections

Cells in lamina IV belong to (1) the spinocervical system, (2) the spinothalamic system, or (3) the propriospinal systems. The projections of lamina IV cells to the lateral cervical nucleus were demonstrated by anatomic reconstructions of microelectrode recording sites,

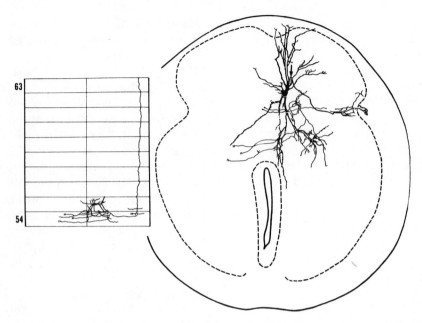

Fig. 3.27. A large neuron located at the boundary of laminae IV and V. Its axonal and dendritic processes were followed in serial sections. Note the dorsal dendrites. Also note how the dendrites of this cell spread over laminae I–VII and on both sides of the spinal cord. (From Mannen, 1975.)

by the intracellular marking of neurons projecting to the lateral cervical nucleus, and by the retrograde transport of horseradish peroxidase that was injected into the lateral cervical nucleus (see Chapter 7). The projections of lamina IV neurons to the thalamus were demonstrated by retrograde chromatolysis, by the anatomic reconstruction of microelectrode recording sites, and by the retrograde transport of horseradish peroxidase injected into appropriate areas of the thalamus (see Chapter 8). The projection of lamina IV neurons to the spinocervical nucleus is mostly ipsilateral. The projection of lamina IV neurons to the thalamus is mostly contralateral. Relatively little is known about any other projections of lamina IV neurons, although it is generally accepted that many of these neurons are propriospinal (Réthelyi and Szentágothai, 1973).

The axonal projections of lamina IV cells, as revealed in Golgi stains, are consistent with the above data. Ramon y Cajal illustrated several cells deep in the dorsal horn, which are probably in lamina IV or V, that send their axons into the white matter of the lateral white column (Figs. 3.2, 3.9, 3.10). Ramon y Cajal also illustrated neurons in this area that sent their axons across the midline in the posterior commissure (Fig. 3.28). Szentágothai (1964) notes that most textbooks state that large dorsal-horn neurons send their axons to the opposite spinothalamic tract through the anterior white commissure. Szentágothai (1964) further notes, however, that he never observed a lamina IV or V neuron in the cat sending its axon into the anterior white commissure. Cells that send their axons into this commissure are located in deeper layers, namely laminae VI, VII, and VIII. It must be remembered, however, that many neurons in laminae IV and V send their axons to the thalamus (see Chapter 7 and Matsushita, 1969). It is not clear whether this implies that the axons do not cross in the anterior white commissure or whether they ascend for a segment or so before crossing, a fact that could not be discerned in the Golgi studies using single sections (Ramon y Cajal, 1909; Szentágothai, 1964).

Scheibel and Scheibel (1968) are confirmatory of earlier work. They note that the axons of lamina IV cells "enter propriospinal bundles either in the lateral or dorsolateral white matter, most often in the central area of Marie." They emphasize the tortuous course of these axons before they get to the white matter. They also point out that the axons often bifurcate, a fact which was also noted by some earlier investigators, and that collaterals of the axons penetrate into deeper laminae.

Matsushita (1969, 1970) takes up the question of the axonal projection of neurons in lamina IV. He notes that "the main axons of lamina IV cells enter the dorsal part of the lateral funiculus," which agrees with earlier work. Before the axons enter the lateral white matter, however, they give off collaterals in the region of the cell body that ramify in laminae III, IV, and V (similar to the lamina III cell in Fig. 3.16), Matsushita (1970) also points out, however, that the axons of some lamina IV neurons travel ventrally into lamina VII before passing

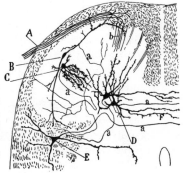

Fig. 3.28. A picture showing that some large cells (D) in the dorsal horn send their axons across the midline in the posterior commissure. Cell B is identified by Ramon y Cajal as a fusiform cell of the substance of Rolando, but its appearance suggests that it might be a marginal cell. (From Ramon y Cajal, 1909.)

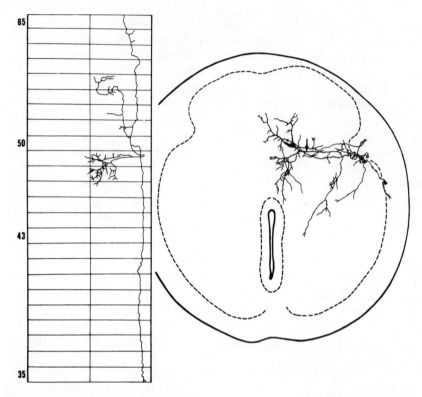

Fig. 3.29. A lamina V cell reconstructed from serial sections of Golgi-impregnated spinal cord. Note that the dendritic spread of this cell is primarily in a horizontal direction and is very wide. Note that the axon has three branches, one passing cranially and one caudally in the white matter of the spinal cord and another ramifying in the gray matter of the dorsal horn. (From Mannen, 1975.)

dorsolaterally to enter the lateral white matter. The question of Golgi type II cells, which are cells whose axons are confined to the gray matter and arborize around the dendrites of the neuron from which they arise, is also considered. Matsushita quotes Ramon y Cajal (1909) and Testa (1964) as doubting the existence of short-axoned cells in this part of the spinal cord. Then, he points out that the axonal collaterals of the lamina IV cells given off before the main axon or axons enter the white matter must be responsible for the activity that is interpreted by physiologists as resulting from inhibitory Golgi type II interneurons.

Matsushita (1970) mentions that the spinothalamic tract is thought to originate from cells in the dorsal horn whose axons pass into the anterior white commissure before ascending to the thalamus. Matsushita noted cells in laminae IV and V whose axons could be followed to the anterior white commissure (Fig. 3.30). Matsushita (1969) also noted a number of cells in intermediate regions and the ventral horn that sent their axons into the anterior white commissure (Fig. 3.30).

Mannen (1975) considers the axonal distributions of Golgi-impregnated lamina IV cells, but in serial sections rather than single sections. He confirms that "Neurons found in the dorsal horn (laminae IV and V) send their axons either to the ipsilateral lateral funiculus . . . or to the ipsilateral lateral funiculus as well as to the contralateral anterior funiculus." Mannen goes on to say about lamina IV cells that "in regard to the terminal area of the axon as well as its collaterals, neurons found in the dorsal horn send their axonal branches into the dorsal half of the intermediate region, including laminae VII and X of the ipsilateral side . . . or contralateral side . . . or both." Thus, the axon collaterals of lamina IV cells (as well as lamina V cells) send numerous branches into deeper laminae of the spinal cord (see also Scheibel and Scheibel, 1966, 1968; Matsushita, 1969, 1970; Mannen, 1975).

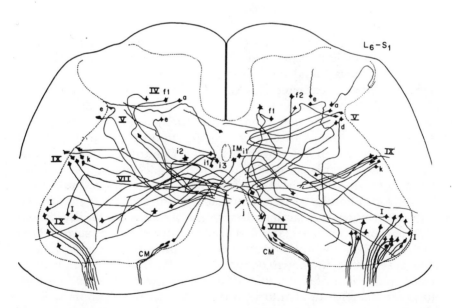

Fig. 3.30. Matsushita's diagram of the axonal projections of neurons in various areas of the L6–S1 segment of spinal cord. Note particularly that cells labeled e and f send their axons across the midline in the anterior white commissure. (From Matsushita, 1970.)

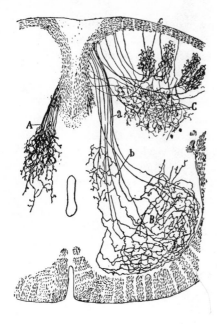

Fig. 3.31. Ramon y Cajal's drawing of some of the different types of primary afferent input into the spinal cord. In particular, the fibers labeled c are the coarse primary afferent collaterals that break up into the flame-shaped arbors in the substantia gelatinosa and those labeled C form the longitudinal plexus to the head of the posterior horn. (From Ramon y Cajal, 1909.)

Primary Afferent Input

When discussing the input from primary afferent fibers into lamina IV, it should be remembered that many of the lamina IV neruons send their dorsal dendrites superficially into laminae II and III. It should also be remembered that the primary afferent input into lamina II and III is by fine afferents that enter from the tract of Lissauer and nearby white matter and from coarse afferents that end in flame-shaped arborizations that enter by coming through the medial part of the dorsal horn and entering from below. Dendrites from the lamina IV cells have never been identified by marking techniques, so it is impossible to be certain about precise synaptic connections, but studies of the dorsal horn after dorsal rhizotomy indicate that there are two types of dendrites in laminae II and III that are contacted by degenerating axonal terminals. The first are the outer dendrites surrounding the central boutons in the glomeruli of laminae I, II, and III; the second are solitary unknown dendrites on which axons end in these laminae. If either of these types of dendrites are from lamina IV cells, then the afferent input into laminae II and III would contact dorsal dendrites of lamina IV neurons. Some of these synaptic connections are generally thought to exist and are depicted in Fig. 3.15.

Other primary afferent axons besides those that enter laminae II and III contact the neurons of lamina IV. For example, numerous axons come from the dorsal parts of the posterior columns to ramify in the head ("*tête*") of the dorsal horn (Ramon y Cajal, 1909) (Figs. 3.17, 3.31). These axons form a longitudinal plexus, and synaptic contacts are made on the cell bodies of the large neurons of the dorsal horn. Ramon y Cajal stated that most of these fibers are the terminal ramifications of large myelinated primary afferent fibers, and he drew them as being separate from the coarse primary afferent fibers that broke up into the flame-shaped arbors (Fig. 3.31). These fibers to the head of the dorsal horn, according to Ramon y Cajal (1909), come through the substance of Rolando, but they give off no obvious collaterals to this substance. Although these collaterals are described as penetrating the substance of Rolando, in Fig. 3.31 they are shown as coming primarily from deeper parts of the posterior white column. From Ramon y Cajal's statement that they do not give off collaterals into the substance of Rolando and from his drawings, it is obvious that he felt that the large, recurring, flame-shaped collaterals and this system were different. Scheibel and Scheibel (1968) also drew the two types of fibers as separate. Ralston (1965), however, pictured both types of fibers as coming from the same parent collateral (Fig. 3.32), and Szentágothai (1964) pictured them as two different collaterals off the same parent

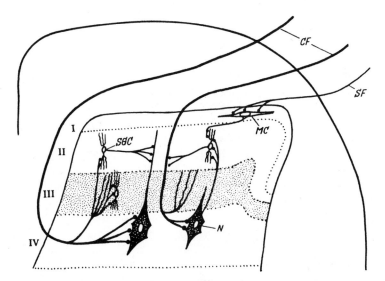

Fig. 3.32. A schematic diagram showing the primary afferent input to the dorsal horn. Note that the terminals of large primary afferent fibers (CF) are diagrammed as ending (1) on the large cell bodies in lamina IV and (2) and as the flame-shaped arborizations, which are here diagrammed as largely being restricted to lamina III. (From Ralston, 1965.)

dorsal root fiber (Fig. 3.15). It is not known with certainty, therefore, whether the same or different fibers give rise to the flame-shaped arbors and the primary afferent longitudinal plexus to the head of the dorsal horn.

Agreement is good but not completely uniform as to the relationship of the Rexed laminae to Ramon y Cajal's (1909) longitudinal plexus to the head of the dorsal horn. Sprague and Ha (1964) state that this plexus is found in lamina IV. By contrast, Réthelyi and Szentágothai (1973) locate the plexus in laminae III, IV, and the upper part of V, and Sterling and Kuypers (1967) show a longitudinal primary afferent axonal plexus in laminae III and IV, but they do not relate it to the plexus of Ramon y Cajal (1909). It seems probable from these results that Ramon y Cajal's (1909) longitudinal plexus to the head of the dorsal horn ramifies primarily in lamina IV, but some components of it may enter laminae III or V.

Scheibel and Scheibel (1968) provide a relatively complex picture of the afferent innervation to lamina IV. These investigators wrote that there are three primary sources of afferents to the cell bodies of lamina IV: (1) primary afferent collaterals, (2) corticospinal fibers, (3) fibers from the cornucommissural bundle of Marie. Scheibel and Scheibel feel that the main primary sensory input to these cells is on the dorsal dendrites that are ascending through the substantia gelatinosa, whereas the corticospinal fibers they feel end on the lateral dendrites of these cells. The dorsal dendrites have longer and more numerous spines than those of the lateral dendrites. The fibers from the cornucommissural bundle intertwine in lamina IV and Scheibel and Scheibel (1968) suggest that they form a "wealth of axoaxonal contacts with resulting possibilities for presynaptic modulation." To the medial dendrites of the lamina IV cells come a more heterogeneous population of afferents: (1) terminal collaterals emerging from the cornucommissural bundle and adjacent white matter, (2) fibers from the contralateral dorsal horn crossing in the posterior commissure, and (3) branches of contralateral primary afferent collaterals (Scheibel and Scheibel, 1968). They do not relate any of these systems to Ramon y Cajal's longitudinal plexus.

The dense longitudinal axonal plexus of the head of the dorsal horn first discussed by Ramon y Cajal (1909) has been given a special name by Réthelyi and Szentágothai (1973), "the central longitudinally oriented axonal plexus of the dorsal horn." These authors point out that this plexus infiltrates laminae III, IV, and the upper part of V, and they feel that this layer defines a nucleus of the dorsal horn. Thus, this part of the dorsal horn, which probably corresponds to the nucleus proprius of most earlier authors, is defined by neuropil architectonics rather than cytoarchitectonics. Kerr (1975a) also provides a special name for this longitudinal axonal plexus. He calls it the "dorsal intracornual tract" and notes that it exists primarily in laminae IV, V, and VI. Kerr (1975a) notes that Ramon y Cajal thought that these fibers were collaterals of primary afferents. Kerr notes, however, that a significant number of these axons remain after dorsal rhizotomy, and thus, many of the fibers must arise from interneurons. Kerr (1975a) speculates that this pathway might possibly be involved in nociceptive sensation, perhaps as "a supplementary pathway in instances of long-term interruptions of nociceptive pathways in the human."

Finally, LaMotte (1977) feels that the large-caliber primary afferents end primarily in laminae IV–VI and fine-caliber afferents in laminae I–III. This is because lesions of the dorsal column produce degeneration primarily in laminae IV–VI. As mentioned before, this finding speaks against the almost universally accepted notion that the flame-shaped afferents, which arborize in laminae II and III, or at least lamina III, come from coarse afferents, but it is in accord with studies showing much primary afferent degeneration in laminae IV–VI.

Organization of the Neuropil

The synaptic architecture of lamina IV is quite different from the synaptic architecture of laminae I–III, but it is indistinguishable from that of laminae V and VI (Ralston, 1968a, 1971; Kerr, 1970a, 1975a). Thus, it is possible to distinguish lamina IV from the laminae dorsal to it on the basis of the morphology of the synapses, but it is not possible to distinguish lamina IV from laminae V and VI on this basis.

The synapses in lamina IV are axosomatic, axodendritic, and axoaxonal (Ralston, 1968a; Kerr, 1970a). The axosomatic synapses, which are almost never seen in laminae II and III, are moderately common in lamina IV, and the glomeruli that characterize laminae I–III are not present (Ralston, 1968a; Kerr, 1970a). Presynaptic terminals can be classified on the basis of their synaptic vesicle content into round vesicle, flat- or pleomorphic-vesicle, and dense-core-vesicle types. The presynaptic endings with round vesicles—the S type endings of Kerr (1970a)—have a very dense "subsynaptic membrane" whereas the flattened vesicle synapse—the F-type ending of Kerr (1970a)—has a much less electron-dense subsynaptic membrane (Ralston, 1968a). In lamina IV, the number of F-type endings is as great as or exceeds the number of S-type terminals (Kerr, 1970a; Ralston, 1977). Ralston (1968a) also notes that some synaptic knobs contain neurofilaments that are often arranged in filamentous rings.

When the dorsal root is cut, there are surprisingly few degenerating terminals (Kerr, 1970b). Ralston (1977) notes that only 3% of the axonal profiles in lamina IV show signs of degeneration. According to Ralston (1968a), the majority of degenerating synaptic knobs appear very electron dense, but some are characterized by an increase in the content of neurofilaments. Kerr (1970b) was not able to confirm the presence of the neurofilamentous type of degeneration, however, nor was he able to find any degenerating terminals on cell bodies. The degenerating knobs, according to Ralston (1968b), are observed primarily in the middle half of laminae IV–VI. This is in accord with the light microscopic data of Sprague and Ha (1964). The degenerating synapses make contact with "the cell bodies and proximal dendrites of the large and medium neurons but not with small . . . cells" (Ralston, 1968b). In addition, degenerating terminals are seen on small dendrites and on other synaptic knobs (Fig. 3.17). This last type of contact is axoaxonal, and for these synapses, Ralston (1968b) makes the important point that "in contrast to lamina III, in which degenerating knobs are presynaptic in axoaxonal contacts, the knobs of dorsal root origin in IV, V and VI are postsynaptic to other knobs" (Fig. 3.7). Kerr (1970b) notes that, when the axoaxonal complex is involved, the normal bouton that is synapsing on the degenerating terminal contains flattened vesicles.

In summary, lamina IV is a thick layer consisting of nerve cells of various sizes, ranging from very small to quite large. The large cells have dendrites that pass dorsally, laterally, and medially. Szentágothai gave special emphasis to the cells with predominately dorsal dendrites and called these the antenna-type neurons. He emphasized that the antenna-type neurons were the output of the substantia gelatinosa. The large cells of lamina IV are thought to project to the lateral cervical nucleus, the thalamus, and other areas of the spinal cord. One part of the afferent input to these cells is the afferent input to the substantia gelatinosa. This input contacts primarily the dorsal dendrites. The other major input seems to be from the longitudinal axonal plexus to the head of the dorsal horn. It is not completely clear whether this plexus arises from the fibers that give rise to the flame-shaped arbors or not. It is also not clear whether this is a primary afferent or a propriospinal system, although the former is probable. The synaptic architecture of the neuropil is different from the synaptic architecture of laminae I–III. In particular, axosomatic synapses are common and the glomeruli are not present. In addition, axodendritic and axoaxonic synapses are seen. When there is a degenerating element in an axoaxonic synapse, the degenerating element is postsynaptic in contrast to the situation in laminae II and III.

LAMINA V

This lamina extends as a rather thick band across the narrowest part of the dorsal horn (Fig. 3.1). It occupies the zone often called the neck of the dorsal horn. It has a sharp boundary on the dorsal funiculus, but its lateral boundary is indistinct because of the many bundles of myelinated fibers coursing through this area. These bundles of myelinated fibers give the lateral part of this lamina a reticulated appearance. Thus, lamina V can be subdivided into a medial and a lateral zone, and the lateral zone usually occupies about one-third of the lamina. The medial zone does not have as many myelinated fibers, so that its appearance is more uniform than that of the lateral part. This lamina can be distinguished cytoarchitectonically from lamina IV because the cells are even more varying in size and shape than in lamina IV and from lamina VI, which consists of a medial zone with small, packed, compact cells and a lateral zone with slightly larger cells that are nevertheless more regular than those in lamina V. A good clue to the location of lamina V is the presence of the reticulated area on its lateral side.

Cell Bodies and Dendritic Organization

The cell bodies in this region are of varying sizes, the smallest of which are 8–10 μm and the largest 30–45 μm. Most of the cells fall in the range of 10–13 by 15–20 μm, however (Rexed, 1952). The cells are large and have clear, distinct nucleoli. Nissl substance is relatively sparse but can clearly be seen, particularly in the large cells.

Ramon y Cajal (1909) did not separate the cells in this region of the dorsal horn on the basis of their dendritic patterns, so that his description of lamina IV cells would apply equally well to the cells of lamina V. Scheibel and Scheibel (1968), however, emphasize that there is a major shift in the axonal and dendritic neuropil when one changes from lamina IV to lamina V. The axonal change will be discussed in a later section of this chapter, and the change in the dendritic neuropil is as follows. The dendrites of the lamina V cells "radiate along the dorsoventral and mediolateral planes with little or no extensions along the longitudinal axis of the cord" (Scheibel and Scheibel, 1968). Thus, the dendritic shapes of these cells can best be described as flattened disks (Fig. 3.7). This contrasts strongly with the longitudinal orientation of most of the neurons in lamina IV.

To our knowledge, only two other studies considered the anatomy of the dendritic systems of lamina V neurons in any detail. The first was by Mannen (1975), who reconstructed the dendritic and axonal trees of sixteen spinal neurons. Three of these neurons were located in lamina V, and although this is too small a sample for any general conclusions, the general impression is that the dendrites spread over large areas in all directions (Fig. 3.29). Nevertheless, although one could not regard these dendrite fields described by Mannen as discoid in shape, as Scheibel and Scheibel (1968) suggest, the dendritic fields are larger in the mediolateral and dorsoventral directions as compared to their craniocaudal extent. The second study was by Proshansky and Egger (1977), who note that the dendritic fields were more widely spread in lamina V neurons as compared to lamina IV neurons and that some of the lamina V cells had radiating dendrites as compared to the bushy dendrites of the lamina IV neurons. This subject has already been discussed in the section on the dendritic organization of the lamina IV neurons, but the observation of Mannen (1975) that the dendritic field of a neuron in this region of the spinal cord cannot be completely visualized unless serial sections are studied should be remembered.

Axonal Projections

As for the lamina IV neurons, the three main projection sites that are suggested for the lamina V neurons are the thalamus, the lateral cervical nucleus, and the gray matter of the spinal cord. The studies identifying spinocervical and spinothalamic cells in lamina V are discussed in Chapters 7 and 8.

There is relatively little work on the axonal projections of lamina V cells as distinct from lamina IV cells. Ramon y Cajal (1909) showed that cells in this region of the spinal cord send their axons into the neighboring white matter that surrounds the dorsal horn or across the posterior commissure to the opposite side of the spinal cord (Fig. 3.28). Ramon y Cajal (1909) was not aware of the Rexed laminae, and so the notion that these neurons are in lamina V is an estimate based on their general position in the spinal cord. Matsushita (1969, 1970) studied the spinal cord with silver and Golgi stains. In his earlier study, Matsushita (1969) noted that it was difficult to distinguish neurons in lamina IV from those in lamina V in sections of spinal cord prepared with the silver stain of Ramon y Cajal, because the axonal pathways of both types of cell are similar. Matsushita did note, however, in addition to the lamina V neurons that sent their axons into the lateral funiculus, there were a number of these neurons that sent their axons ventrally to cross in the anterior commissure (Fig. 3.30). These cells fulfill, therefore, the classic descriptions of spinothalamic cells. One other finding mentioned by Matsushita is that some lamina V cells "give thick myelinated axons to the motoneuron groups." Also, there are large dorsal commissural cells "in the lateral part of lamina V and in the central part of lamina VI of the cervico-thoracic and the lumbar cord." These could presumably be the same cells that Ramon y Cajal described as sending axons into the posterior commissure. In his second paper (1970), Matsushita essentially confirms his earlier work and emphasizes that some cells in laminae V and VI send their axons across the spinal cord in the anterior commissure. Matsushita (1970) also emphasizes that the axons of the medium-sized neurons in lamina V give off collaterals to areas surrounding the cell body. These collaterals reach ventrally as far as lamina VII and dorsally into lamina III and IV. The importance of these cells for Matsushita is that they may subserve the function of Golgi type II cells, even though these cells have at least one process that leaves the region of the cell body.

To summarize, it would appear that many lamina IV and V cells have a similar axonal organization with collaterals ramifying in the gray matter around the cells and at least one primary axon passing into the white matter of the lateral funiculus. In addition, some of the neurons, particularly in lamina V, send axons into the anterior commissure, where they presumably pass to the thalamus on the opposite side of the spinal cord.

Primary Afferent Input

Ramon y Cajal (1909), as usual, made many of the important early observations on the primary afferent input into the base of the dorsal horn. It is difficult to be certain about the laminar location of his primary afferent collaterals, but the axons of Ramon y Cajal's longitudinal plexus to the head of the dorsal horn may well ramify to some extent in lamina V. These axons have been discussed in the section on primary afferent fibers in lamina IV.

Sprague and Ha (1964) studied primary afferent degeneration with silver stains for degenerating axons and noted that there was a heavy degeneration in laminae I–IV in the same segment of the spinal cord where the dorsal root was cut. Many of the large fibers then turn ventrally to end in the medial part of lamina V and to a lesser extent lamina VI. Thus, Sprague and Ha (1964) regard the plexus in lamina V as primarily oriented in a dorsoventral direction, in contrast to the primarily longitudinal orientation of the primary afferent plexus in lamina IV. They also point out that the degeneration is confined to the central area of lamina V.

Sterling and Kuypers (1967) have a view similar to that of Sprague and Ha (1964). They note the very prominent longitudinal orientation of the degenerating primary afferent axons in lamine III and IV and contrast it to the primary dorsoventral or vertical orientation of the fibers in laminae V and VI. They also noted the central location of the terminals in lamina V. They point out that the terminals of the primary afferent axons in laminae V and VI are not somatotopically organized as they are in laminae III and IV.

Scheibel and Scheibel also agree that there is a marked change in the orientation of the axonal neuropil at the junction of laminae IV and V, the orientation changing from longitudinal to dorsoventral. Scheibel and Scheibel (1968) note that the dorsoventral orientation of these fields corresponds to the dorsoventral orientation of the dendritic system of the neurons in this area.

Szentágothai and Réthelyi (1973) support the view of Scheibel and Scheibel (1968) and state that the axonal neuropil of lamina V is organized in transversely oriented sheets or disks. "Relatively few axon arborizations . . . depart from the transversal plane of arborization" (Szentágothai and Réthelyi, 1973).

In a long and excellent review article, Réthelyi and Szentágothai take up in succession the six groups of primary afferent collaterals to the spinal cord originally described by Ramon y Cajal (1909). The collaterals to the center of the dorsal horn are described as having a horizontal course before breaking up into the dense neuropil in the medial part of the neck and bend of the dorsal horn, which they equate with laminae IV and V. Thus, in contrast to most other investigators, they identify a prominent horizontal afferent axonal plexus in laminae IV and V. In a later section of this same chapter, where they are discussing the structure of the dorsal horn proper (Réthelyi and Szentágothai, 1973, p. 232), they state that "The longitudinally oriented axonal plexus, mainly of primary afferent origin (Sterling and Kuypers, 1967) . . . corresponds to lamina III, IV and the upper part of V." Thus, there are presumably two overlapping plexuses, one horizontal and the other longitudinal.

Kerr (1975a) mentions that the longitudinal plexus "that Cajal concluded . . . were either all ascending or descending collaterals of primary afferents" extended through the entire nucleus proprius, by which he meant laminae IV, V, and VI. This conclusion is similar to that of LaMotte (1977), who stated that the large primary afferents degenerated in and were thus distributed to laminae IV, V, and VI. There was no mention of longitudinal or vertical systems of afferents by LaMotte (1977).

It is difficult to summarize the ideas about the primary afferent input to lamina V, because there are some divergent opinions (see above) about the mode of termination of the axons. Presumably, filling individual identified axons with a visualizable material (Light and Perl, 1977; Brown, 1977) may begin in a new era in the understanding of the primary afferent input into lamina V.

In summary, the cells of lamina V are even more heterogeneous than those of lamina IV. In addition, the lateral third of lamina V is heavily myelinated and thus has a reticulate appearance. The dendritic organization of lamina V cells is not markedly different from the dendritic organization of the cells in lamina IV, except that the general orientation of the lamina V cell is vertical as contrasted to the predominately longitudinal orientation of the lamina IV neuron. The axonal projections seem to be to the thalamus, the lateralcervical nucleus, and the spinal cord. Many authors report that there is a major shift in the orientation of the primary afferents to this area, as compared with lamina IV, the primary afferents to lamina V being vertically organized, which contrasts to the longitudinal plexus that characterizes lamina IV. The neuropil does not differ greatly from that of lamina IV.

LAMINA VI

This layer exists only in the cervical and lumbosacral enlargements of the spinal cord (Fig. 3.1). The cells in this layer are smaller and more regular in their arrangement than those in lamina V. The smallest cells are 8–8 μm and the largest are 30–35 μm. There is more Nissl substance in these cells than in the cells of laminae V and VII. Thus, lamina VI has a darker appearance than laminae V and VII in Nissl-stained sections. Lamina VI is divided into two halves, the medial half consisting of a compact group of small or medium-sized heavily staining cells and a lateral half of larger well-stained triangular or star-shaped cells. In this layer are the major parts of the internal and external basal nuclei of Ramon y Cajal (1909).

Cell Bodies and Dendritic Patterns

Relatively few investigators have been particularly concerned with the dendritic pattern of lamina VI neurons. Scheibel and Scheibel (1968) point out that these cells are arranged much like those in lamina V, with dendrites that radiate in dorsoventral and mediolateral planes but with almost no extension in the longitudinal axis of the cord. Thus, these dendritic domains are in the shapes of flattened disks (Fig. 3.7). Proshansky and Egger (1977) noted that these neurons were isodendritic, with long, straight, relatively unbranched dendrites. Proshansky and Egger also noted that the dendritic spread was wider than the dendritic spread of the laminae IV and V neurons.

Finally Szentágothai and Réthelyi (1973) and Réthelyi and Szentágothai (1973) note that the general dendritic organization of many cells in the middle parts of laminae V–VIII form a cylinder. The functional implications of this cylinder is not known.

Axonal Projections

As with the dendritic fields, there has been little work done on the axonal projections of these cells as determined by anatomic means. It is clear from the various labeling experiments described in Chapters 7 and 8 that some of these cells project to the thalamus or to the lateral cervical nucleus, and the majority of these cells are probably propriospinal. Matsushita (1969) points out that the small cells in the medial part of lamina VI possess the most "abundantly ramifying axon collaterals in the spinal cord." These axon collaterals seem to end primarily in lamina IV, V, VI, and VII, and recurrent collaterals end near the parent cell and in neighboring neurons.

Primary Afferent Input

The primary afferent input to lamina VI is complex. Many collaterals from primary afferent axons destined to reach ventral horn cells end in this area (Ramon y Cajal, 1909; Scheibel and Scheibel, 1968). A particularly prominent group of terminals from Ia fibers is found in the center of lamina VI. There are also several systems of descending fibers ending in this area.

CONCLUSIONS

1. The majority of the dendrites of marginal cells travel tangentially over the surface of the dorsal horn, but some penetrate into the substance of the dorsal horn.

2. The axons of the marginal cells project to the thalamus or to other regions of the spinal cord.

3. The afferent input of the marginal cells comes from the marginal plexus, which arises as fine collaterals from axons in the tract of Lissauer and nearby white matter. These fibers are presumably a mixture of primary afferents plus propriospinal axons, with the latter predominating.

4. Primary afferent degeneration is characterized by degenerating

boutons on small dendrites. Propriospinal degeneration is characterized by degenerating boutons on cell bodies or proximal dendrites.

5. The substantia gelatinosa is an area of the spinal cord consisting of small, closely packed neurons and few myelinated axons. There has been debate as to whether only lamina II or both laminae II and III constitute the substantia gelatinosa of early investigators.

6. Two cell types were identified in the substantia gelatinosa by Ramon y Cajal—the central cells and the "cellules limitrophes." It is probable, however, that this subdivision is not justified and that there are a few cells on the outer border of the gelatinosa with dendritic arborizations that resemble the arborizations of both marginal cells and central cells.

7. The dendrites of lamina II cells are primarily organized in a radial direction. Furthermore, although the cells are small, the dendrites of these cells have an extensive arborization.

8. The axons of lamina II cells project either into the tract of Lissauer or into the dorsolateral fasciculus proprius or they remain confined to the gray matter of the substantia gelatinosa.

9. The axons of lamina II cells end in the substantia gelatinosa.

10. It is generally agreed that coarse collaterals to the substantia gelatinosa arise from large axons in the dorsolateral white matter of the dorsal horn. These curve ventrally around the medial edge of the dorsal horn, enter the substantia gelatinosa from below, and then break up into the characteristic flame-shaped arbors. It is not certain whether the flame-shaped arbors span both laminae II and III or just lamina III.

11. The coarse collaterals are of primary afferent origin, and the receptive fields of these fibers respond preferentially to the movement of hair.

12. Fine fibers into the gelatinosa arise primarily as collaterals from axons in the tract of Lissauer or nearby white matter.

13. It is not clear whether these fine fibers are of primary afferent or propriospinal origin, but recent opinion is that they are predominantly propriospinal.

14. Other sources of fine fibers into the substantia gelatinosa have been suggested. They are: (1) from posterior commissure axons, (2) from more ventral parts of the lateral funiculus than the dorsolateral fasciculus proprius, (3) from deeper parts of the dorsal horn, and (4) from the cornucommissural bundle of Marie.

15. The most striking structures in the neuropil of lamina II are the glomeruli.

16. The glomeruli consist of a central bouton surrounded by a variable number of peripheral processes.

17. The origin of the central bouton is usually thought to be a primary afferent fiber; the origin of the various peripheral processes is unknown.

18. The nonglomerular neuropil consists primarily of axodendritic and axoaxonal synapses. Axosomatic synapses are rare.

19. The origin of a few of the presynaptic axon terminals in the axodendritic and axoaxonal synapses are from primary afferent fibers; the origin of the majority of the terminals is unknown.

20. The cell bodies, dendrites, and axonal projections of lamina III cells are generally similar to those of laminae II cells, except the dendritic and axonal arborizations of lamina III cells are somewhat more extensive.

21. Because the axons of lamina II and lamina III neurons are thought to synapse only in the substantia gelatinosa, the substantia gelatinosa is regarded as a closed system.

22. Regardless of general validity of conclusion 21, recent work has demonstrated that axons of some lamina III cells travel in laminae deep to II and III before the axons end in the substantia gelatinosa.

23. The primary afferent input into lamina III is generally described as being similar to that of lamina II, except for recent evidence suggesting that the coarse collaterals end in lamina III and fine collaterals in lamina II.

24. The neuropil of lamina III is similar to that of lamina II.

25. Lamina IV is a thick band across the center of the dorsal horn, and it consists of cells of widely varying sizes, some of which are very large.

26. The dendrites of the large cells of lamina IV pass dorsally, medially, and laterally.

27. Primary attention has focussed on the dorsal dendrites of lamina IV cells, because they are most numerous and because they penetrate the substance of the substantia gelatinosa.

28. Cells with prominent dorsal dendrites are called antenna-type neurons, and they represent the output of the substantia gelatinosa.

29. The axons of the large lamina IV cells project to the thalamus, the lateral cervical nucleus, and other areas of the spinal cord.

30. Primary afferent input to the large neurons of lamina IV comes from the afferents to the substantia gelatinosa, which presumably contact the dorsal dendrites of the lamina IV cells, and from the longitudinal axonal plexus to the head of the dorsal horn.

31. The neuropil of lamina IV consists of axosomatic, axodendritic, and axoaxonal synapses. Glomeruli are not seen.

32. Primary afferent degeneration is manifested by occasional

degenerating axonal boutons on cell bodies and dendrites and as the postsynaptic element in axoaxonal terminals.

33. Lamina V is a broad band across the dorsal horn and its lateral third is reticulate because of the presence of numerous myelinated fibers.

34. The dendritic organization of the lamina V cell is predominately in a dorsoventral plane, as opposed to the longitudinal orientation for lamina IV cells.

35. The axonal input into lamina V is also primarily dorsoventral in orientation, as opposed to the longitudinal orientation of the afferent input into lamina IV.

36. The axonal projections of lamina V cells are to the thalamus, the lateral cervical nucleus, and other areas of the spinal cord.

37. The neuropil of lamina V does not differ from that of lamina IV.

38. The cells of lamina VI project to the lateral cervical nucleus, the thalamus, and other areas of the spinal cord.

4 Functional Organization of Dorsal Horn Interneurons

Sensory processing in the spinal cord involves the interaction between primary afferent fibers bearing information from the sensory receptors, interneurons, ascending tract cells conveying sensory messages to the brain, and descending tract cells modulating cord circuits. Such interactions are complex and still poorly understood. In this chapter, evidence will be discussed concerning the interactions between primary afferents and spinal interneurons and also between the descending tracts and interneurons. The organization of the ascending tracts and also their descending control will form the subject matter of Chapters 5–8.

FIELD POTENTIALS

As a first approximation, the distribution of activity evoked by primary afferent fibers in the spinal cord can be gauged by recordings of electrical field potentials. The field potentials reflect in part the excitation of interneurons of the dorsal horn. Field potentials can be recorded either from the surface of the spinal cord with a gross electrode (the "intermediary cord potentials" or "cord dorsum potentials") or from within the cord with a microelectrode.

The potentials that can be recorded from the cord dorsum in response to a volley in cutaneous afferents following electrical stimulation of a peripheral nerve include an afferent volley, and then one or more negative waves, and finally a positive wave (Gasser and Gra-

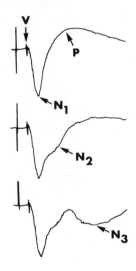

Fig. 4.1. Field potentials recorded from the dorsal surface of the monkey spinal cord in response to stimulation of a cutaneous nerve. The stimulus strength was progressively increased from above down. V= afferent volley; N_1, N_2, and N_3= negative field potentials; P= positive field potential. (From Beall *et al.*, 1977.)

ham, 1933; Bernhard, 1953; Bernhard and Widen, 1953; Lindblom and Ottoson, 1953a,b; Austin and McCouch, 1955; Willis *et al.*, 1973; Beall *et al.*, 1977). In monkey, there is a sequence of three negative waves (Fig. 4.1), the N_1, N_2, and N_3 potentials (Beall *et al.*, 1977). The N_1 wave is due to activity evoked by $A\alpha\beta$ fibers, while the N_3 wave is produced by $A\delta$ fibers.

Recordings from within the spinal cord gray matter show that the negative waves reach a maximum in the middle layers of the dorsal horn and reverse to become positive in the ventral horn (Fig. 4.2) (Howland *et al.*, 1955; Coombs *et al.*, 1956; Fernandez de Molina and Gray, 1957; Willis *et al.*, 1973; Beall *et al.*, 1977).

Since the area of peak negativity corresponds to a region that contains many interneurons activated by the cutaneous nerve volley, it can be presumed that the negativity reflects excitatory processes. Negativity would be expected from the direction of current flow in the extracellular space into the sinks produced at the somata and dendrites of interneurons by excitatory postsynaptic potentials and action potentials (see below) (see Fig. 6.19). The area of positivity in the ventral part of the cord would represent current sources distributed along the axons of interneurons projecting ventrally. It should be pointed out that neurons can also be found in the ventral part of the cord that are excited by the afferent volley. The extracellular potentials represent the summed activity of many neurons, and the negativity around excited cells in the ventral part of the cord is swamped by the positivity caused by the many more dorsally situated neurons producing a source in the same region.

It is interesting that in the monkey the $A\alpha\beta$ fibers produce a maximum negative wave in laminae IV and V (Fig. 4.2A), whereas the $A\delta$ fibers have their greatest effect in two separate foci (Fig. 4.2C), one along the dorsal border of the dorsal horn and the other in laminae V and VI (Beall et al., 1977). This implies that interneurons should be identified in laminae IV and V that are strongly excited by $A\alpha\beta$ fibers and that there should be cells in laminae I and V–VI that are powerfully excited by $A\delta$ fibers.

The positive wave (or P wave) that follows the N waves is a reflection of the depolarization of primary afferent fibers and corresponds to the negative dorsal-root potential (Barron and Matthews, 1938; Lloyd and McIntyre, 1949; Lloyd, 1952; Koketsu, 1956; J. C. Eccles and Krnjević, 1959; J. C. Eccles et al., 1962c; J. C. Eccles et al., 1963a). Primary afferent depolarization is thought to be responsible for the process known as presynaptic inhibition (J. C. Eccles, 1964; Schmidt, 1971). The P wave evoked by stimulation of cutaneous nerves reverses to negativity in the dorsal horn. It is thought that a depolarization is generated by axoaxonal synapses in the regions of termination of the

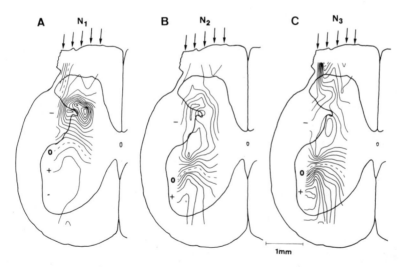

Fig. 4.2. Isopotential contour plots of the field potentials evoked in the monkey spinal cord by afferent volleys in cutaneous fibers. The stimulus strength was graded, so that the potentials produced by small myelinated afferents could be determined by subtraction of the field potentials produced by large afferents. The measurements were made at fixed time intervals corresponding to the peaks of the N_1, N_2, and N_3 waves recorded at the depth at which the potentials were maximal. The contour plot in A shows the spatial distribution of the field potential equivalent to the N_1 wave; B corresponds to the N_2 wave, and C to the N_3 wave. (From Beall et al., 1977.)

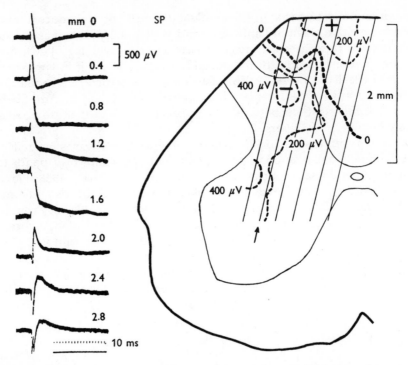

Fig. 4.3. Field potentials produced by stimulation of the superficial peroneal nerve are shown in the column at the left (negativity upward). The P wave is seen to reverse at a depth between 0.4 and 0.8 mm from the surface of the cord. The contour plot at the right was constructed based on measurements of the field potential 40 ms after the afferent volley. The records at the left were from the track indicated by the arrow. Note that the P wave in surface recordings becomes negative in the dorsal horn; the dipoles generating the field potentials are oriented in a dorsomedial to ventrolateral direction. (From J. C. Eccles *et al.*, 1962a.)

primary afferent fibers. The axoaxonal synapses are made by interneurons that synapse with the terminal boutons of the primary afferents (see below). A negative extracellular field potential would be produced by sinks resulting from activity at the axoaxonal synapses, while sources developing along the primary afferent axons situated dorsally would explain the positive field recorded near the surface of the cord (Fig. 4.3) (see J. C. Eccles *et al.*, 1962c; J. C. Eccles *et al.*, 1962a).

Muscle afferents also evoke field potentials. The N waves due to group I fibers are best recorded in the cat by an electrode inserted into the deep layers of the dorsal horn or the intermediate region (Fig. 4.4), since only small cord dorsum N waves are seen with recordings from the surface of the cord (J. C. Eccles *et al.*, 1954; Coombs *et al.*, 1956;

Lucas and Willis, 1974). Larger early and late N waves are produced when high-threshold muscle afferents are stimulated (Bernhard, 1953; Mendell, 1972), and these can easily be seen in cord dorsum recordings. At least a portion of the N waves evoked by high-threshold muscle afferents is a reflection of primary afferent hyperpolarization (Mendell, 1972). Muscle afferents also produce P waves, especially when nerves to flexor muscles are stimulated repetitively (J. C. Eccles *et al.*, 1962c).

In summary, negative field potentials can be recorded from the cord dorsum or from the dorsal horn in response to stimulation of cutaneous af-

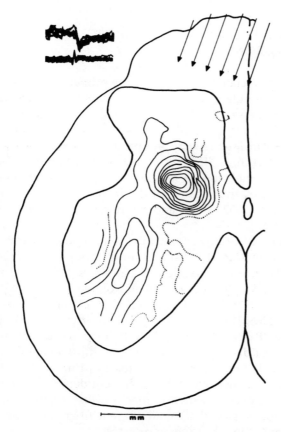

Fig. 4.4. Contour plot of the field potential produced by group I muscle afferents in the cat. Measurements were made at the time of the peak negativity measured from the record made at the depth where the potential was maximal. The inset shows the field potential (above) and the afferent volley recorded from the dorsal root entry zone (below). (From Lucas and Willis, 1974.)

ferents. The N_1 wave is due to input in $A\alpha\beta$ fibers and the N_3 wave in $A\delta$ fibers. The N waves reflect the excitation of dorsal horn interneurons. The N_1 wave is largest in laminae IV and V and the N_3 wave in laminae I, V, and VI. A positive field potential near the dorsal surface of the cord reflects primary afferent depolarization. Large muscle afferents produce a negative field potential in the base of the dorsal horn and intermediate region; they also evoke a positive cord dorsum potential, especially if stimulated repetitively. High-threshold muscle afferents evoke large field potentials, which reflect a combination of interneuronal excitation, primary afferent depolarization, and primary afferent hyperpolarization.

SYNAPTIC EXCITATION AND INHIBITION OF INTERNEURONS

A better appreciation of the response properties of interneurons is obtained with single-unit recordings, whether extracellular or intracellular. Interneurons can be distinguished from afferent fibers on the basis of their response characteristics and spike configuration in extracellular recordings and by the presence of synaptic potentials in intracellular recordings. They can be distinguished from tract cells or motoneurons by their failure to show antidromic activation following stimulation of the white matter of the cord or of motor axons (Woodbury and Patton, 1952; Frank and Fuortes, 1956; Wall, 1959; J. C. Eccles et al., 1960).

Intracellular recordings from interneurons demonstrate excitatory postsynaptic potentials (EPSPs) and inhibitory postsynaptic potentials (IPSPs) in response to activation of pathways impinging upon these cells (Fig. 4.5) (Haapanen et al., 1958; Kolmodin and Skoglund, 1958; Hunt and Kuno, 1959a,b; J. C. Eccles et al., 1960; Kostiuk, 1960; Hongo et al., 1966; Price et al., 1971). When primary afferents are stimulated, the EPSPs may be monosynaptic or polysynaptic, whereas the IPSPs are at least disynaptic, indicating an interneuronal relay (Hongo et al., 1966). This implies that the action of primary afferents is exclusively excitatory. However, such a judgment depends on measurement of the timing of events, which is practical just for the large afferents. Thus, it cannot be said that small afferent fibers must necessarily be just excitatory, although it seems probable.

There is a good possibility that the excitatory synaptic transmitter released by at least the large primary afferents is glutamic acid (Curtis et al., 1960; Graham et al., 1967; Duggan and Johnston, 1970; J. L. Johnson and Aprison, 1970; Haldeman and McLennan, 1972; J. L.

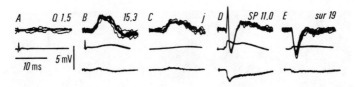

Fig. 4.5. Excitatory and inhibitory postsynaptic potentials recorded from an interneuron at a depth of 1.4 mm from the dorsal surface of the cat spinal cord. There was no effect when just group I afferents of the quadriceps nerve (Q) were stimulated (A), but high-threshold muscle afferents (B) and joint afferents (C) produced an EPSP. The superficial peroneal nerve (SP) evoked a monosynaptic EPSP (D), followed by an IPSP and a late EPSP. The sural nerve (SUR) was responsible for an IPSP (E). The intracellular recordings are in the upper traces and the cord dorsum recordings are in the second traces of each set. The lower traces in B–E were taken with the microelectrode in a position just extracellular to the neuron, using comparable afferent volleys to those that evoked the intracellular responses. (From Hongo *et al.*, 1966.)

Johnson, 1972; Roberts *et al.*, 1973; however, cf. Roberts and Keen, 1974).

Evidence is increasing that some small primary afferents contain substance P (Figs. 4.6 and 4.7) and others somatostatin; it is possible that these polypeptides are transmitters (Konishi and Otsuka, 1974; Saito *et al.*, 1975; Takahashi and Otsuka, 1975; Hökfelt *et al.*, 1975, 1976; Henry, 1976; Pickel *et al.*, 1977; Randić and Miletic, 1977).

Both γ-aminobutyric acid (GABA) and glycine are candidate transmitters to account for IPSPs in dorsal horn interneurons resulting from stimulation of primary afferents (Graham *et al.*, 1967; Bruggencate and Engberg, 1968; Curtis *et al.*, 1968, 1971a,b; Davidoff *et al.*, 1969; Game and Lodge, 1975). These amino acids would presumably be released by inhibitory interneurons.

In addition to the production of postsynaptic potentials in interneurons, afferent volleys result in the generation of primary afferent depolarization (PAD). This can be demonstrated by intracellular recordings from primary afferents (Koketsu, 1956; J. C. Eccles and Krnjević, 1959; J. C. Eccles *et al.*, 1962, 1963a), by tests for changes in the excitability of afferent terminals (Wall, 1958; J. C. Eccles *et al.*, 1962c, 1963a), as well as by the recording of dorsal root and field potentials (see above). A rather specific organization has been found for afferent fiber types giving or receiving PAD (see review by Schmidt, 1971; see also Whitehorn and Burgess, 1973). For instance, among cutaneous afferents, the slowly adapting mechanoreceptors preferentially produce PAD in the terminals of other slowly adapting mechanoreceptors (Fig. 4.8), whereas rapidly adapting receptors tend to produce PAD in the afferents of other rapidly adapting receptors (Jänig *et al.*, 1968b). PAD

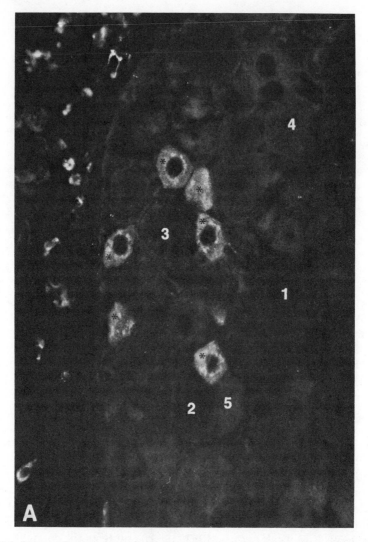

Fig. 4.6. Immunofluorescence micrographs of sections through a dorsal-root ganglion. The sections were adjacent and show the same neurons. The labeled cells on the left were positive for somatostatin, but not substance P, while the labeled cells on the right were positive for substance P but not for somatostatin. Note that the labeled cells are small and that large cells, such as 1 and 3, did not label. (From Hökfelt *et al.*, 1976.)

is believed to cause presynaptic inhibition by reducing the amount of excitatory transmitter released by afferent terminals (J. C. Eccles, 1964; Schmidt, 1971).

PAD has been attributed to the activity of axoaxonal synapses (Gray, 1963; Khattab, 1968; Ralston, 1965, 1968a,b; Conradi, 1969;

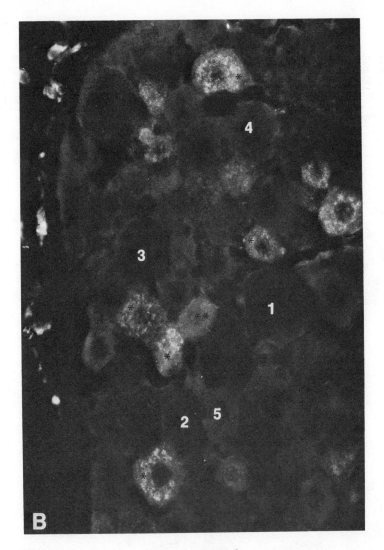

Fig. 4.6 continued.

Réthelyi and Szentágothai, 1969; McLaughlin, 1972). There is evidence that the synaptic transmitter involved is γ-aminobutyric acid (Fig. 4.9) (J. C. Eccles *et al.*, 1963b; Schmidt, 1963; Curtis *et al.*, 1971a, 1977; Levy *et al.*, 1971; Davidoff, 1972; Benoist *et al.*, 1972, 1974; Levy and Anderson, 1972; DeGroat *et al.*, 1972; Barker and Nicoll, 1973; Levy, 1974, 1975; McLaughlin *et al.*, 1975; however, cf. Curtis and Ryall, 1966; Repkin *et al.*, 1976). An alternative possibility is that K^+ liberated into the extracellular space mediates PAD (Vyklický *et al.*, 1972, 1975, 1976; Kríz *et al.*, 1974, 1975; Syková *et al.*, 1976; Deschenes *et al.*,

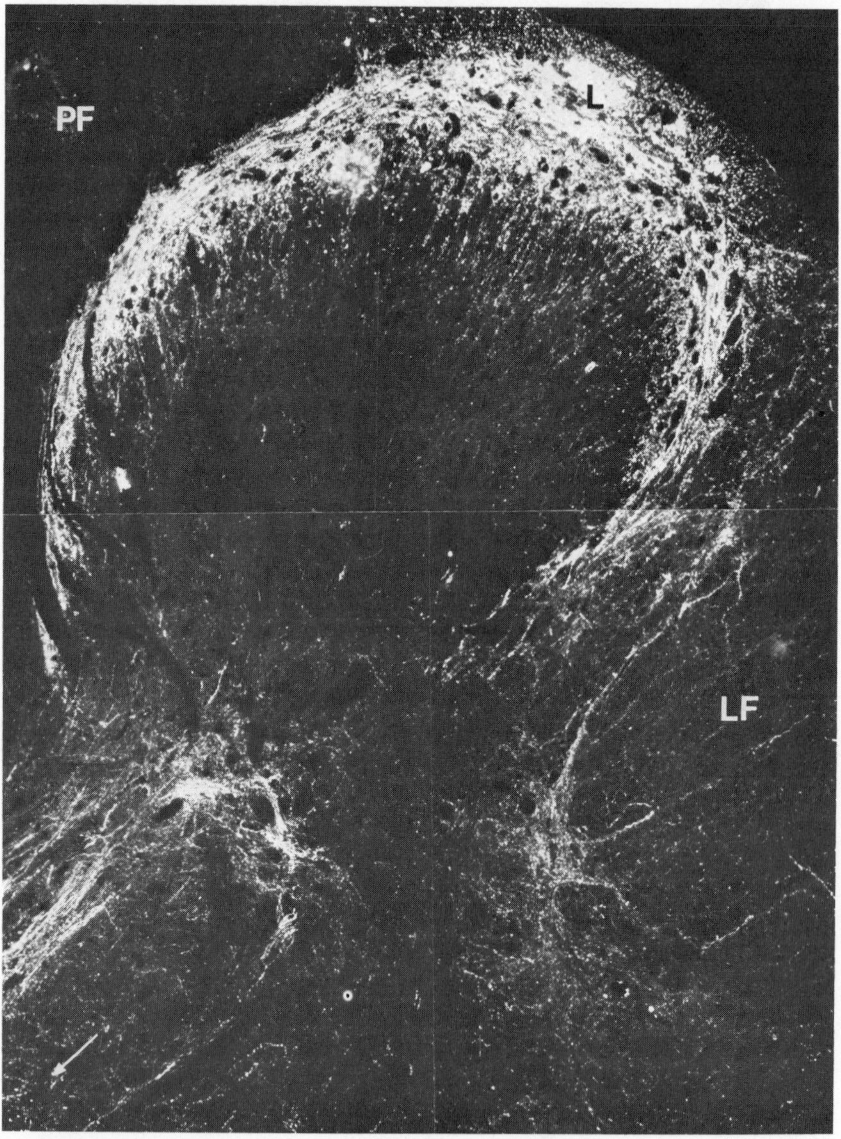

Fig. 4.7. Dorsal horn of cat demonstrating by immunofluorescence the distribution of substance P. Abbreviations: L=Lissauer's fasciculus, PF=posterior funiculus, LF=lateral funiculus. Arrow indicates the central canal. (From Hökfelt *et al.*, 1975.)

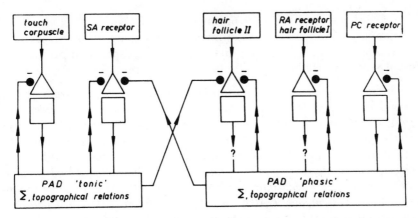

Fig. 4.8. The organization of the cutaneous PAD systems. The diagram indicates that the PAD produced by slowly adapting cutaneous mechanoreceptors acts chiefly upon slowly adapting receptors, and the PAD produced by rapidly adapting mechanorecep-tors acts chiefly upon rapidly adapting receptors, although there is some cross-talk. (From Jänig *et al.*, 1968b.)

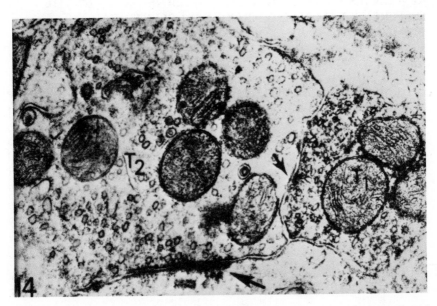

Fig. 4.9. Axoaxonal synapse in lamina II. A terminal positively stained for glutamic acid decarboxylase (T_1) is seen at the right. It is making synaptic contact with another end-ing, T_2, which does not contain glutamic acid decarboxylase and which is synapsing upon a dendrite. (From McLaughlin *et al.*, 1975.)

1976; Deschenes and Feltz, 1976; however, cf. Bruggencate *et al.*, 1974; Somjen and Lothman, 1974; Lothman and Somjen, 1975). An intriguing recent finding is that there may be opiate receptors on primary afferent terminals (LaMotte *et al.*, 1976) (see Chapter 9).

In summary, intracellular recordings show that interneurons of the dorsal horn generate excitatory and inhibitory postsynaptic potentials when afferent pathways to them are stimulated. The EPSPs produced by large primary afferents can be either monosynaptic or polysynaptic, while the IPSPs are polysynaptic. The excitatory synaptic transmitter utilized by larger primary afferents may be glutamic acid. Substance P and somatostatin are candidate transmitters for some small afferents. Possible inhibitory transmitters include GABA and glycine. Primary afferent depolarization (PAD) is thought to produce presynaptic inhibition by reducing the amount of excitatory transmitter released by afferents. The mechanism of PAD may involve axoaxonal synapses and the release of GABA. Alternatively, PAD may result from an accumulation of K^+ in the extracellular space.

RESPONSES OF DORSAL HORN INTERNEURONS IN THE DIFFERENT LAMINAE OF REXED TO ELECTRICAL STIMULATION

Lamina I

Christensen and Perl (1970) found that most cells in lamina I of the cat spinal cord were activated by Aδ- and/or C-sized afferents, but not by A$\alpha\beta$ afferents. This observation was confirmed for cats and extended to monkeys by Kumazawa *et al.* (1975). However, Kumazawa and Perl (1976, 1978) concluded that the chief input to cells in lamina I is from Aδ fibers, although some C fiber input could be demonstrated as well. Cervero *et al.* (1976) confirmed that there is convergence of input from Aδ and C fibers onto many cells of lamina I. Some cells were excited in addition by larger myelinated fibers. These cells may have received an input from the fraction of the Aδ nociceptor population which conducts at velocities over 30 m/s (Kumazawa and Perl, 1978; cf. Burgess and Perl, 1967; Georgopoulos, 1976).

Laminae II–III

Very few studies report successful recordings from neurons of the substantia gelatinosa. Kumazawa and Perl (1976, 1978) found that the cells they were able to investigate in this region are activated primarily by C fibers, although there was often an Aδ input as well. Yaksh *et al.* (1977) found a convergent input from A and C fibers onto all the cells in their large sample of substantia gelatinosa neurons. Gregor and Zimmermann (1972) illustrate the activity of a cell that appeared to be in lamina III and that responded only to C fiber input.

Laminae IV–VI

A population of cells can be found along the medial part of laminae IV–VI that is monosynaptically excited by stimulation of the medial plantar nerve and also by weak mechanical stimulation of the plantar surface of the foot (Armett *et al.*, 1961).

The interneurons of laminae IV–VI may be responsive just to stimulation of A fibers or they may respond also to C fibers (Mendell and Wall, 1965). The cells of these two populations appear to be intermingled with no areas of concentration (Gregor and Zimmermann, 1972; Menétrey *et al.*, 1977). Graded stimulus strengths often demonstrate a convergence of Aαβ, Aδ, and C fibers upon the same neuron (Wagman and Price, 1969). Repetitive stimulation of C fibers at rates of 1 per 3 s or greater produces an enchancement of the discharge rate of many interneurons, a phenomenon called "windup" (Mendell and Wall, 1965; Mendell, 1966; Wagman and Price, 1969).

In the thoracic cord, cells in lamina V receive a convergent excitatory input from cutaneous afferents and from Aδ visceral afferents of the splanchnic nerve and sympathetic chain (Pomeranz *et al.*, 1968; Selzer and Spencer, 1969). In the lumbosacral enlargement, comparable cells are activated by both cutaneous afferents and by group III muscle afferents (Pomeranz *et al.*, 1968).

Many neurons near the base of the dorsal horn in lamina VI (and also lamina VII) receive monosynaptic excitatory connections from group I muscle afferents (J. C. Eccles *et al.*, 1956, 1960; R. M. Eccles, 1965; Lucas and Willis, 1974). The same interneurons may also be polysynaptically excited by cutaneous afferents (J. C. Eccles *et al.*, 1960; R. M. Eccles, 1965).

In summary, interneurons in laminae I–III are excited chiefly by small afferents, either of the Aδ or C categories. Cells in lamina IV can be excited either by just the large Aαβ fibers or by a convergent input from A and C fibers. Lamina V cells often show a convergent input from cutaneous afferents of all sizes, and they may in addition be activated by group III muscle afferents or by Aδ visceral afferents. Interneurons of lamina VI can be excited by group I muscle afferents, as well as by cutaneous afferents.

RESPONSES OF DORSAL HORN INTERNEURONS TO NATURAL FORMS OF STIMULATION

Lamina I

Christensen and Perl (1970) found several kinds of responses to natural stimuli in recordings from neurons of lamina I of the cat. One group of cells could be activated only by Aδ mechanical nociceptors (Fig. 4.10). A second group was excited by intense mechanical stimulation of the skin or by noxious heat. Since both Aδ and C fibers converged on these cells, it was suggested that the receptors involved are Aδ mechanical nociceptors and C polymodal nociceptors. A third group of cells could be activated by innocuous temperature changes as well as by intense mechanical and thermal stimuli.

Kumazawa *et al.* (1975) extended these findings to the monkey and also demonstrated that some lamina I cells projected contralaterally to the upper cervical cord; this observation is consistent with the findings of Trevino *et al.* (1973) and Willis *et al.* (1974) that some spinothalamic tract cells are located in lamina I (see Chapter 8). Some recordings were also made by Kumazawa *et al.* (1975) from cells that were specifically activated by innocuous cooling or warming. Kumazawa and Perl (1978) subdivided their population of lamina I cells in the monkey into three categories: (1) cells activated only by intense mechanical stimulation (and only Aδ afferents), (2) cells excited by innocuous skin cooling (and Aδ afferents), and (3) a few cells that were discharged by noxious mechanical and thermal stimuli (C polymodal afferents).

Cervero *et al.* (1976) confirmed the finding that a high proportion

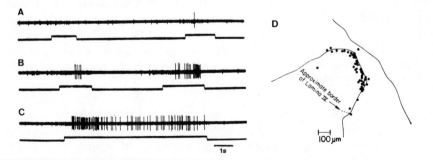

Fig. 4.10. (A) Responses of lamina I neuron to stroking skin with glass rod; (B) squeezing skin with smooth-surfaced forceps; and (C) squeezing skin with serrated forceps. The locations of lamina I neurons responsive to strong mechanical stimuli or strong mechanical stimuli and noxious heat are shown in D. (From Christensen and Perl, 1970.)

of cells in lamina I can be excited just by intense stimuli. However, some of their lamina I cells had a wide dynamic range of responsiveness, indicating that the lamina I population is not homogeneous. Specific nociceptive cells in lamina I could be excited either just by Aδ nociceptors or both by Aδ nociceptors and C thermal nociceptors (polymodal nociceptors), as in the experiments of Perl's group. Only the cells with C fiber input could be driven by noxious heat stimuli as well as by noxious mechanical stimuli. The cells with a convergent input from cutaneous Aδ and C fibers could usually also be activated by group III and IV muscle afferents.

Substantia Gelatinosa

Kumazawa and Perl (1976, 1978) recorded from a number of neurons that were shown by dye marks to be in the substantia gelatinosa. They were inclined to believe that the cells were among the population of larger neurons sometimes observed in this region, since their recordings were more stable than would be expected if the cells were very small. None of these cells tested could be antidromically activated from the cervical cord (Kumazawa et al., 1975). Input to them was chiefly from C fibers. Many were activated by C polymodal nociceptors; some were excited by C mechanoreceptors (Kumazawa and Perl, 1976, 1978).

Yaksh et al. (1977) recorded from neurons in the substantia gelatinosa that were either spontaneously active or that could be antidromically or orthodromically activated by stimulation of Lissauer's fasciculus. Many of the cells had small receptive fields (less than 1.5 cm²), although other cells located deeper in the substantia gelatinosa had somewhat larger fields, which could encompass those of the more dorsal cells. Repeated stimuli often revealed habituation of the responses. Many cells showed a prolonged discharge, lasting seconds to minutes, following a single brush stimulus. The prolonged discharge was blocked by barbiturate anesthesia. Most cells responded to hair movement or other weak mechanical stimuli, but some cells required intense pressure or pinch before responding.

Cervero et al. (1977b) also used a volley in the isolated Lissauer's tract as a search stimulus for neurons of the substantia gelatinosa. Cells were either antidromically or orthodromically activated by such a volley. One criterion that was used to identify neurons intrinsic to the substantia gelatinosa was that the responses had to differ from those known to characterize cells in laminae I and IV, so that recordings from dendrites could be ruled out; this restriction would of course eliminate from the sample any substantia gelatinosa cells that behaved like the neighboring cells. Another restriction was that the extracellular spikes should show an inflexion on the rising phase. The records to date that met these criteria indicate that neurons of the substantia gelatinosa have a high background discharge rate, most are inhibited by cutaneous stimulation, and some show prolonged discharges (seconds) after brief periods of stimulation.

Laminae IV–VI

The activity of interneurons in the neck and base of the dorsal horn of the cat in response to natural forms of stimulation has been surveyed by Wall and his associates. Wall (1960) found that the receptive fields of cells in this area were ovoid and larger than the receptive fields of primary afferents (average of 63 by 32 mm for the cells). The central part of the receptive field was the most sensitive. Strong stimuli applied to the skin adjacent to the excitatory field could produce inhibition. Cells were typically activated both by rapidly adapting tactile receptors and also by slowly adapting pressure receptors. Noxious stimuli added to the response. Cells of this kind were later described as having a "wide dynamic range of response" (Mendell, 1966). Convergence of input from a number of receptor types upon dorsal horn interneurons was confirmed by Wall and Cronly-Dillon (1960).

Wall (1967) later found that the response properties of neurons in different laminae could be distinguished. Cells in lamina IV received a convergent input from mechanoreceptors. They could often be excited by hair movement, touch, and stimulation of tactile domes. Some cells, but not all, could be excited additionally by pressure and pinch. Thus, lamina IV was found to contain "narrow"- and "wide-dynamic-range cells." There was no input from deep receptors. The effects of descending pathways were also examined, as discussed later. Many narrow-dynamic-range cells developed a wide dynamic range after the cord was blocked by cold. Neurons in lamina V had larger receptive fields than did those of lamina IV, and the latency for activation was longer by an average of 1.5 ms. Responses were to touch and pressure. Again, no input was noticed from deep receptors. Spinal cord block lowered the threshold for cutaneous stimulation and expanded the receptive field size. Neurons in lamina VI responded to both cutaneous stimulation and to joint movement. The receptive fields were similar to those of cells in lamina V, but response latencies were longer still. Spinal block increased the excitability to cutaneous stimuli and reduced it to proprioceptive stimuli; thus, activity descending from the brain could act as a switch to shift the responsiveness of cells to lamina VI between cutaneous or proprioceptive inputs. A somatotopic organization was described for laminae IV and V in which the toes were represented medially and the lateral aspect of the foot and more proximal regions were represented laterally. It was suggested that cells in lamina IV excite those in lamina V and that cells in lamina V excite those in lamina VI in a cascade arrangement. Lamina VI neurons would in addition receive a direct input from proprioceptors.

Hillman and Wall (1969) investigated further the properties of cells located in the region of lamina V. The cells had larger receptive fields than did cells characteristic of lamina IV. The receptive fields consisted of three concentric zones. In the center of the receptive field, the movement of hair was sufficient to activate the neuron. Pressure or pinch were required when the stimuli were applied more peripherally. In the surrounding area of skin, tactile stimuli produced inhibition. Electrical stimulation of the dorsal columns or of dorsal roots other than those carrying the excitatory afferents produced inhibition of neurons in lamina V.

The results of these pivotal studies will be compared with the findings of other investigators. There have been numerous reports that neurons in the region of lamina IV can be found that are activated just by weak mechanical stimuli (Kolmodin and Skoglund, 1960; Armett et al., 1962; Fetz, 1968; Wagman and Price, 1969; Gregor and Zimmermann, 1972; Heavner and DeJong, 1973; Tapper et al., 1973; Price and Browe, 1973; Price and Mayer, 1974; Handwerker et al., 1975; Besson et al., 1972; Fields et al., 1977a; Menétrey et al., 1977). A convergent input from several types of receptor is typical, although neither invariable nor random (P. B. Brown, 1969; Heavner and DeJong, 1973; Tapper et al., 1973).

Wide-dynamic-range cells have also been reported by various investigators (Kolmodin and Skoglund, 1960; Fetz, 1968; Wagman and Price, 1969; Besson et al., 1972; Gregor and Zimmermann, 1972; Price and Browe, 1973; Price and Mayer, 1974; Heavner and DeJong, 1973; Handwerker et al., 1975; Fields et al., 1977a; Menétrey et al., 1977).

However, several groups have found that there are dorsal horn interneurons in addition to those in lamina I which respond just to intense stimuli (Kolmodin and Skoglund, 1960; Gregor and Zimmermann, 1972; Heavner and DeJong, 1973; Price and Browe, 1973; Menétrey et al. 1977; see also Pomeranz, 1973).

Thus, it can be concluded that the dorsal horn contains not only narrow-dynamic-range interneurons responsive to weak mechanical stimuli and wide-dynamic-range interneurons, but also interneurons that are specifically responsive to intense stimuli.

The presence of cells in the deepest part of the dorsal horn that receive a proprioceptive input has been confirmed by several groups

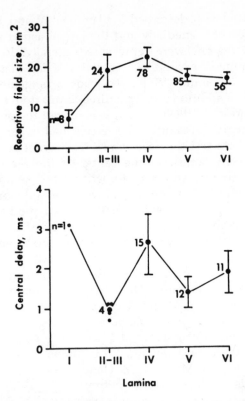

Fig. 4.11. The graphs show the relationship between the location of dorsal horn inter-neurons in the different laminae of Rexed and receptive field size (top) and the central delay for evoking the first spike by tactile stimuli (bottom). Each point represents the mean of the number of trials indicated, and the bars show standard errors. (From P. B. Brown *et al.*, 1975.)

(Heavner and DeJong, 1973; Willis *et al.*, 1974; Fields *et al.*, 1977b; Menétrey *et al.*, 1977). However, such neurons are not confined to lamina VI, but rather extend from laminae V to VIII.

The progressive increase in receptive field size that Wall (1967) found for cells at progressively greater depths in laminae IV–VI was not confirmed by P. B. Brown *et al.* (1975), nor was the progressively greater latency of response (Fig. 4.11). P. B. Brown *et al.* (1975), there-fore, dispute the idea of a cascade excitation of interneurons in the deeper layers of the dorsal horn by cells located more superficially. However, Applebaum *et al.* (1975) found a progressive increase in the sizes of the receptive fields of primate spinothalamic neurons in lam-inae I, IV, and V.

The somatotopic organization described by Wall (1967) for interneurons of laminae IV and V was dissimilar to that found by Bryan *et al.* (1973) for spinocervical tract neurons. However, P. B. Brown and Fuchs (1975) demonstrated a somatotopic arrangement (Fig. 4.12) that is in reasonable agreement with both that suggested by Wall and that by Bryan *et al.* Brown and Fuchs found both distoproximal and ventrodorsal gradients in the receptive fields of interneurons located across the mediolateral extent of the dorsal horn. The recent observation (Devor and Wall, 1976) that cells placed laterally in the dorsal horn may have very proximal receptive fields is consistent with the proposal of Brown and Fuchs.

The inhibitory effect of stimulation of the dorsal columns (Hillman and Wall, 1969) upon spinal interneurons has been confirmed (Handwerker *et al.*, 1975; Foreman *et al.*, 1976a,b).

In summary, interneurons in lamina I are often activated just by intense mechanical stimuli or by intense mechanical and thermal stimuli. Comparable cells are also found in deeper layers of the dorsal horn. Some cells in lamina I are responsive to activity in specific thermoreceptors, while others have a wide dynamic range of responsiveness to mechanical stimuli. Cells of the substantia gelatinosa appear to receive an input from a variety of receptors having C-fiber afferents, including nociceptors, thermoreceptors and mechanoreceptors. There is often a convergent input from myelinated afferents as well. A striking finding is that cells in the substantia gelatinosa may continue to discharge for a prolonged period of time after stimulation. Lamina IV contains cells that are activated by weak mechanical stimuli or by weak and strong mechanical stimuli. Wide-dynamic-range interneurons are also present in laminae V and VI. There is an input from high-threshold muscle afferents and also visceral afferents onto lamina V interneurons and from proprioceptors onto lamina VI interneurons. There is some evidence that the sizes of the receptive fields increase for interneurons in progressively deeper laminae, although this is disputed. The suggestion that cells in lamina IV excite those in lamina V and that those in lamina V excite those in lamina VI has not been proved. The interneurons in the dorsal horn have a somatotopic organization.

CLASSIFICATION OF DORSAL HORN INTERNEURONS

Several attempts have been made to develop a system of classification for dorsal horn interneurons, but none of the approaches suggested to date is completely satisfactory. A major difficulty is that the projection path of interneurons is generally unknown, and so the only

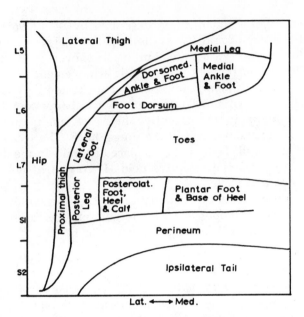

Fig. 4.12. The diagram above shows a scheme of the somatotopic organization of the dorsal horn in the lumbosacral enlargement of the cat. The abscissa indicates the lateral to medial extent of the dorsal horn, while the ordinate shows the segmental level. Receptive fields at each segmental level between L5 and S1 are shown in the four summary diagrams at right. Note that all of the diagrams are in the horizontal plane. (From P. B. Brown and Fuchs, 1975.)

information available about the cell may be its location in the spinal cord and its response properties to peripheral (or central) stimulation.

J. C. Eccles *et al.* (1960) described the responses of interneurons in the region of the intermediate nucleus. The nomenclature introduced by them was based on monosynaptic inputs from group Ia, group Ib, or cutaneous afferents to type A, B, and C interneurons, respectively. The inference could be drawn that there are no other significant peripheral inputs to these cells, yet many receive strong polysynaptic effects from afferent fiber types other than those making monosynaptic connections. It is not at all clear that monosynaptic connections reflect the most important connections during the normal operation of interneuronal pathways, although presumably monosynaptic pathways are likely to be subject to minimal interference. Another objection to this nomenclature is that the C interneurons would include cells receiving an input from a wide variety of cutaneous receptors (Tapper *et al.,* 1973); thus, the use of a single category for cells having a cutaneous input would tend to obscure a diversity of functions. J. C. Eccles *et al.*

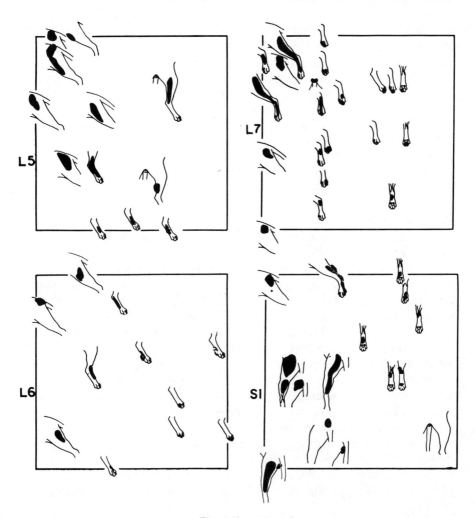

Fig. 4.12 continued.

(1960) did subdivide the C class into C and CT, the latter being tract cells (presumably spinocervical tract cells).

The alphabetical list of interneuronal classes was expanded by J. C. Eccles *et al.* (1962a). They describe a set of interneurons, labeled D, which have the properties that would be suitable for the interneurons responsible for producing primary afferent depolarization. Type D interneurons are not activated monosynaptically by primary afferents, and so the taxonomy of these cells is based upon other criteria, including convergence of certain kinds of input and the time course of discharge in response to single and repetitive input volleys.

Wall (1967) found that interneurons in laminae IV, V, and VI of the dorsal horn tend to have different properties. Many of the cells in lamina IV respond exclusively to tactile stimuli. Cells in lamina V typically respond both to tactile and to noxious stimuli. Interneurons of lamina IV often behave like those in lamina V, but in addition they may receive a proprioceptive input. An informal nomenclature developed as a result of these observations. An interneuron that responded exclusively to tactile stimulation was called a "lamina IV cell," while an interneuron that responded both to tactile and noxious stimulation was called a "lamina V cell" (e.g., Hillman and Wall, 1969; Besson *et al.*, 1975), irrespective of the actual location of the interneuron. However, even in the 1967 paper, Wall points out that interneurons can be found in lamina IV that have a convergent input from tactile receptors and nociceptors. Presumably such neurons in lamina IV should not be called "lamina V cells."

Gregor and Zimmermann (1972) determined whether dorsal horn interneurons were excited just by myelinated cutaneous afferents or by both myelinated and unmyelinated fibers. They also determined whether the connections from the A fibers were monosynaptic or polysynaptic. Interneurons could then be categorized as activated just by A fibers with mono- or polysynaptic connections (MA and PA classes) or by A plus C fibers with mono- or polysynaptic connections (MC and PC classes). One of the cells in their sample did not fit the scheme, since it was activated just by C fibers. A major flaw in this approach is the difficulty in correlating the responses to electrical stimulation of peripheral nerves with the responses to natural forms of stimulation of the skin. The only correlations observed by Gregor and Zimmermann between a C fiber input and the response to natural stimuli seemed to be negative ones, e.g., PA units were not activated when intense stimuli were applied to the skin and they had little or no background discharge.

Willis *et al.* (1974) categorized spinothalamic tract neurons according to the weakest form of stimulation that would effectively excite the cells. They recognized cells excited following hair movement or tactile stimulation of the skin; other cells required intense mechanical stimulation of the skin; still others responded to stimulation of subcutaneous receptors. A major difficulty with this approach is that some neurons respond just to tactile stimuli, while others respond both to tactile and to intense stimuli. Thus, a hair-activated cell, according to the above scheme, might or might not respond additionally to a noxious stimulus.

A system of classification that takes into account the intensity "bandwidth" was introduced by Mendell (1966). Interneurons that respond just to tactile stimuli were called "narrow-dynamic-range" cells, while interneurons that could be activated both by tactile and by intense stimuli were said to have a "wide dynamic range." Although high-threshold interneurons were not widely recognized in 1966, they can be accommodated in this scheme as another form of narrow-dynamic-range cell.

Price and Browe (1973) and Price and Mayer (1974) evaluated the responses of dorsal horn interneurons to touch, to pressure, and to pinch. The cells were then subdivided into five classes: (1) touch units, (2) touch–pressure units, (3) touch–pressure–pinch units, (4) pressure–pinch units, and (5) pinch units. Class 3 is essentially equivalent to the wide-dynamic-range category, while the other classes represent cells having narrow or intermediate dynamic ranges. This system of classification can become more complicated if the responses to thermal stimuli are also taken into account. Furthermore, it is easy to extend this approach to include many more permutations of response to mechanical stimuli. For example, Heavner and DeJong (1973) were able to identify nineteen different kinds of responses to such stimulus modes as hair movement, prick, pinch, pressure, vibration, and proprioception. Tapper et al. (1973) sought the convergence of input from four cutaneous receptor types that they could activate selectively and found cells representing all sixteen possible combinations.

A simplified terminology was suggested by Handwerker et al. (1975). They suggested that cells excited by myelinated afferents only be called class 1 cells and that cells excited by myelinated and unmyelinated fibers be called class 2 cells. Class 1 cells would include both the MA and PA units of Gregor and Zimmermann (1972). The effective receptors could be either sensitive mechanoreceptors of the skin or proprioceptors. Class 2 cells in addition respond to C fibers and to noxious heating of the skin. They include both the MC and PC units of Gregor and Zimmermann (1972). Cutaneous receptors that activate these cells include several types of hair-follicle afferents and the rapidly and slowly adapting tactile receptors of the foot pads. Class 1 cells are equatable with narrow-dynamic-range cells that respond to weak stimuli, and class 2 cells are comparable to wide-dynamic-range cells.

Cervero et al. (1976) expanded the terminology of Handwerker et al. (1975) to include another kind of cell, class 3. Class 3 cells respond only to noxious stimuli. Two subtypes are recognized, class 3a and class 3b. The class 3a cells receive an input from $A\delta$ nociceptors, chiefly the $A\delta$ mechanical nociceptors. Thus, most of these cells fail to respond to noxious heat. The class 3b cells are excited by $A\delta$ and C nociceptors. Thus, they are activated by noxious heat via the discharges of C polymodal nociceptors. In addition, some class 3b cells can be excited by group III and IV muscle afferents.

The most recent classification scheme is that of Menétrey *et al.* (1977). Four classes of dorsal horn neuron are recognized. Class 1 cells are excited by innocuous stimuli. Two subclasses include 1A (activated by hair movement and/or touch only) and 1B (hair movement and/or touch and pressure or pressure only). Class 2 cells are excited by innocuous and noxious stimuli. Again, there are two subclasses, 2A (hair movement and/or touch, pressure, pinch and/or pinprick) and 2B (pressure, pinch and/or pinprick). Class 3 cells are excited just by noxious stimuli (pinch and/or pinprick). Class 4 cells respond to joint movement or deep pressure.

Table 4.1 summarizes the various schemes for classifying dorsal horn interneurons. It appears that the most useful approaches at present are those that reflect both stimulus intensity and bandwidth. However, it seems likely that it will be necessary to specify the receptor types that activate (and inhibit) particular neurons and also the distribution of the axonal projections before the functional roles of dorsal horn interneurons can be determined.

In summary, attempts to classify interneurons of the dorsal horn have been based either on responses to electrical stimulation or to natural stimulation. One system subdivides interneurons by pathways that connect monosynaptically to the cells. Another subdivides interneurons receiving cutaneous afferent connections according to whether just A fibers or A and C fibers excite the cells and whether the A fiber connections are monosynaptic or polysynaptic. An elaboration of this scheme adds tests using natural stimuli to determine if the cell is activated by innocuous and/or noxious stimuli. A simple approach using natural stimuli defines the bandwidth of the input; narrow-dynamic-range cells receive inputs from mechanoreceptors or from nociceptors, whereas wide-dynamic-range cells are excited by both. Other classification schemes subdivide the wide- and narrow-dynamic-range categories to different extents, according to either the kinds of stimuli utilized for testing the response properties or the receptor types that connect with the cells. Eventually it will be necessary to know what receptors excite or inhibit an interneuron and also what its axonal projections are before it will be possible to assign a functional role to a given interneuron.

GATE THEORY OF PAIN

In 1965, Melzack and Wall published a model for the dorsal horn circuitry responsible for pain transmission. They called the model the

TABLE 4.1.   Classification of Dorsal Horn Interneurons

Interneuronal classes	Responses	References
Systems Based on Electrical Stimulation		
Type A	Monosynaptically excited by group Ia muscle afferents	J. C. Eccles *et al.*, 1960
Type B	Monosynaptically excited by group Ib muscle afferents	J. C. Eccles *et al.*, 1960
Type C	Monosynaptically excited by cutaneous afferents	J. C. Eccles *et al.*, 1960
Type D	Polysynaptically excited	J. C. Eccles *et al.*, 1962a
Type MA	Monosynaptically excited by A fibers	Gregor and Zimmermann, 1972
Type PA	Polysynaptically excited by A fibers	Gregor and Zimmermann, 1972
Type MC	Like MA, but also excited by C fibers	Gregor and Zimmermann, 1972
Type PC	Like PA, but also excited by C fibers	Gregor and Zimmermann, 1972
Systems Based on Electrical and Natural Stimulation		
Class 1	Excited by A fibers and by either sensitive mechanoreceptors or proprioceptors	Handwerker *et al.*, 1975
Class 2	Excited by A and C fibers and by sensitive mechanoreceptors and by heat nociceptors	Handwerker *et al.*, 1975
Class 3a	Excited by A fibers and by noxious mechanical (but usually not noxious thermal) stimuli	Cervero *et al.*, 1976
Class 3b	Excited by A and C fibers and by noxious mechanical and thermal stimuli; also by group III and IV muscle afferents in many cases	Cervero *et al.*, 1976
Systems Based on Natural Stimuli		
Hair activated	Activated by hair movement (often also by nociceptors)	Willis *et al.*, 1974
Low threshold	Activated by touch (often also by nociceptors)	Willis *et al.*, 1974
High threshold	Require intense stimuli	Willis *et al.*, 1974
Deep	Excited by proprioceptors or other subcutaneous receptors	Willis *et al.*, 1974
Narrow dynamic range	Excited just by weak stimuli (or just by strong stimuli)	Mendell, 1966
Wide dynamic range	Excited both by weak and by strong stimuli	Mendell, 1966

(continued)

TABLE 4.1. (*continued*)

Interneuronal classes	Responses	References
Class I	Excited by touch	Price and Browe, 1973; Price and Mayer, 1974
Class II	Excited by touch-pressure	Price and Browe, 1973; Price and Mayer, 1974
Class III	Excited by touch–pressure–pinch	Price and Browe, 1973; Price and Mayer, 1974
Class IV	Excited by pressure–pinch	Price and Browe, 1973; Price and Mayer, 1974
Class V	Excited by pinch	Price and Browe, 1973; Price and Mayer, 1974
Class 1A	Activated just by hair movement and/or touch	Menétrey *et al.*, 1977
Class 1B	Hair movement and/or touch and pressure or pressure only	Menétrey *et al.*, 1977
Class 2A	Hair movement and/or touch; pressure; pinch and/or pinprick	Menétrey *et al.*, 1977
Class 2B	Pressure, pinch and/or pinprick	Menétrey *et al.*, 1977
Class 3	Pinch and/or pinprick	Menétrey *et al.*, 1977
Class 4	Joint movement or deep pressure	Menétrey *et al.*, 1977

"gate control system." The gate theory has stimulated a great deal of research during the ensuing decade, and as a consequence, we know much more about spinal cord physiology and pain transmission. Because of the importance of this theory and its wide currency in clinical circles, the evidence that led to the development of the theory and the present status of the theory will be discussed (see also review by Nathan, 1976).

The starting point for the gate theory was the belief of Melzack and Wall that neither the specificity theory (that pain has its own peripheral and central neural apparatus) nor the pattern theory (that pain resulted from intense stimulation of nonspecific receptors) could account for what is known about pain. Clinical observations which are difficult to account for by the specificity theory include (1) the failure of surgical lesions to produce permanent pain relief, (2) the production of pain by innocuous stimuli in some patients, (3) the spread of pain and of trigger zones to areas of the body uninvolved in pathology, and (4) the slow onset of pain in hyperalgesic skin coupled with continuation of pain for a long period after stimulation is terminated. Psychological evidence is also not in agreement with a one-to-one relationship between pain perception and stimulus intensity. For instance, motivational factors influence pain perception dramatically. Physiological evidence at the time was lacking for significant numbers of nociceptive afferents in peripheral nerve. Furthermore, cells in the dorsal horn responded to a wide range of stimulus intensity, rather than specifically to noxious strengths (Wall, 1960; Wall and Cronly-Dillon, 1960). Although neurons were observed in the posterior thalamic nuclei that appeared to signal noxious inputs (Poggio and Mountcastle, 1960), comparable cells in unanesthetized animals responded to innocuous stimuli (Casey, 1966). On the other hand, the pattern theory of Weddell (1955) and Sinclair (1955) was based on the notion that sensory receptors other than hair-follicle afferents lacked specificity. This is not in keeping with the observations of many physiologists studying the properties of cutaneous sensory receptors. Another possibility is a theory based upon the properties of a central summation mechanism (e.g., Livingston, 1943; Hebb, 1949; Gerard, 1951). If there were a system that normally prevented summation, then its destruction could account for pathological pain. The gate theory proposes that activity in large fibers inhibits synaptic transmission in a system otherwise activated by small afferents carrying the signal for pain. A similar proposal was made by Noordenbos (1959) based on clinical findings.

Melzack and Wall made a specific proposal concerning the organization of a spinal cord gating mechanism (Fig. 4.13). Since afferent input activated cells of the substantia gelatinosa and the "first central transmission (T) cells in the dorsal horn," as well as dorsal column fibers, Melzack and Wall proposed that the substantia gelatinosa acts as a gating mechanism to control afferent input before it affects the T cells. The dorsal column fibers trigger brain mechanisms, which, in turn, influence the gate. The output of the T cells results in activation of the neural mechanisms causing responses and perception. Evidence for the involvement of the substantia gelatinosa in the control of afferent input came from the experiments of Wall (1962) and Mendell and Wall (1964) on dorsal root potentials. Recordings from dorsal horn neurons (candidate T cells) showed that large afferents produce a short lasting excitation, whereas the addition of small-fiber activity results in greatly increased activity (Wall, 1958, 1959; Mendell and Wall, 1965; Mendell, 1966). Negative and positive feedback loops were proposed

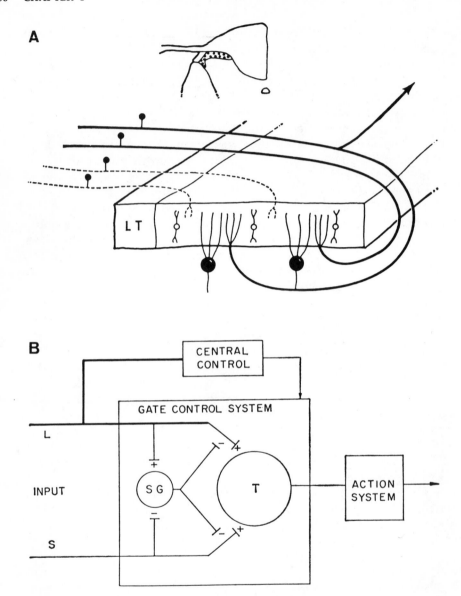

Fig. 4.13. (A) Representation of the manner in which small (dashed lines) and large (heavy lines) afferent fibers terminate in the substantia gelatinosa. Some of the large afferents also give off collaterals, which ascend in the dorsal column (arrow). The substantia gelatinosa contains small intrinsic neurons (somata shown by open circles) and the dendrites of neurons whose cell bodies are in deeper laminae. (B) The Melzack–Wall proposal for a gating circuit that might determine the output in the "action system." (From Melzack and Wall, 1965.)

to account for the different responses (Melzack and Wall, 1965). The feedback was thought to occur at a presynaptic level, although post-synaptic actions were not excluded. For the gate to operate properly, there would need to be (1) on-going activity in small myelinated and unmyelinated fibers, (2) stimulus-evoked activity, and (3) a relative balance of activity in large versus small fibers. The tonic activity in small fibers would keep the gate partly open, while an input over large fibers would close the gate, limiting the discharge of the T cells. An increased stimulus intensity would shift the balance of large and small fiber inputs, thereby increasing the output through the T cells. A pro-longed stimulus would result in adaptation of the large afferents, and the small fibers would get the upper hand, opening the gate further. The gate could be returned toward a closed position by adding a large-fiber input. Descending pathways could alter the gate control system. The activity in such pathways needs to be appropriate to the situation, and so a central control trigger was proposed. The dorsal column pathway and the spinocervicothalamic pathway were considered as likely candidates to provide the discriminative information needed for a central decision to alter the sensitivity of the gate mechanism. Some of the clinical and psychological observations mentioned as difficulties for the specificity and pattern theories were accounted for in terms of the gate theory.

Criticism of the gate theory center around new findings in three areas: (1) the properties of cutaneous receptors, (2) the dorsal root po-tentials produced by large and small afferents, and (3) the response characteristics of dorsal horn neurons.

Although the proportions of afferent fibers in peripheral nerve that could be called nociceptive was thought to be small in 1965, fur-ther investigations have shown that there are in fact large numbers of such fibers, both in the small myelinated and the unmyelinated size range (Burgess and Perl, 1967; Perl, 1968; Bessou and Perl, 1969; Iggo and Ogawa, 1971; Georgopoulos, 1976).

The circuit proposed to explain the negative and positive feedback in the operation of the gate control mechanism is shown in Fig. 4.13B. The neurons of the substantia gelatinosa were thought to be excited by large afferents, but they then produced presynaptic inhibition of the large afferents and so limited the excitation of the T cells. The presyn-aptic depolarization produced in large cutaneous afferents by the ac-tivity in other large afferents is in keeping with this model (Koketsu, 1956; J. C. Eccles and Krnjević, 1959; J. C. Eccles et al., 1963a; Hodge, 1972; Whitehorn and Burgess, 1973). However, small afferents were suggested by Melzack and Wall to inhibit the tonic activity of gela-tinosa neurons and so to cause presynaptic disinhibition. The dorsal root potential associated with such an event would be positive, instead of the usual negative wave. Positive dorsal root potentials have been described by a number of investigators (Lloyd, 1952; Wall, 1964; Andén *et al.*, 1966b; Dawson *et al.*, 1970; Mendell, 1970, 1972, 1973; Burke *et al.*, 1971; Hodge, 1972). The activation of unmyelinated afferent fibers has been generally associated with the production of negative dorsal root potentials (Zimmermann, 1968; Franz and Iggo, 1968; Jänig and Zimmermann, 1971; Gregor and Zimmermann, 1973), although sometimes a positive dorsal root potential results (Dawson *et al.*, 1970; Hodge, 1972). Significantly, the activation of C fibers connected with thermal nociceptors produces a negative dorsal root potential (Fig. 4.14) (Burke *et al.*, 1971), even though positive dorsal root potentials can be evoked in the same animal, ruling out the condition of the preparation as a factor. Since many small myelinated and C fibers are connected with sensitive mechanoreceptors, the finding of negative dorsal root potentials when a natural noxious stimulus is used appears to be more meaningful than the finding of positive dorsal root potentials following electrical stimulation of small fibers. Further evidence concerning the presynaptic modulation of afferent fibers comes from the investigation of Whitehorn and Burgess (1973). They showed that the excitability of the terminals of large afferents was increased whether stimulation was at an innocuous or a noxious level of intensity. Primary afferent hyperpolarization was not seen, except as an off response. Noxious mechanical stimuli produced primary afferent depolarization of small myelinated nociceptive afferents, although noxious heat had little effect.

The other major finding since the introduction of the gate theory has been the dorsal horn interneuronal population in lamina I, which is specifically responsive to intense levels of stimulation (Christensen and Perl, 1970; Kumazawa *et al.*, 1975). In addition to confirming the high-threshold responsiveness of the lamina I cells in the monkey, Willis *et al.* (1974) showed that these cells project to the contralateral diencephalon and that similar neurons can be found within the deeper parts of the dorsal horn. It thus appears that specific nociceptive neurons occur both at the primary afferent levels and at the level of the spinothalamic tract.

Evidence that supports the gate theory has been reviewed by Wall (1973). The fact that many cells in the dorsal horn receive convergent input has been amply documented (Wall, 1967; Pomeranz *et al.*, 1968; Selzer and Spencer, 1969; Hillman and Wall, 1969; Wagman and Price, 1969). Many spinothalamic tract cells in the monkey show such a convergent input (Willis *et al.*, 1974). The value of stimulating large afferents in relieving pain has received major attention in recent years

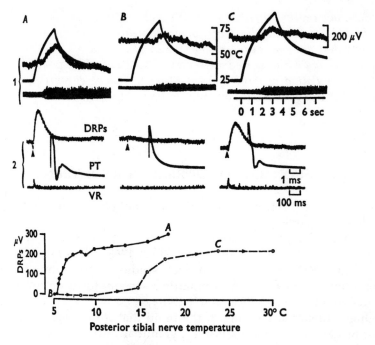

Fig. 4.14. The top traces in A–C are dorsal root potentials (negativity upward). The middle traces in 1 are temperature measurements from the skin, while those in 2 are neurograms from the plantar nerve before (A), during (B), and after (C) cold block of the nerve. The lower traces show activity in the ventral root. The graph below shows the size of the plantar nerve A fiber volley during (A) and after (C) application of the cold block. Heat pulses applied to the foot pad by a radiant heat source evoked negative dorsal root potentials. At least part of this effect was mediated by C fibers, since the blockage of conduction in A fibers did not eliminate the DRP produced by the heat pulses. (From Burke *et al.*, 1971.)

(Wall and Sweet, 1967; Shealy *et al.*, 1970; Nashold and Friedman, 1972; Nielson *et al.*, 1975). Wall (1973) admits that the weight of the evidence obtained since 1965 requires a modification of some of the details of the gate theory, but that it still provides a useful model. The question is whether or not the model is still recognizable in a testable form.

In summary, the gate theory of pain was proposed to account for a number of clinical observations that seem difficult to explain on the basis of a specificity theory of pain. However, several of the lines of evidence on which the details of the gate circuitry were based have been challenged. Peripheral nerves are now known to contain large numbers of afferents from nociceptors. Although small afferent fibers may evoke positive dorsal root potentials, nociceptive afferents produce negative dorsal-root potentials. Finally, in addition to wide-dynamic-range interneurons, the dorsal horn contains cells that are specifically responsive to intense forms of stimulation. Although the gate theory led to several important clinical applications based on stimulation of large afferent fibers to relieve chronic pain, it is doubtful that the gate model continues to be a satisfactory basis for future experiments.

DESCENDING CONTROL OF DORSAL HORN INTERNEURONS

There have been many studies of the effects of descending pathways from the brain that influence the activity of interneurons (e.g., Lloyd, 1941a,b; Lindblom and Ottosson, 1957; Suda *et al.*, 1958; Koizumi *et al.*, 1959; Lundberg *et al.*, 1962, 1963; Vasilenko and Kostyuk, 1965, 1966). A difficulty in such studies is to distinguish between interneurons that serve primarily a sensory function from those that are chiefly involved in motor activity.

One pathway originating in the brain that influences the activity of dorsal horn interneurons is the pyramidal tract. It is well known that some corticospinal axons terminate in the dorsal horn (Nyberg-Hansen and Brodal, 1963; Liu and Chambers, 1964; Petras, 1967; Coulter and Jones, 1977). Corticospinal terminals can be found in the dorsal horn of the monkey in laminae III–VI, but not in laminae I or II; projections to discrete regions of the dorsal horn originate from cytoarchitectonic regions 4, 3a, 3b, 1, 2, and 5 (Coulter and Jones, 1977). In addition to these direct projections, the cerebral cortex can affect spinal neurons by way of activity relayed in the brainstem (Carpenter *et al.*, 1963b; Hongo and Jankowska, 1967).

The reports of Wall (1967) and of Fetz (1968) can be taken as representative of studies concerning the influence of the pyramidal tract upon dorsal horn interneurons. Wall (1967) was unable to find any effect of stimulation of the pyramidal tract while recording from interneurons in the area of lamina IV, whereas comparable stimuli produced excitation or inhibition of most cells in lamina V and VI. Inhibition was more prominent in lamina V and excitation in lamina VI. Fetz (1968), on the other hand, observed that two-thirds of the cells in lamina IV were inhibited by pyramidal tract volleys and other cells showed an excitation followed by inhibition. About one-third of cells in lamina V were inhibited, one-third excited, and one-fifth excited and then inhibited. Of cells in lamina VI, two-thirds were excited, but some showed either mixed effects or inhibition. Thus, Fetz is in agreement with Wall that inhibition is more prominent dorsally and excitation ventrally.

In addition to the excitation and inhibition of interneurons, corticospinal volleys have been shown to produce primary afferent depolarization of cutaneous afferents and also group Ib and II muscle afferents (but not group Ia muscle afferents) (Carpenter et al., 1963b; Andersen et al., 1964e).

Several other pathways originating from subcortical nuclei are known that affect dorsal horn interneurons or that produce primary afferent depolarization. One pathway, called the "dorsal reticulospinal system" by Lundberg's group, arises from the medial portion of the lower brainstem and descends in the dorsolateral fasciculus of the spinal cord (Holmqvist and Lundberg, 1959, 1961; Engberg et al., 1968b,c,d). The "dorsal reticulospinal system" is responsible for a tonic inhibition of transmission through the spinal flexion reflex pathways (Job, 1953; R. M. Eccles and Lundberg, 1959b; Kuno and Perl, 1960; Holmqvist and Lundberg, 1959, 1961; Holmqvist et al., 1960a; Carpenter et al., 1963a; Engberg et al., 1968a,b,c,d; Chambers et al., 1970). Interruption of the tonic descending inhibitory system not only produces many of the motor-release phenomena seen in the spinal animal, but it also results in an enhanced responsiveness of spinal interneurons and ascending tract cells to peripheral input, especially to noxious input (Fig. 4.15) (R. M. Eccles and Lundberg, 1959b; Holmqvist and Lundberg, 1959; Holmqvist et al., 1960a; Carpenter et

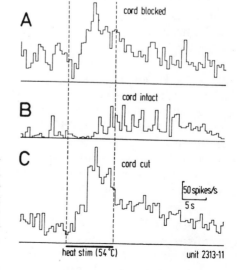

Fig. 4.15. Background discharge and response of a wide-dynamic-range dorsal horn interneuron to noxious heat. (A) The transmission of signals descending from the brain was blocked by cold; (B) the cord was intact; (C) the cord was transected. (From Handwerker et al., 1975.)

al., 1965; Wall, 1967; A. G. Brown, 1970, 1971; Besson *et al.*, 1975; Handwerker *et al.*, 1975; Cervero *et al.*, 1976, 1977a). Spinal transection also results in an enhancement of the flexion reflex afferent contribution to primary afferent depolarization (Carpenter *et al.*, 1963a).

Pharmacological studies suggested that at least a part of the tonic descending inhibition might be mediated by a monoamine synaptic transmitter, probably 5-hydroxytryptamine (serotonin) (Andén *et al.*, 1966a; Engberg *et al.*, 1968a,b). Since it was known that there is a projection descending in the dorsolateral fasciculus from the raphe nuclei (Brodal *et al.*, 1960a), a region rich in serotonin-containing neurons (Dahlström and Fuxe, 1965), it was natural to consider the possibility that the tonic descending inhibitory pathway originates from the raphe nuclei. However, Engberg *et al.* (1968b) concluded that this was only in part the case. Lesions that destroyed essentially all of the raphe nuclei of the caudal brainstem reduced but did not completely eliminate the tonic descending inhibition. Furthermore, stimulation of axons in the dorsolateral fasciculi produce inhibition having a latency consistent with a myelinated pathway conducting at about 30 m/s, whereas monoamine axons are thought to be unmyelinated (Dahlström and Fuxe, 1965). It was concluded that the tonic descending inhibition is due both to a descending tryptaminergic pathway from the raphe nuclei and to a dorsally located reticulospinal path (Engberg *et al.*, 1968b).

Recent studies confirm that there is a spinal projection from the raphe nuclei of the lower brainstem (Kuypers and Maisky, 1975; Basbaum *et al.*, 1976; Martin *et al.*, 1977, 1978; Basbaum and Fields, 1977). The nucleus raphe magnus projects to the dorsal horn through the dorsolateral fasciculus (Basbaum *et al.*, 1976; Martin *et al.*, 1977, 1978; Basbaum and Fields, 1977). Fluorescence histochemistry reveals the presence of numerous serotonin-containing neurons in the raphe magnus nucleus of several species (Dahlström and Fuxe, 1965; Pin *et al.*, 1968; Felten *et al.*, 1974; Hubbard and DiCarlo, 1974). Stimulation in the region of the raphe magnus nucleus produces inhibition of many dorsal horn interneurons (Basbaum *et al.*, 1976; Fields *et al.*, 1977a; Guilbaud *et al.*, 1977b; Willis *et al.*, 1977), as well as primary afferent depolarization (Proudfit and Anderson, 1974). Iontophoretic application of serotonin onto spinal interneurons often produces a depression of their activity (Engberg and Ryall, 1966; Weight and Salmoiraghi, 1966; Randić and Yu, 1976). Further evidence concerning the inhibitory action of the raphe–spinal pathway will be considered in relation to the spinothalamic tract in Chapter 8 and to the intrinsic analgesia system in Chapter 9.

However, in addition to raphe–spinal axons, the dorsolateral fasciculus also contains descending projections originating in other brainstem nuclei, including an ipsilateral projection from the hypothalamus, the region of the Edinger–Westphal nucleus, the nucleus subcaeruleus, and the magnocellular reticular nucleus; a bilateral projection from the nucleus paragigantocellularis, locus caeruleus, parabrachialis, retroambiguus, and solitary nucleus; and a crossed projection from the red nucleus and a parabrachial portion of the pontine reticular formation (Basbaum and Fields, 1977). Thus, if there is a non-serotonergic contribution to the tonic descending inhibitory system, there are a number of candidate sources for the "dorsal reticulospinal" projection. However, the lesion studies of the Lundberg group limit the candidate nuclei to those found within the medial portion of the lower brainstem.

The argument that the tonic descending inhibitory pathway is not exclusively serotonergic because it includes axons that conduct at rates up to 30 m/s needs to be reevaluated. The evidence that the monoamine axons are all unmyelinated is based on the examination in the light microscope of axons in freeze-dried material prepared for fluorescence histochemistry (Dahlström and Fuxe, 1965); such material is hardly optimal for the detailed study of small fibers. Furthermore, the work by Dahlström and Fuxe utilized the rat, which may differ from the cat or the monkey with respect to the lack of myelination of the raphe–spinal projection. Evidence that tends to support the notion that many raphe–spinal axons are myelinated comes from experiments in which the conduction velocities of raphe–spinal axons were determined from the latencies of antidromic spikes evoked by stimulation of the axons at a spinal level (Menzies, 1976; Anderson et al., 1977; West and Wolstencroft, 1977). The conduction velocities of the axons of neurons in the raphe magnus nucleus range from 5 to 67 m/s (West and Wolstencroft, 1977). A major reservation is that there may be non-serotonergic neurons within the raphe nuclei. It would be helpful to know what proportion of raphe neurons contain serotonin and also whether cells labeled in some fashion for serotonin contents have myelinated axons.

Undoubtedly, many other descending pathways are capable of influencing, either directly or indirectly, the activity of interneurons of the dorsal horn. For instance, stimulation of the vestibular nerve has been shown to excite interneurons not only in the ventral horn but also in the dorsal horn (Erulkar et al., 1966). This action could be mediated by way of either vestibulospinal or reticulospinal tracts. Furthermore, stimulation either of the eighth cranial nerve or of medial and descending vestibular nuclei evokes primary afferent depolarization of cutaneous afferents as well as of group Ia muscle afferents (Cook et al., 1969a,b). Stimulation within the reticular formation, part of the cerebellar cortex, or of the fastigial nucleus of the cerebellum will also result in primary afferent depolarization at a lumbar level (Carpenter *et al.*, 1966; Cangiano *et al.*, 1969). Thus, even pathways that are generally regarded as a part of the motor system produce actions at the spinal cord level that must have consequences for sensation.

In summary, a number of pathways descending from the brain influence the activity of spinal cord interneurons. The pyramidal tract inhibits many cells in laminae IV and V and excites many cells in laminae V and VI. A pathway originating in the nucleus raphe magnus of the lower brainstem and descending in the dorsolateral fasciculi inhibits many interneurons. This pathway forms at least part of the "dorsal reticulospinal system" of Lundberg, which is responsible for a tonic descending inhibition of the spinal cord flexion reflex pathway.

ACTIVITY OF DORSAL HORN INTERNEURONS IN UNANESTHETIZED, BEHAVING ANIMALS

The activity of interneurons is influenced by the presence or absence of anesthetic drugs and also by several pathways descending from the brain. Before it will be possible to relate the activity of particular classes of interneurons to behavioral events, it will be necessary to evaluate the discharge patterns of such neurons in unanesthetized animals. However, the usual experimental preparations available that avoid anesthesia (decerebrate or spinalized animals) have the drawback that there is an abnormal set in the activity of the descending control systems. For example, decerebrate animals have an increased activity in the brainstem pathways that produce a tonic inhibition of flexion reflex pathways (e.g., R. M. Eccles and Lundberg, 1959b), whereas spinalized animals completely lack such descending control.

An approach to the solution of this kind of problem is to record from unanesthetized, behaving animals. Such an approach has been very successful for studies of the activty of neurons in the brain. Technical difficulties have prevented widespread application of this approach to the spinal cord. However, studies by Wall *et al.* (1967), Courtney and Fetz (1973), and Bromberg and Fetz (1977) suggest that such investigations may become more profitable in future.

CONCLUSIONS

1. Negative field potentials recorded from the dorsal surface of the spinal cord or in the dorsal horn reflect the excitation of interneurons by cutaneous afferents.

2. In the monkey, the N_1 wave is due to activity in $A\alpha\beta$ fibers and

the N_3 wave to Aδ fibers. The N_1 wave is largest in laminae IV and V, while the N_3 wave is maximal in laminae I, V, and VI.

3. A positive field potential recorded from the dorsalmost part of the cord in response to cutaneous volleys is associated with primary afferent depolarization.

4. The negative field potentials resulting from stimulation of large muscle afferents are small in recordings from the cord dorsum and maximal in the base of the dorsal horn and intermediate region.

5. Large muscle afferents can produce a positive field potential associated with primary afferent depolarization, especially when repetitively stimulated.

6. Intracellular recordings reveal that interneurons of the spinal cord generate excitatory and inhibitory postsynaptic potentials in response to stimulation of afferent pathways.

7. Large primary afferents excite interneurons monosynaptically or polysynaptically. Inhibition is polysynaptic.

8. Candidate excitatory synaptic transmitters include glutamic acid (large afferents) and the polypeptides substance P and somatostatin (small afferents).

9. Candidate inhibitory transmitters include γ-aminobutyric acid and glycine.

10. Primary afferent depolarization is thought to cause presynaptic inhibition by reducing the amount of excitatory transmitter released by afferent terminals.

11. Axoaxonal synapses may produce primary afferent depolarization by means of the release of γ-aminobutyric acid. Alternatively, a build-up of the concentration of extracellular potassium ions may be responsible.

12. The following types of afferent fibers have been found to excite interneurons in the different laminae of Rexed:

Lamina	Afferent types
I, II, III	Chiefly Aδ and C
IV	A$\alpha\beta$ or A and C
V	A, C cutaneous; group III muscle; Aδ visceral
VI	A, C, group I muscle

13. The following types of natural stimuli activate interneurons in the different laminae of Rexed:

Lamina	Adequate stimuli
I, II, III	Intense mechanical and thermal; specific thermal; innocuous mechanical
IV	Innocuous mechanical; wide dynamic range
V	Wide dynamic range; intense mechanical
VI	Wide dynamic range; proprioceptive

14. Receptive field sizes may be larger for interneurons in progressively deeper laminae, at least for certain types of cells. However, this is controversial.

15. The suggestion that cells in lamina IV excite those in lamina V and that cells in lamina V excite those in lamina VI is controversial.

16. There is a topographic relationship between receptive field distribution and the locations of interneurons in the dorsal horn. For a mediolateral gradient of interneurons in the dorsal horn, the receptive fields have distoproximal and ventrodorsal gradients on the hind limb.

17. Dorsal horn interneurons can be inhibited by electrical stimulation of the dorsal columns.

18. A number of systems have been devised for classifying dorsal horn interneurons. These depend either on the responses of the cells to electrical stimulation or to natural stimuli. No system is completely satisfactory. One problem is a lack of complete knowledge of either the input or of the axonal projections of these cells.

19. The gate theory of pain stresses interactions between inputs over large and small primary afferents. Several of the experimental observations upon which the gate theory was based have been superceded by new information, and so it is questionable if the gate theory should still be considered a viable model.

20. Interneurons are subject to descending control from the brain by pathways that include the pyramidal tract, a raphe–spinal tract, and reticulospinal tracts.

21. It is likely that the raphe–spinal pathway, which originates from the nucleus raphe magnus, is at least in part coextensive with the "dorsal reticulospinal system" of Lundberg, which is responsible for the tonic descending inhibition of spinal cord flexion reflex pathways.

22. In future, more information is needed about the activity of dorsal horn interneurons in unanesthetized preparations. Decerebration or spinalization so alter the set of the descending control systems that such preparations provide no better insight into the normal activity of interneurons than do anesthetized preparations. It seems possible that studies using unanesthetized, behaving animals will be helpful in this regard.

5 Ascending Sensory Pathways in the Cord White Matter

INFORMATION TRANSMITTED BY THE ASCENDING PATHWAYS

Clues about the function of the sensory pathways come both from clinical and from animal studies. The clinical evidence is of particular importance, since the human patients can provide a subjective report of alterations in their sensory experience, and objective tests of changes in reaction to particular sensory stimuli can be used to confirm the subjective information. The difficulty with clinical studies is that most disease processes do not produce sufficiently localized damage to allow the assignment of a particular deficit to the interruption of a particular neural pathway in an unambiguous fashion, even when postmortem examination is possible. Lesion studies in animals have the advantage of precision in the surgical interruption of specific neural structures and in the postmortem verification of the area damaged, but the role of an ascending pathway in sensory experience can be evaluated only indirectly. Two ways in which the effects of lesions in animals can be investigated are studies of behavioral changes that are produced by lesions and recordings of alterations in neuronal activity. The discussion to follow will consider the evidence concerning the sensory pathways that ascend in the dorsal columns, the dorsolateral fasciculus, and the ventral quadrant of the spinal cord.

CLINICAL STUDIES

The traditional view of the function of the dorsal column is that the ascending fibers of this structure are responsible for the transmission of the information required for discriminative touch, vibratory sensibility, and position sense (Head and Thompson, 1906; Calne and Pallis, 1966). The history of this viewpoint and some of the clinical and experimental evidence that contradicts it have been reviewed by Wall (1970). For example, a variety of clinical cases have shown a distinct loss of vibratory sense with preservation of position sense or vice versa (Davison and Wechsler, 1936; Weinstein and Bender, 1947; Fox and Klemperer, 1942; Netsky, 1953; see also Calne and Pallis, 1966).

The development of the traditional concept of dorsal column function can be attributed to the sensory deficits that occur in disease states, such as the Brown–Sequard syndrome from cord hemisection, tables dorsalis, Friedreich's ataxia, and subacute combined degeneration. In none of these is there an isolated destruction of the dorsal column, and, therefore, the interpretation of the sensory deficit as the consequence of loss of dorsal column function alone must be held suspect. Wall (1970) points out, for instance, that in the Brown–Sequard syndrome, not only is the dorsal column interrupted but also the dorsolateral fasciculus. As will be discussed in Chapter 6, the dorsolateral fasciculus contains an important pathway for somatic sensation from the ipsilateral body, the spinocervical tract, and there is reason to believe that this pathway is present in man. Tabes dorsalis has been used as a model of dorsal column disease, since the loss of many of the fibers of the dorsal columns in neuropathologic material is striking. However, the disease process appears to affect the dorsal roots and dorsal-root ganglia and is not restricted to large fibers (Calne and Pallis, 1966). The loss of dorsal column fibers is accompanied by the loss of afferents that do not ascend the dorsal column to the medulla but that do provide sensory input to other ascending pathways, including the spinocervical, spinothalamic, spinoreticular, spinotectal, and other ascending tracts. Similarly, Friedreich's ataxia and subacute combined degeneration affect other pathways in addition to the dorsal column (Calne and Pallis, 1966).

More specific lesions of the dorsal columns have been made surgically (Browder and Gallagher, 1948; Rabiner and Browder, 1948; Cook and Browder, 1965) in an attempt to relieve phantom limb pain. In the study by Cook and Browder (1965), a total of eight patients had dorsal cordotomies, five in the upper thoracic cord and three in the upper cervical cord (Fig. 5.1). Of the patients with thoracic dorsal cordotomies, two had a transient and minimal reduction in tactile sensibil-

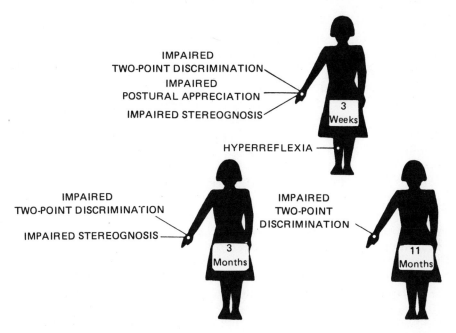

Fig. 5.1. Sensory deficits at various times after dorsal cordotomy at a cervical level. (From Cook and Browder, 1965.)

ity, one had a temporary slight decrease in appreciation of passive movement, and two had a disturbance of sphincter function that lasted some months. The patients with cervical dorsal cordotomies also showed little deficit. One had a short-lived zone of hypersensitivity of the arm and upper thorax. Another had a slight transient decrease in the sense of passive movement. The third patient had a permanent reduction in two-point discrimination and a temporary reduction in stereognosis and position sense. There was no loss in vibratory sensibility. A serious weakness in this study was the lack of postmortem confirmation of the extent of the lesions. If even a small number of fibers remained intact in the dorsal columns, it is conceivable that there would be little clinical deficit on the basis of the partial interruption. In cats, over 90% of the cross-sectional area of the dorsal columns must be sectioned before motor and sensory deficits can be demonstrated (Dobry and Casey, 1972a). Only a small part of the dorsal column in the monkey can prevent the appearance of a tactile deficit when the rest of the dorsal column plus the spinothalamic tract are cut (Vierck, 1974). Furthermore, it is now known that in cats, at least, the relay neurons of the dorsal column nuclei can be activated by fibers ascending in the dorsolateral fasciculus (Dart and Gordon, 1973). If the same is true of the human spinal cord, then it may be impossible to draw any conclusions about the function of the dorsal columns from the negative results of dorsal column lesions.

Additional evidence about the function of the dorsal columns in man can be obtained from stimulation of fibers in the dorsal columns. In recent years, a technique has been developed for the relief of pain by use of a chronically implanted electrode for stimulating the dorsal columns (Shealy et al., 1967, 1970). This is discussed elsewhere with reference to pain transmission (Chapter 9). For the present, the sensory effects of dorsal column stimulation per se will be considered. During dorsal column stimulation at high frequencies, patients report a buzzing or tingling sensation that radiates down the body to the feet (Shealy et al., 1970; Nashold et al., 1972). With low frequencies, the sensation is described as beating or thumping. High stimulus intensities produce an unpleasant sensation that patients wish to avoid but that is not described as painful (Nashold et al., 1972). Dorsal column stimulation does not consistently interfere grossly with tactile, position, or vibratory sensibility or with pain elicited by pinprick on clinical testing (Shealy et al., 1967, 1970; Nashold and Friedman, 1972), but a blunting or even suppression of awareness of touch, mild pinprick, and passive movement of the toes can be demonstrated in many cases (Nashold et al., 1972). Since the rate generally chosen by patients employing dorsal column stimulation is 100–200 Hz (Shealy et al., 1970), a case can be made that the buzzing sensation felt by such patients is due to the activation of afferents within the dorsal column connected with Pacinian corpuscles, which are responsive to high rates of vibration (Hunt, 1961; McIntyre, 1962; McIntrye et al., 1967; Silfvenius, 1970; see also Calne and Pallis, 1966). However, there is no reason to believe that such an unnatural form of stimulation would result in a pattern of neural discharge that would be interpreted in terms of a normal sensation. Furthermore, it is unlikely that sensory experiences produced by dorsal column stimulation result just from the ascending traffic of impulses within the dorsal column itself. The same fibers give off collaterals at the segmental level that excite neurons of the spinocervical tract (Taub and Bishop, 1965) and the spinothalamic tract (Foreman et al., 1976a), and so dorsal column stimulation would presumably activate at least some neurons in all of the major sensory pathways.

Nothing can be said from clinical evidence about the function of the pathways in the dorsolateral fasciculus (spinocervical or spinomedullothalamic tracts) in man. However, a great deal has been deduced about the role of the pathways in the anterolateral quadrant (including the spinothalamic, spinoreticular, and spinotectal tracts). The fact that pain and temperature transmission depends upon ascending fibers in the anterolateral white matter of the cord was demonstrated by Spiller (1905). A patient had lost pain and temperature sensation over the lower half of the body, but tactile sensibility was preserved. Spiller found at autopsy that the patient had spinal tuberculomas that disrupted the anterolateral quadrants bilaterally. This finding led to the first cordotomy for pain relief (Spiller and Martin, 1912). Several previous clinical reports were consistent with Spiller's observation (Müller, 1871; Gowers, 1878, Petrén, 1902). Since the early 1900s there have been numerous reports of clinical experiences with cordotomy (e.g., Frazier, 1920; Horrax, 1929; Grant, 1930, 1932; Kahn, 1933; Hyndman and Van Epps, 1939; Hyndman and Wolkin, 1943; Falconer and Lindsay, 1946; White et al., 1950, 1956; Nathan, 1963). Some neurosurgeons have interrupted the spinothalamic tract in the brainstem (Schwartz and O'Leary, 1941; White, 1941; Walker, 1942a), but the success rate decreases for higher levels of lesions (White and Sweet, 1955). More recently, the technique of percutaneous cordotomy has been introduced, with a resultant lowering of the operative mortality and postoperative morbidity (Mullen et al., 1963; Rosomoff et al., 1965, 1966; Mullen, 1966).

Cordotomies have provided information about the distribution of pain and temperature fibers within the cord, the effects of interruption of these fibers upon various sensory modalities, and the sensory experiences produced by stimulation in the anterolateral quadrant. Early results with cordotomy suggested that the pain pathway is a compact bundle in the lateral funiculus (Fig. 5.2A,B). However, it is now recognized that adequate pain relief requires an incision to within a few millimeters of the ventral sulcus (Kahn and Peet, 1948; White et al., 1956; White and Sweet, 1969). There is a somatotopic arrangement (Fig. 5.2C–F and 5.3), with the sacral and lumbar fibers lying laterally and dorsally and the thoracic and cervical fibers medially and ventrally at a high cervical level (Walker, 1940; White and Sweet, 1969). However, some mixing of the fibers from all levels is thought to occur (Nathan, 1963; White and Sweet, 1969). The pain pathway generally takes at least two segments to cross and move laterally (White et al., 1956), although Foerster and Gagel (1931) felt it crossed the midline within one segment. The discrepancy between the level of sensory loss and that of the cordotomy can be accounted for, in part, by the ascent of pain afferents in Lissauer's fasciculus from segments caudal to the cordotomy (Hyndman, 1942), rather than to a requirement for axons of the pain pathway to ascend before decussating. Although primary afferents ascend only one to two segments in Lissauer's fasciculus before

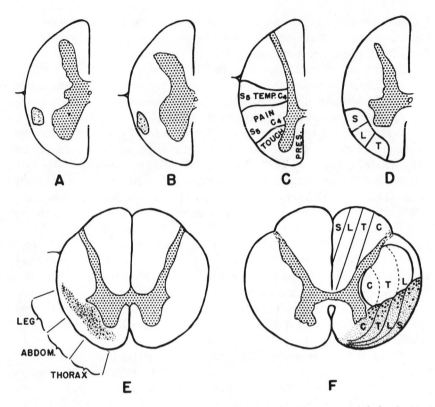

Fig. 5.2. Location and somatotopic organization of the human spinothalamic tract within the spinal cord according to a variety of authors. (From White and Sweet, 1969.)

terminating (Earle, 1952), second-order connections in cells of the substantia gelatinosa could provide an additional ascending link.

When a cordotomy is properly performed, the patient loses pain and temperature sensation completely on the contralateral side of the body. In a few rare cases, the sensory loss is ipsilateral (French and Peyton, 1948; Sweet *et al.*, 1950; Voris, 1951, 1957). The level of sensory loss depends upon the level of the cordotomy (Fig. 5.3); a high cervical cordotomy produces a sensory loss as high as the upper cervical dermatomes (but in some only to the upper thorax), while an upper thoracic cordotomy results in a sensory loss to a level between the nipple and the umbilicus (White and Sweet, 1969). The sensory loss persists for one or more years in over half of the patients, but in many cases, analgesia is replaced by hypalgesia or the pain may in fact recur. The reason for recurrence is a matter of speculation. Among the suggestions are regeneration of the sensory tract (unlikely) and the development of other sensory channels for pain information, such as ipsilateral spinothalamic tract fibers or other pathways (White and Sweet, 1969).

Following cordotomy, visceral pain is lost as well as somatic pain, and pain from pressure on bone is reduced (White and Sweet, 1969). It is possible, however, to elicit pain in patients with successful unilateral cordotomies by electrical stimulation of the skin, by testicular compression, and by distention of the renal pelvis (Hyndman and Wolkin, 1943; White et al., 1950). Bilateral cordotomy eliminates the pain of testicular compression and of renal pelvis distention (Hyndman and Wolkin, 1943). Itch is lost following cordotomy (Hyndman and Wolkin, 1943; White et al., 1950), suggesting that itch is related to pain. Tickle may (Foerster and Gagel, 1931; Schwartz and O'Leary, 1941) or may not (Hyndman and Wolkin, 1943; White et al., 1950) be lost. Position sense is unchanged (White et al., 1950).

In addition to the loss of pain sensation, patients who have cordotomies lose thermal sensation (Frazier, 1920; Hyndman and Wolkin, 1943). Thermanesthesia is generally more complete than is analgesia, and thermal sense is less likely to recur (White and Sweet, 1969).

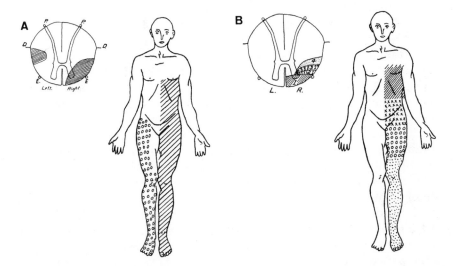

Fig. 5.3. Results of partial cordotomies. (A) The cross-hatched area on the left side of the body is devoid of pain and temperature sense due to the lesion of the right side of the cord, while the circles indicate a partial loss of these sensations on the right side of the lower extremity following the more restricted lesion on the left side of the cord. (B) Complete loss of pain and temperature sensation over the area below the left nipple. The different symbols show the progressive increment in the sensory loss as the cordotomy was extended. (From Hyndman and Van Epps, 1939.)

Shivering is abolished as well (Hyndman and Wolkin, 1943). There is some evidence for a differential distribution of pain and temperature fibers within the anterolateral quadrant. For example, some lesions result in a preferential loss of pain sensation (Wilson and Fay, 1929; Stookey, 1929; F. C. Grant, 1930; Foerster and Gagel, 1931; Sherman and Arieff, 1948; Kuru, 1949). Most of the results could be explained if the temperature fibers lay deep to the pain fibers; however, Stookey (1929) suggested the opposite arrangement. The regions of analgesia and thermanesthesia following cordotomy are generally superimposable (Fig. 5.3) (White and Sweet, 1955).

Bilateral cordotomy may abolish erection, ejaculation, or orgasm in the male, orgasm in the female, as well as libidinous sensations (Foerster and Gagel, 1931; Hyndman and Wolkin, 1943), although such changes are not necessarily found with unilateral cordotomy (White et al., 1950). Touch is not dramatically affected by cordotomy, although there is a slight increase in tactile threshold on careful testing (Foerster and Gagel, 1931; Kuru, 1949; White et al., 1950). Vibratory sense, position sense, tactile localization, stereognosis, and graphesthesia are little if at all affected (Hyndman and Van Epps, 1939; Hyndman and Wolkin, 1943; White et al., 1950; White and Sweet, 1969). Two-point discrimination is impaired when the compass points are sharp, but there is only a slight deficit when the points are blunt (White et al., 1950).

Stimulation of the fibers within the anterolateral white matter in man results in sensations of pain and/or of temperature (Foerster and Gagel, 1931; Sweet et al., 1950; Mayer et al., 1975). The sensations are generally referred to the contralateral side of the body, although on occasion the referral is to the same side or bilaterally.

The stimulus parameters required to produce pain in humans by stimulation within the anterolateral white matter have recently been described by Mayer et al. (1975). The data were collected during percutaneous cordotomy in conscious subjects. The threshold stimulus strengths were generally below 300 μA for the electrode configuration used (unipolar electrode 0.5 mm in diameter without insulation over last 2 mm). No pain was produced by stimulus rates of 5 Hz or less when the stimulus was at a painful intensity for higher rates, although some patients reported tingling or warmth. Raising the intensity at 5 Hz did not always result in a pain report, although it did in some cases. Stimuli below pain threshold and at rates of 50–500 Hz produced a tingling paresthesia. By using a double-pulse technique, it was possible to estimate the refractory period of the fibers carrying pain information. Usually, a value between 1.0 and 1.5 ms was obtained. On the basis of a comparison of the data with results using monkeys to determine the refractory periods of different classes of spinothalamic tract neurons, it was suggested that the axons of spinothalamic tract cells in laminae IV–VI and having a wide dynamic range are sufficient to cause pain (Price and Mayer, 1975). This assumes that the observations in monkeys are immediately applicable to man.

Recently, a unique case was reported by Noordenbos and Wall (1976). The patient had been stabbed in the back with a knife, with the result that all of the cord was transected except for the left anterolateral quadrant. The lesion was verified at surgery (Fig. 5.4). Since the patient was intelligent, cooperative, and knowledgeable about neuro-

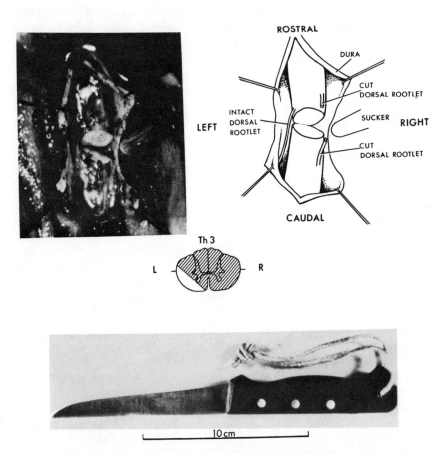

Fig. 5.4. The photograph and the sketch show the spinal cord after surgical exposure. The drawing of the spinal cord in cross-section indicates the extent of the lesion. The weapon is shown below. (From Noordenbos and Wall, 1976.)

logical disease (she was an occupational therapist), the case gave an unusual opportunity to test for those sensory functions that can be mediated by the anterolateral quadrant in isolation. After a period of recovery, it was found that the patient could detect touch and pressure bilaterally below the level of the lesion, although the threshold was generally higher than normal. Localization was rather good. Position sense was accurate to within 5° for the left knee and ankle, but it was lost for the left toes and for the right lower extremity. Vibratory sense was absent. Temperature sensation was lost on the left side of the body but intact on the right. Pinprick applied to the left side was unpleasant, but lacked the pricking quality and tendency to radiate that resulted when pinprick was applied on the right. It can be concluded that a single anterolateral quadrant can transmit sufficient information to permit touch and pressure sensations bilaterally. It should be noted that pinprick and temperature were intact for the right side, while position sense was partially intact on the left, indicating decussation of pain and temperature paths but not of proprioceptive fibers.

The clinical evidence is thus very clear that there is a major pathway for pain and temperature sensations in the ventral quadrant of the human spinal cord on the side contralateral to the sensory input. It is generally assumed that this pathway is the spinothalamic tract. However, some authors include other pathways in this term (cf., Nathan, 1963) or refer to the "anterolateral" pathways, which would include the spinoreticular and spinotectal tracts.

In summary, clinical evidence concerning the function of the dorsal columns is inconclusive. The traditional view that the dorsal columns are responsible for discriminative touch, vibratory sensibility, and position sense was originally based on disease states that do not produce a pure loss of dorsal column function. Even the negative evidence in cases in which the dorsal columns were cut surgically is insufficient in the absence of autopsy verification of the extent of the lesions. Stimulation of the dorsal columns produces a "buzzing sensation," but sensory data would reach the brain in such cases over several different sensory pathways. Evidence concerning the pain and temperature pathway in the human is more secure. Cordotomy cases show that the major pain and temperature path is a crossed one, ascending in the anterolateral quadrant. The fact that pain often recurs, sometimes more than a year after cordotomy, suggests that there are other minor pain pathways in man. Cordotomies also produce slight changes in tactile sensibility. The presence of a tactile pathway in the anterolateral quadrant is confirmed in a patient who had a lesion involving all of the spinal cord except one anterolateral quadrant. Touch and pressure sensations were present bilaterally in this patient, and position sense was partially in-

tact on the side ipsilateral to the functioning anterolateral quadrant. A crossed deficit in pain and temperature sensation was present, as expected.

ANIMAL STUDIES: ALTERATIONS IN BEHAVIORAL MEASURES

Animal experiments that bear a resemblance to clinical entities that affect sensation involve lesions that interrupt one or more of the ascending sensory pathways of the spinal cord. Such experiments have the advantage that the lesions can be made in discrete regions of otherwise healthy individuals, the effect of additional lesions can be determined, and postmortem evaluation of the extent of the lesions can be done readily. However, changes in the sensory experience of animals must be judged on the basis of behavioral tests, and inferences from such tests can be misleading.

Experiments designed to determine the functions of the sensory pathways of the spinal cord have included studies in which transections of any of the following have been made: the dorsal column, all of the cord but the dorsal column, the dorsolateral fasciculus, the dorsal column and the dorsolateral fasciculus, the ventrolateral quadrant.

Dorsal Column

A number of investigations of the effects of interruption of the dorsal columns have found either no change, minimal changes, or only transient changes in the behavioral responses examined. The behavioral measures in such investigations included tactile placing (Lundberg and Norrsell, 1960), tactile localization (Diamond *et al.*, 1964), and roughness discrimination in cats (Kitai and Weinberg, 1968); conditioned reflexes to tactile stimuli in dogs (Norrsell, 1966b); weight discrimination (DeVito and Ruch, 1956; DeVito *et al.*, 1964), proprioceptive and tactile placing (Christiansen, 1966), two-point discrimination (Levitt and Schwartzman, 1966); limb position (Vierck, 1966; Schwartzman and Bogdonoff, 1969), vibration (Schwartzman and Bogdonoff, 1968, 1969), tactile discrimination (A. S. Schwartz *et al.*, 1972), and ramp or ballistic movements in monkeys (Eidelberg *et al.*, 1976).

One explanation for these negative findings is that other sensory pathways, in addition to the dorsal columns, can transmit the information needed for the behavioral responses that were tested. An alternative approach to a lesion of the dorsal column is to see what functional capabilities remain after interruption of all of the cord except the dorsal columns. Wall (1970) tried this in rats. The animals became paraplegic. Intense stimulation of the hindlimb failed to produce orientation, vocalization, or changes in respiration in awake animals; similar stimuli did not awaken the sleeping animal. Wall suggests that the dorsal columns are particularly important for exploratory behavior; an absence of responses to stimuli that are received passively is in keeping with such a role. However, different conclusions were reached when a similar experiment was done in the cat (Myers *et al.*, 1974; Frommer *et al.*, 1977). Sensation was tested by operant conditioning in the study by Myers *et al.* (1974) and found to return to normal soon after surgery. Frommer *et al.* (1977) trained cats to do a tactile discrimination task. Following transection of all of the spinal cord except the dorsal columns, the cats were still able to discriminate between tactile stimuli. However, like Wall's rats, the cats that had cord lesions sparing only the dorsal columns did not show orienting responses to somatic stimuli applied below the level of the lesion. It seems likely that orientation and arousal reactions require input to the reticular formation and that such input is lacking in animals whose ventral white matter is interrupted.

Other investigations in which the dorsal columns have been cut have shown more striking changes on behavioral testing. Ferraro and Barrera (1934) reported that monkeys had a deficit in grasping movements, in position sense, and in placing and hopping reflexes; after lesions of the dorsal columns at a cervical level, the deficit was more severe for the upper than for the lower extremities. The deficit in grasping and in contact playing was confirmed by DeVito *et al.* (1964). Gilman and Denny-Brown (1966) found similar deficits in their animals and concluded that dorsal column lesions produce a severe disorder in exploratory movements. A lack of attention was also found to be characteristic of monkeys with transected dorsal columns (Schwartzman and Bogdonoff, 1968, 1969).

Recent experiments using more rigorous tests of sensory and motor performance have demonstrated alterations in both spheres. Dobry and Casey (1972a) found a deficit in roughness discrimination in cats, provided that more than 90% of the cervical dorsal columns was interrupted. Electrical recordings from neurons in the somatosensory cortex in the same animals revealed changes in the response properties of the neurons from normal (Dobry and Casey, 1972b). It seems likely that an insufficient interruption of the dorsal columns contributed to some of the negative results in previous investigations.

A dorsal column lesion alone did not impair the performance of monkeys in a movement-detection test (Vierck, 1974). However, the dorsal column lesion eliminated the ability of the monkey to distinguish the direction of a stimulus moved across the skin (Fig. 5.5).

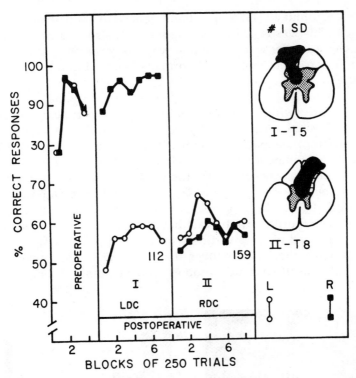

Fig. 5.5. The abscissa shows the times of testing before and after the two lesions indicated in the column at the right. The ordinate shows the proportion of correct responses in a stroke-direction task performed by the monkey subject. Left and right extremities are indicated by the open circles and filled squares, respectively. (From Vierck, 1974.)

Since the deficit was in discrimination of a passively detected stimulus, the role of the dorsal column is evidently not limited to exploratory activity.

Azulay and Schwartz (1975) required their monkey subjects to discriminate between plastic disks of various geometric patterns. The animals had to palpate the disks actively in order to distinguish between them. Lesions of the dorsal columns made it very difficult or impossible to make the discrimination. It was concluded that the dorsal columns play a unique role in the discrimination of tactile stimuli requiring sequential or spatiotemporal analysis.

Other studies emphasize the part played by the dorsal columns in motor activity. Melzack and Bridges (1971) found that dorsal column lesions interfered with the ability of cats to perform coordinated walking and turning on a narrow beam or to jump to a moving target. Melzack and Southmayd (1974) also found deficits in "anticipatory" motor behavior. This was tested by having the animals use a conveyor belt. Sometimes a barrier was placed part way along the belt. After a dorsal column lesion, a cat that would normally get on and off the belt and jump the barrier without difficulty would now experience problems in stepping onto the belt and would often be carried by the belt into the barrier before trying to jump over it. These experiments suggested that the information carried by the dorsal columns is needed for selecting the appropriate motor programs. Visual information alone did not seem to be adequate for such "anticipatory" motor behavior.

Experiments consistent with the work of Melzack and his associates have been done by Dubrovsky *et al.* (1971) and Dubrovsky and Garcia-Rill (1973). They showed a considerable deficit in the performance of serial-order acts by cats having dorsal column lesions. The cats were trained to jump vertically to release a piece of liver attached to a rotating wheel placed over them (Fig. 5.6). Performance was judged in terms of efficiency (proportion of successful attempts), accu-

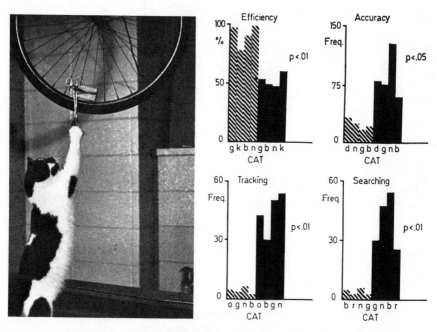

Fig. 5.6. The behavioral task is shown at the left. The cat releases a piece of liver from a clip attached to a revolving wheel. Performance judgements were evaluated in terms of efficiency, accuracy, tracking, and searching. The control levels are shown by the hatched bars in the graphs at the right. The performance after a dorsal column lesion is shown by the black bars. (From Dubrovsky and Garcia-Rill, 1973.)

racy, tracking of the falling liver, and searching when the cat failed to release the liver. All of these measures showed a deficit after a dorsal column lesion (Fig. 5.6), although the efficiency rating could be improved by overtraining before surgery. It was suggested that the deficits were due to the interruption of proprioceptive input from the forelimbs with a resultant incoordination.

A proprioceptive deficit was also found by Reynolds *et al.* (1972) in dogs following a dorsal column lesion. The dogs were trained to maintain a symmetrical stance, but their ability to do this was impaired after the lesion. However, the dogs responded in the same way to perturbations whether or not they had a dorsal column lesion.

Dorsolateral Fasciculus

There is less evidence concerning the behavioral changes which result from lesions of the dorsolateral fasciculus. Kennard (1954) found that cats having bilateral lesions of the dorsal quadrants showed hypalgesia, indicating that some nociceptive information is transmitted in the dorsal regions of the cord (however, cf. Ranson and Hess, 1915). Since responses to pain were unaltered by dorsal column section, the nociceptive pathway was presumably in the dorsolateral fasciculus.

The tactile placing reaction was abolished by a lesion of the dorsolateral fasciculus, but not by lesions in either the dorsal column or the ventrolateral quadrant (Lundberg and Norrsell, 1960). However, the pathway involved proved not to be the spinocervical tract, since there was no deficit in tactile placing when the cervicothalamic tract was interrupted at C1 (Norrsell and Voorhoeve, 1962).

A lesion of the dorsolateral fasciculus produced a transient reduction in the conditioned response to tactile stimulation in the dog (Fig. 5.7), whereas there was no change following just a dorsal column lesion (Norrsell, 1966b); however, a combined lesion produced a severe deficit.

Two-point discrimination was impaired in monkeys following a combined lesion of the dorsal column and dorsolateral fasciculus, whereas there was no change with just a dorsal column lesion or with combined lesions of the dorsal column and ventrolateral quadrant (Levitt and Schwartzman, 1966).

Changes in proprioceptive and tactile placing in monkeys were more lasting following a lesion of the dorsal column and dorsolateral fasciculus than with a lesion just of the dorsal column (Christiansen, 1966).

Tactile roughness discrimination in cats was severely impaired following a lesion of the cervicothalamic tract or a combination lesion of

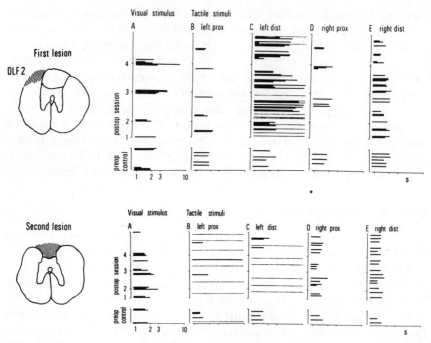

Fig. 5.7. Responses of a dog to conditioned stimuli before and after lesions of the dorsolateral fasciculus and of the dorsal columns. The lesions are shown at the left. The responses are indicated by horizontal bars, with successive trials starting at the bottom of each column. The lines are interrupted at a point corresponding to the latency of the response, unless there was no response within 10 s, in which case the horizontal line is a dotted one. There was no change in the responses to control stimuli (visual; tactile stimuli applied to the right lower extremity, either proximally or distally). In the first part of the experiment (top) a lesion of the dorsolateral fasciculus produced an impairment in the response to stimulation of the distal part of the left hind limb, but there was little change in the response to more proximal stimuli. However, when the dorsal columns were also sectioned (bottom), there was a severe deficit in conditioned responses to tactile stimulation of either the distal or proximal left hind limb. (From Norrsell, 1966b.)

this pathway and the dorsal column, but they were minimally affected by just a dorsal column lesion (Kitai and Weinberg, 1968).

Cats trained in a conditioned avoidance paradigm to respond to activation of a single tactile dome (type I slowly adapting receptor) showed an unaltered response when the dorsal column was sectioned, but they no longer responded to tactile stimuli after a combined lesion of the dorsal column and dorsolateral fasciculus (Tapper, 1970).

Vierck (1973) examined the ability of monkeys to discriminate between different-sized plastic cylinders. After a combined lesion of the dorsal column and dorsolateral fasciculus, the threshold for discrimination remained elevated, whereas a lesion just of the dorsal column produced a change of threshold with recovery to preoperative levels after several months.

In summary, behavioral evidence suggests that both the dorsal column and the dorsolateral fasciculus are involved in a number of sensory functions, often in a parallel fashion. One of the technical difficulties in these lesion studies is that most of the dorsal column must be interrupted to produce a deficit; however, a concomitant danger is that an overambitious dorsal column lesion may also damage the dorsolateral fasciculus. Therefore, the conclusions drawn by many investigators must be accepted with caution. Among the functions of the dorsal columns are roughness discrimination, recognition of stimulus movement, and discrimination of stimuli resulting from tactile exploration; in addition, the dorsal columns provide information needed for the performance of skilled, sequential movements and for "anticipatory" motor behavior. Deficits in motor behavior may be in part due to interruption of the flow of proprioceptive information in the dorsal columns, particularly from the forelimbs. The dorsolateral fasciculus of the cat may be involved in nociception. However, most studies have emphasized its role in mechanoreception. Fibers in the dorsolateral fasciculus of the cat are required for tactile placing (but these are not the spinocervical tract). Conditioned responses to tactile stimuli depend more on the dorsolateral fasciculus, but this function is shared with the dorsal columns. Two-point discrimination, proprioceptive and tactile placing, and spatial discrimination in the monkey depend on the dorsolateral fasciculus, perhaps in addition to the dorsal column. Tactile roughness discrimination and responses to type I slowly adapting receptors appear to result primarily from transmission through the dorsolateral fasciculus.

Ventral Quadrant

Transection of the ventral quadrant of the spinal cord in the dog produced an increased threshold for nociception (Cadwalader and Sweet, 1912). This observation was used as experimental support for the introduction of cordotomy for the treatment of pain in humans (Spiller and Martin, 1912).

It is interesting that reactions to painful stimuli applied to one side of the body in cats are not prevented by hemisecting the contralateral cord (Ranson and Hess, 1915; Kennard, 1954) and that the dorsolateral fasciculus appears to be more important for the transmission of nociceptive information than is the ventral quadrant in this animal (Kennard, 1954; however, cf. Ranson and Hess, 1915). One difference between the cat and the dog may be a more prominent spinothalamic tract in the latter (Hagg and Ha, 1970). However, nociceptive information does seem to be transmitted in the ventral quadrants of the cat spinal cord. Kennard (1954) found that the analgesia immediately following bilateral lesions of the dorsal quadrants diminished to hypalgesia with time, indicating that nociceptive information must be able to reach the brain through the ventral white matter. Neither Ranson and Hess (1915) nor Melzack *et al.* (1958) observed alterations in response to noxious stimuli following lesions of the dorsal half of the cord in cats.

Several investigators have found that ventrolateral cordotomy produced analgesia contralaterally in monkeys (Yoss, 1953; Kennard, 1954; Christiansen, 1966; Vierck *et al.*, 1971). A lesion of the dorsolateral fasciculus of the monkey did not result in analgesia in the experiments of Vierck *et al.* (1971). On the contrary, there was an increased reaction to noxious stimulation. A possible explanation for this might be the interruption of fibers descending in the dorsolateral fasciculus that inhibit transmission of nociceptive information.

The ventral quadrant of the spinal cord also seems to contain fibers that contribute in monkeys to weight discrimination (DeVito and Ruch, 1956; DeVito *et al.*, 1964) and position sense (Vierck, 1966).

In summary, pathways ascending in the ventral quadrant of the spinal cord are important in nociception, especially in the primate. In addition, the ventral quadrants make a contribution to several other varieties of somatic sensation, including weight discrimination and position sense in monkeys.

ANIMAL STUDIES: ALTERATIONS IN NEURAL ACTIVITY

The effects of lesions that interrupt one or more of the sensory pathways of the spinal cord have also been studied by recordings of activity at either the thalamic level or in the cerebral cortex.

Evoked Potentials

Cortical evoked potentials have been used by a number of investigators to monitor the effects of lesions that interrupt the dorsal column, the dorsolateral fasciculus (including the spinocervical and spinomedullothalamic tracts), or the ventral quadrant (including the spinothalamic, spinoreticular, and spinotectal tracts). Although some early reports suggested that sectioning the dorsal columns eliminates the potentials evoked in the sensorimotor cortex by peripheral nerve stimulation (Ruch *et al.*, 1952; Bohm, 1953), most later reports indicate that small changes at most are seen following transection just of the dorsal column.

The spinal pathways carrying information from cutaneous receptors, as revealed by evoked potential studies combined with selective lesions, will be discussed first. Pathways responsible for information from other receptors will then be considered.

In the cat, the shortest latency cortical potentials evoked by stimulation of cutaneous afferents depend partly on the dorsal column pathway and partly on the dorsolateral fasciculus (Gardner and Haddad, 1953; Morin, 1955; Catalano and Lamarche, 1957; Mark and Steiner, 1958; Norrsell and Voorhoeve, 1962; Andersson, 1962; Norrsell and Wolpow, 1966; Oscarsson and Rosén, 1966). The same is true for the dog (Gambarian, 1960; Norrsell, 1966a). Interestingly, when the dorsolateral fasciculus is cut (Fig. 5.8), the potentials evoked by stimulating hindlimb cutaneous nerves increase in latency, whereas no change in latency occurs following a lesion of the dorsal column (Mark and Steiner, 1958; Norrsell and Voorhoeve, 1962; Andersson, 1962; Norrsell and Wolpow, 1966). This indicates that the overall conduction velocity of the pathway in the dorsolateral fasciculus (presumably the spinocervicothalamic pathway, see Chapter 7) is faster than that of the dorsal column pathway, despite the presence of an extra synapse. However, the latencies of the potentials evoked via the two pathways are the same when forelimb nerves are stimulated (Andersson, 1962) or the dorsal column path is faster (Oscarsson and Rosén, 1966). Evi-

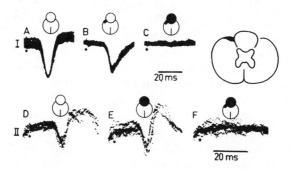

Fig. 5.8. Evoked potentials recorded in the right SI region following hair movement on the left hind limb. For the animal in A–C, the first lesion interrupted the dorsolateral fasciculus and the second the dorsal columns. In the other animal, D–F, the initial lesion was of the dorsal column, followed by the dorsolateral fasciculus. The drawing at the upper right shows the extent of the smallest lesion needed to interrupt the tactile tract of the dorsolateral fasciculus. Note the latency difference for the evoked potentials in B and A. (From Norrsell and Voorhoeve, 1962.)

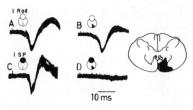

Fig. 5.9. Evoked potentials recorded from the right SI cortex in response to stimulation of the left radial nerve, A and B, and of the left superficial peroneal nerve, C and D. Lesions interrupted the dorsal columns at a midthoracic level and then the right ventral funiculus at C1 (shown in drawing at right). The hindlimb evoked potential was not greatly affected by the dorsal column lesion, but it was abolished by the addition of the lesion of C1, which interrupted the cervicothalamic pathway. (From Norrsell and Voorhoeve, 1962.)

dence that the potentials evoked via the dorsolateral fasciculus depend on the spinocervicothalamic path (Fig. 5.9) comes from experiments in which the potentials disappear following a combined lesion of the dorsal column and of the cervicothalamic tract (Morin, 1955; Norrsell and Voorhoove, 1962).

Recent studies that dispute the finding that cortical evoked potentials following cutaneous nerve stimulation depend upon pathways in both the dorsal columns and the dorsolateral fasciculus are those of Whitehorn *et al.* (1969) and Ennever and Towe (1974). Towe's group found that a complete transection of the dorsal column essentially eliminated the short latency potentials evoked by cutaneous stimulation. Direct stimulation of the dorsal column produced an evoked potential like that which results from cutaneous stimulation, but direct stimulation of the dorsolateral fasciculus had a minimal effect, provided that a mica sheet was inserted between the dorsal column and the dorsolateral fasciculus to reduce stimulus spread. Most cortical units sampled responded to dorsal column stimulation, but only about one-fourth responded to stimulation of the dorsolateral fasciculus, and these were mostly wide-field, rather than small-field. Previous studies were thought to be in error in not having complete lesions of the dorsal columns. However, Andersson and Leissner (1975) were able to evoke a cortical potential by stimulating the dorsolateral fasciculus, even though stimulus spread was minimized by placing a Teflon sheet between the dorsolateral fasciculus and the dorsal column. They suggest that the failure of Towe's group to produce a cortical evoked potential via the spinocervical tract was due to damage of the dorsolateral fasciculus or of the lateral cervical nucleus.

There is evidence that cortical potentials evoked by particular receptor types may utilize one or the other of these pathways. For example, McIntyre (1962) found that the potential evoked in SII by stimulation of large fibers in the interosseous nerve of the hindlimb disappears when the dorsal column is cut (see also Norrsell and Wolpow, 1966). He gave evidence that this potential was due to excitation of afferents from Pacinian corpuscles. This supposition was supported by a later study (McIntyre *et al.*, 1967) in which it was demonstrated that individually dissected Pacinian corpuscles could produce detectable cortical evoked potentials when mechanically stimulated (Fig. 5.10). These findings were confirmed and extended to the forelimb (Silfvenius, 1970). High-threshold fibers of the interosseous nerves still produce evoked potentials after dorsal column lesions, but not after dorsal quadrant lesions (McIntyre, 1962; Norrsell and Wolpow, 1966; Silfvenius, 1970).

Lesions interrupting a part of the dorsal column were found by Mann *et al.* (1972) not to alter the cortical evoked potential produced by activation of a single type I slowly adapting receptor, whereas a discrete lesion in the part of the dorsolateral fasciculus that contains the spinocervical tract eliminates the evoked potential.

Although cutaneous short-latency cortical evoked potentials are abolished by lesions interrupting both the dorsal columns and the dorsolateral fasciculi, it is possible to observe in cats small, late evoked potentials due to conduction in more ventrally located pathways (Norrsell, 1966a; Norrsell and Wolpow, 1966; Oscarsson and Rosén, 1966).

The results of similar studies in monkeys reveal that short-latency cortical evoked potentials in primates depend not only on the dorsal column and the dorsolateral fasciculus but also on the ventral quadrant (Gardner and Morin, 1953, 1957; Eidelberg and Woodbury, 1972; An-

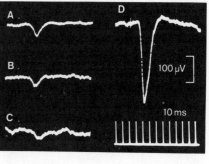
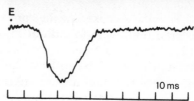
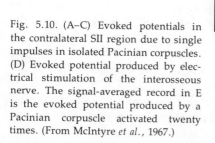

Fig. 5.10. (A–C) Evoked potentials in the contralateral SII region due to single impulses in isolated Pacinian corpuscles. (D) Evoked potential produced by electrical stimulation of the interosseous nerve. The signal-averaged record in E is the evoked potential produced by a Pacinian corpuscle activated twenty times. (From McIntyre *et al.*, 1967.)

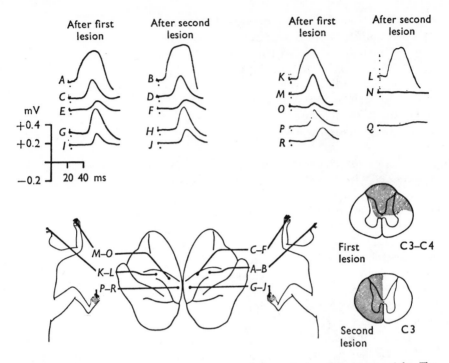

Fig. 5.11. Averaged evoked potentials after the lesions shown at the bottom right. The records above at the left were recorded from the right cerebral hemisphere and those at the right from the left cerebral hemisphere; in each case, stimuli were applied contralaterally at the sites indicated in the drawing. There was no change in the responses to stimulation of the face (A, B, K, L), nor of the left forelimb (C–F) or hind limb (G–J). However, the evoked potentials produced by stimulation of the right forelimb and hind limb (M–Q) were abolished. The pathways available to the left limbs were in the contralateral ventral quadrant. (From Andersson et al., 1972.)

dersson et al., 1972). The pathways in the dorsal part of the cord are ipsilateral to the stimulus, while that in the ventral cord is contralateral (Fig. 5.11). By contrast with the cat, the major early evoked potentials transmitted outside the dorsal column in the monkey are due to fibers in the contralateral ventral quadrant, presumably in the spinothalamic tract (Eidelberg and Woodbury, 1972; Andersson et al., 1972).

Potentials evoked in the cortex by stimulation of muscle nerves of the hind limb were found not to depend on the dorsal column in the cat (Gardner and Noer, 1952; Gardner and Haddad, 1953). However, this appears to be true just of the lowest-threshold muscle afferents, since high-threshold muscle afferents can produce cortical evoked potentials by way of either the dorsal column or the dorsolateral fasciculus (Norrsell and Wolpow, 1966). The observation that high-threshold muscle afferents can utilize the dorsal column pathway seems firm, since a cortical evoked potential was elicited even in an animal that had all of the cord sectioned except the dorsal column (Norrsell and Wolpow, 1966); since no afferents of this kind have been found to project directly up the dorsal columns, it seems likely that second-order dorsal column fibers are responsible. The absence of cortical evoked potentials due to activity transmitted in the dorsal column from low-threshold muscle afferents is consistent with evidence cited later that proprioceptive information from the hind limb in the cat is transmitted in the spinomedullothalamic pathway, which ascends in the dorsolateral fasciculus.

By contrast to the findings concerning low-threshold muscle afferents of the hind limb, it has been shown that group I muscle afferents of the cat forelimb produce evoked potentials in SI and SII by means of information transmitted in the dorsal column (Fig. 5.12) (Oscarsson and Rosén, 1963, 1966). The group I fibers include Ia fibers from muscle spindles, although group Ib fibers from Golgi tendon organs were not excluded.

Large visceral afferents in the splanchnic nerve of the cat pro-

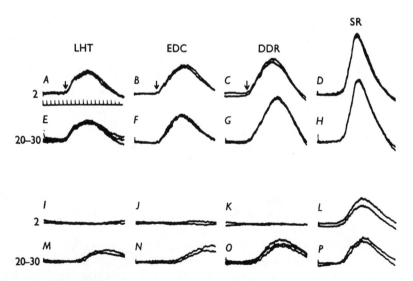

Fig. 5.12. Evoked potentials recorded from the right SI region before and after transection of the dorsal columns at C3. The potentials resulted from stimulation of large afferents (strength of stimulus two times threshold for the nerve) or of large and small afferents (twenty to thirty times threshold). The upper records (A–H) were taken before the lesion, and the lower records afterward (I–P). (From Oscarsson and Rosén, 1963.)

duced evoked potentials that were often abolished by a lesion of the dorsal column (Amassian, 1951; Gardner et al., 1955), but in other cases, there seemed to be a pathway for such activity in the lateral funiculus as well (Gardner et al., 1955). No early evoked potentials could be recorded in the monkey cortex following splanchnic nerve stimulation, presumably because of the small number of large myelinated fibers in this nerve in the monkey (Gardner et al., 1955). Small myelinated splanchnic nerve afferents evoked potentials by way of the ventrolateral quadrants as well as the dorsal column (Amassian, 1951).

In experiments utilizing a different approach, Curry and Gordon (1972) tried to determine what ascending pathways were responsible for evoking potentials in the posterior nuclear complex of the thalamus in the cat. They stimulated the dorsal column, the dorsolateral fasciculus, or the ventral quadrant after making suitable lesions to prevent spread of activity in other pathways. The dorsal column produced evoked potentials both in the ventral posterior lateral nucleus (VPL) and in the medial part of the posterior complex (PO_m). The dorsolateral fasciculus produced smaller evoked potentials in the same nuclei. The ventral quadrant inconsistently produced small evoked potentials in PO_m.

In summary, most investigators agree that the short-latency cortical evoked potentials due to stimulation of cutaneous afferents can be transmitted by activity in both the dorsal column pathway and the dorsolateral fasciculus. A similar evoked potential can also result from activation of a ventral quadrant pathway in the monkey. Some kinds of afferents have a preferential projection in one pathway—Pacinian corpuscle afferents in the dorsal column and type I slowly adapting receptors in the dorsolateral fasciculus. Group I muscle afferents from the hind limb project in the dorsolateral fasciculus, while those from the forelimb utilize the dorsal column.

Unit Activity

There have been several studies of the effects of interruption of sensory pathways of the cord upon the responses of neurons in the thalamus or cortex in cats and monkeys.

Following transection of the dorsal columns, it is still possible to find units in the thalamus or sensory cortex that can be activated by innocuous or by strong stimulation of the skin (Gaze and Gordon, 1955; Andersson, 1962; Levitt and Levitt, 1968; Dobry and Casey, 1972b; Millar, 1973b; Dreyer et al., 1974). Some units can be excited by subcutaneous receptors (Andersson, 1962; Millar, 1973b). However, the proportion of cells in the sensory cortex responding to weak mechanical stimuli decreases and the responses change in pattern (Levitt and Levitt, 1968; Dobry and Casey, 1972b; Dreyer *et al.*, 1974; but cf. Eidelberg *et al.*, 1975).

When all of the cord is cut except the dorsal columns, neurons can be found in the thalamus and cortex that respond to hair movement, vibration, tap, or stimulation of subcutaneous receptors. The cells may have small contralateral receptive fields and demonstrate surround inhibition (Fig. 5.13A), or they may have large receptive fields and be activated by both weak and strong stimuli (Gaze and Gordon, 1955; Andersson, 1962; Levitt and Levitt, 1968; Curry, 1972). Altered receptive field locations are seen after chronic lesions of all of the cord but the dorsal columns (Frommer *et al.*, 1977).

Following a selective lesion of the dorsolateral fasciculus, units can be found in the thalamus that respond to hair movement, tap, or pressure (Curry, 1972), and neurons in much of the sensory cortex of the monkey behave normally (Dreyer *et al.*, 1974). When combined lesions are used to permit conduction only in one dorsolateral fasciculus, units can be found that have small (Fig. 5.13B) or large contralateral receptive fields and that can be activated either just by weak mechanical stimuli, by weak and strong cutaneous stimuli, or by stimulation of subcutaneous receptors (Andersson, 1962). No surround inhibition is seen. There is an increase in the proportion of cortical units that respond to tap in such preparations (Levitt and Levitt, 1968).

Combined lesions of the dorsal columns and one or both dorsolateral fasciculi produce more drastic changes in unit activity (Levitt and Levitt, 1968). Nevertheless, units can still be found in the thalamus and cortex that are activated by somatic stimuli (Gaze and Gordon, 1955; Whitlock and Perl, 1959, 1961; Perl and Whitlock, 1961; Andersson, 1962; Levitt and Levitt, 1968; Curry, 1972; Dreyer *et al.*, 1974; Andersson *et al.*, 1975). The responses seen are often just to strong stimuli, but neurons activated by weak stimuli, such as hair movement, touch, tap, or stimulation of subcutaneous receptors, can be found. Such units (Fig. 5.14) may have restricted contralateral receptive fields (Perl and Whitlock, 1961; Andersson *et al.*, 1975).

In summary, transection of the dorsal column appears to produce some changes in the proportion of units in the sensory cortex responding to somatic stimuli, but many normally behaving units remain. Responses with just the dorsal columns intact are generally like those seen normally, including surround inhibition. A lesion of the dorsolateral fasciculus does not produce an obvious change. Interruption of all of the cord except the dorsolateral fasciculus alters the response properties of cortical neurons. One

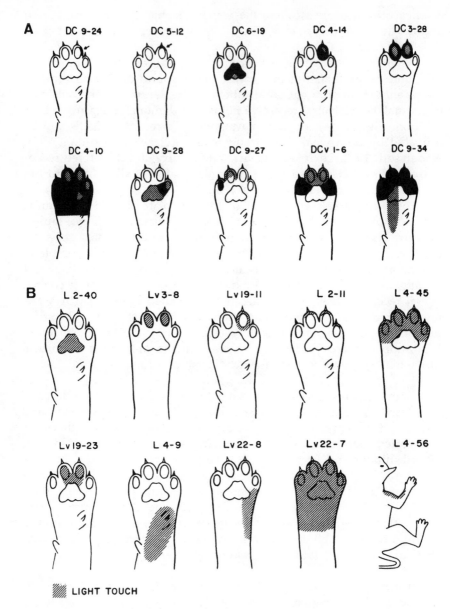

Fig. 5.13. Receptive fields (hatched areas) of neurons in SII in animals with just the dorsal columns intact (A) and in animals with the dorsolateral fasciculus, but not the dorsal columns, intact (B). The neurons in A have inhibitory receptive fields (black areas), often of the surround type. (From Andersson, 1962.)

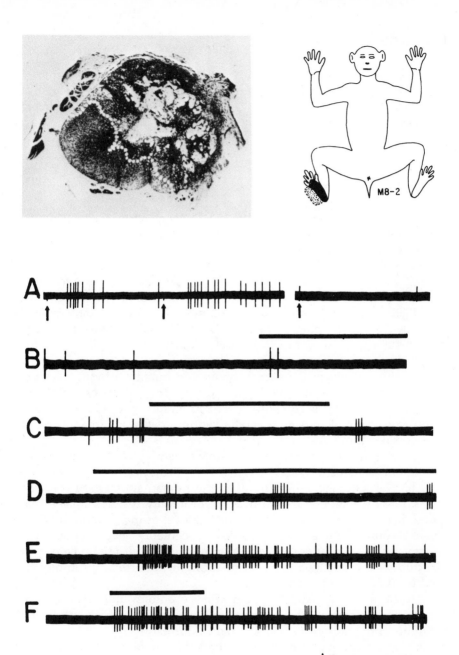

Fig. 5.14. Top left is a lesion of all of the cord but one ventral quadrant at a high cervical level. The top right drawing shows the receptive field of a thalamic neuron in a monkey with such a lesion. The records in A–F show the responses of the neuron to (A) electrical stimulation of the right and left plantar nerves, (B and C) tactile stimulation of the right sole, (D) pressure applied to the right sole, and (E and F) pinch of the right sole. (From Whitlock and Perl, 1961; Perl and Whitlock, 1961.)

result is the absence of surround inhibition. Despite lesions that transect both the dorsal columns and dorsolateral fasciculi, units can still be found in the thalamus and cortex that have small, contralateral receptive fields and that are activated by weak mechanical stimuli.

CONCLUSIONS

1. The traditional concept that the dorsal columns are responsible for discriminative touch, vibratory sensibility, and position is based on inconclusive evidence from disease states that do not produce a selective loss of dorsal column function.

2. Surgical lesions of the dorsal columns in man produce only minimal sensory deficits. However, the lesions may have been incomplete. Furthermore, the dorsal column nuclei can be activated (in cats) by fibers ascending in the dorsolateral fasciculus. Thus, the negative results in clinical cases of purely dorsal column lesions are inconclusive.

3. Stimulation of the dorsal columns in humans produces a buzzing sensation. This may be due to the ascending effects of dorsal column fibers, but not necessarily, since retrograde volleys in dorsal column afferents will activate several ascending pathways in addition to the dorsal column.

4. Nothing is known about possible sensory pathways in the dorsolateral fasciculus in man.

5. The anterolateral quadrant of the human spinal cord contains the pain and temperature pathways. Cordotomy results indicate that these pathways cross near the segmental level of their input and they have a somatotopic arrangement (lower segmental levels represented dorsolaterally and upper levels ventromedially). Itch is also conveyed by this same route. Tactile sensation is slightly affected by cordotomy, but position sense is not.

6. Recovery of pain sensation after cordotomy indicates the potential for pathways in other parts of the cord than the contralateral anterolateral quadrant to transmit pain information.

7. Stimulation of the human anterolateral quadrant results in pain sensation. The fibers responsible have a 1- to 1.5-ms refractory period, suggesting that their cells of origin are relatively rapidly conducting.

8. A human case with a transection of all of the spinal cord except one anterolateral quadrant shows that this part of the cord carries sufficient information to permit touch and pressure sensation bilaterally, pain and temperature sensations from the opposite side of the body, and position sense at some joints ipsilaterally.

9. Interruption of the dorsal columns in animals produces surprisingly little alteration in a number of behavioral tests of sensation, including tactile localization, tactile placing, tactile conditioned reflexes, two-point discrimination, vibratory sensibility, roughness discrimination, proprioceptive placing, weight discrimination, and limb position.

10. Cutaneous stimulation below a lesion interrupting all of the cord but the dorsal columns results in the transmission of sensory information but fails to evoke orienting responses or arousal.

11. Dorsal column lesions have been found to impair both sensory and motor functions when the lesions are sufficiently large and when appropriate tests are used. Sensory deficits that have been found include decreases in position sense, tactile placing, roughness discrimination, recognition of stimulus movement direction, and tactile discrimination requiring spatiotemporal analysis. Motor deficits include impairment of grasping movements, hopping reflexes, exploratory movements, coordinated walking and turning, "anticipatory" motor behavior, serial-order acts, and maintenance of a symmetrical stance. There is also typically a loss of attention in monkeys.

12. The dorsolateral fasciculus appears to contain pathways that transmit information similar to that conveyed in the dorsal column or in the ventral quadrant. The dorsolateral fasciculus of the cat contains at least part of the pain system in that animal. It is also responsible for tactile placing and for information from type I receptors. The dorsal column and the dorsolateral fasciculus both seem to contribute to tactile conditioned reflexes, two-point discrimination, tactile and proprioceptive placing, roughness discrimination, and size discrimination.

13. The ventral quadrant contains at least part of the nociceptive pathway in cats and much of it in monkeys. It also includes the thermoreceptive system, and it contributes to weight discrimination and position sense in monkeys.

14. Short-latency cortical evoked potentials due to stimulation of cutaneous nerves depend both on the dorsal column and the dorsolateral fasciculus in the cat and on these plus the ventral quadrant in the monkey. However, potentials evoked in cats by Pacinian corpuscles depend just on the dorsal column, while those produced by type I receptors depend only on the dorsolateral fasciculus.

15. Short-latency cortical evoked potentials due to stimulation of group I muscle afferents in the cat depend upon the dorsolateral fasciculus for hindlimb nerves and upon the dorsal columns for forelimb nerves. High-threshold muscle afferents of the hind limb can, however, evoke a cortical potential via the dorsal column (perhaps by way of second-order fibers).

16. Short-latency cortical evoked potentials due to stimulation of large visceral afferents of the splanchnic nerve depend on the dorsal and lateral columns. Those due to small visceral afferents depend on the ventral quadrant as well as the dorsal column.

17. Short-latency thalamic evoked potentials in cats due to stimulation of the dorsal columns or the dorsolateral fasciculus can be recorded in the ventral posterior lateral and the medial part of the posterior (PO_m) nuclei, whereas stimulation of the ventral quadrant produces only a small evoked potential in PO_m.

18. The activity of single units with small, contralateral receptive fields to tactile stimulation can be recorded in the thalamus or sensory cortex after lesions of the dorsal columns, dorsolateral fasciculi, or both. However, surround inhibition is absent when the dorsal columns are cut. Interruption of the dorsal half of the cord reduces the number of responsive units drastically.

6 Sensory Pathways in the Dorsal Columns

THE DORSAL COLUMN PATHWAY

The best-studied sensory pathway of the spinal cord is the dorsal column pathway. The part of this pathway that is actually within the cord consists chiefly of the ascending branches of primary afferent fibers entering through the dorsal roots. The dorsal column is subdivided into two components known as the fasciculus gracilis and the fasciculus cuneatus. The fasciculus gracilis includes the ascending branches of afferents from the midthoracic region and caudally, while the fasciculus cuneatus consists of the branches of afferents from midthoracic to upper cervical levels. The fasciculi gracilis and cuneatus terminate in nuclei of the caudal medulla of the same names, nucleus gracilis and nucleus cuneatus. Collectively, these nuclei are often called the dorsal column nuclei (along with the lateral cuneate nucleus). The nuclei gracilis and cuneatus project (among other places) to the contralateral thalamus via the medial lemniscus. For this reason, the dorsal column pathway is sometimes referred to as the dorsal column–medial lemniscus pathway (Fig. 6.1). Although the dorsal column nuclei are sometimes called "relay" nuclei, this term should not be taken to imply a simple organization or function (G. Gordon, 1973). The dorsal columns also contain axons ascending from tract cells in the spinal cord gray matter (second-order dorsal column pathway), and other second-order neurons project to the dorsal column nuclei via the dorsolateral fasciculus.

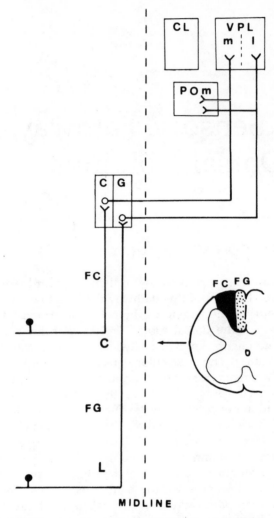

Fig. 6.1. The dorsal column pathway. Axons of primary afferents are shown entering the cord over cervical (C) and lumbar (L) dorsal roots and turning rostrally to ascend in the fasciculus cuneatus (FC) or fasciculus gracilis (FG) to end in the nucleus cuneatus (C) or nucleus gracilis (G). The second-order neurons in the dorsal column nuclei then project contralaterally through the medial lemniscus to end in the medial part of the posterior complex (PO$_m$) and in the ventral posterior lateral nucleus (VPL). The nucleus cuneatus projects to the medial and the nucleus gracilis to the lateral portions (m, l) of VPL. The drawing of a cross-section of the cord indicates the locations of the FC and FG.

PHYLOGENY AND ONTOGENY

The dorsal column pathway is developed to its greatest extent in mammals. A dorsal column pathway does exist in other vertebrates, including amphibia, reptiles, and birds (Craigie, 1928; Kruger and Witkovsky, 1961; Goldby and Robinson, 1962; Ebbesson, 1967, 1969; Hayle, 1973; Silvey et al., 1974; Lasek et al., 1968), but it is most prominent in mammals. Its absence in fish suggests that it may have evolved initially with the emergence from an aquatic environment, where much of the sensory stimulation of the body surface is processed by the lateral line system, while its prominence in mammals suggests further evolution along with the sensory apparatus of hairy skin. All orders of mammals that have been studied in this respect appear to have a substantial dorsal column pathway, including the aquatic mammals (Kappers et al., 1936; Clezy et al., 1961; Lund and Webster, 1967a; J. I. Johnson et al., 1968; Woudenberg, 1970; Jane and Schroeder, 1971; Schroeder and Jane, 1971; Rockel et al., 1972; Hamilton and Johnson, 1973; Walsh and Ebner, 1973).

The ontogenesis of the dorsal column pathway has been examined for the human embryo by A. Hughes (1976). The fasciculus cuneatus appears prior to the fasciculus gracilis. The fasciculus cuneatus is first recognizable at 8 weeks at the same time that the dorsal root ganglion cells of the cervical and thoracic segments differentiate. The tract can be seen to terminate on a cell mass at the level of the obex by 9 weeks. This cell mass later forms the dorsal column nuclei.

DORSAL COLUMN TRACTS AND THEIR PROJECTION ONTO THE DORSAL COLUMN NUCLEI

The dorsal column pathway in the spinal cord consists chiefly of the ascending branches of myelinated primary afferent fibers that enter the cord over the dorsal roots. The fibers course medially from the dorsal roots until they reach the dorsal column, where they bifurcate, sending a branch rostrally and another caudally (Ramon y Cajal, 1909; Réthelyi and Szentágothai, 1973). The branches give off collaterals into the spinal gray matter at the same and at adjacent segmental levels (Ramon y Cajal, 1909; Sprague and Ha, 1964; Sterling and Kuypers, 1967; Carpenter et al., 1968; Shriver et al., 1968; Imai and Kusama, 1969; Réthelyi and Szentágothai, 1973). The distance over which an ascending collateral ascends in the dorsal column depends upon the receptor type to which it is connected peripherally (Fig. 6.2). Three

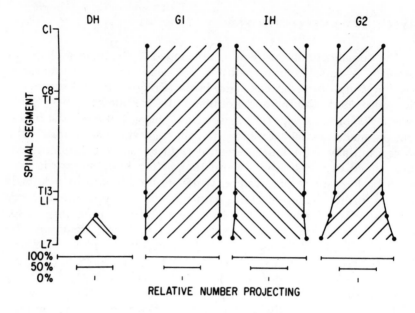

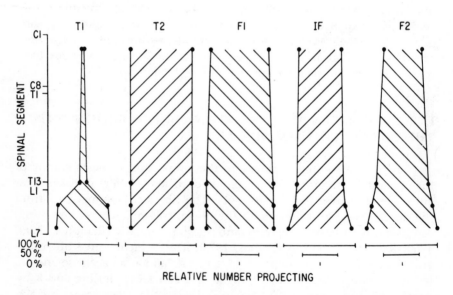

Fig. 6.2. Proportions of various types of mechanoreceptors that project to different levels of the spinal cord through the dorsal column. Abbreviations: DH = D hair-follicle receptors; G1, IH, and G2 = G1, intermediate, and G2 hair-follicle receptors; T1 and T2 = type I and type II slowly adapting receptors; F1, IF, and F2 = F1, intermediate, and F2 field receptors. (From Horch *et al.*, 1976.)

systems of fibers from the hind limb can be described: a short system, an intermediate system, and a long system (Horch *et al.*, 1976). The short system terminates within one or two segments. Myelinated afferents of the short system are the Aδ fibers (both from D hair receptors and nociceptors). The short system obviously acts on segmental circuitry. The intermediate system projects rostrally from four to twelve segments. The afferents are A$\alpha\beta$ fibers. The cutaneous fibers of this system supply type I slowly adapting receptors, G2 hair receptors, intermediate and F2 field receptors, and A$\alpha\beta$ sized nociceptors (Horch *et al.*, 1976). The intermediate system also includes muscle stretch receptors and slowly adapting joint receptors (Lloyd and McIntyre, 1950; Clark, 1972). One site of termination of the intermediate system is in Clarke's column upon neurons giving rise to the dorsal spinocerebellar tract. The long system projects all the way to the medulla to synapse in the dorsal column nuclei (Horch *et al.*, 1976). The properties of these axons will be considered in detail later in this chapter.

It is important to note that the conduction velocities of axons in both the intermediate and the long dorsal column systems slow near the point of their entry into the cord from the dorsal roots, suggesting that the fibers narrow as collaterals are given off at this level. Furthermore, the long-system axons slow again near the level of the cervical enlargement, suggesting that collaterals are given off here as well. Thus, the intermediate system can presumably affect segmental neurons as well as neurons of more rostral levels, such as those of Clarke's column, and the long system from the hind limb can act segmentally and also on the neural machinery controlling the forelimb (Horch *et al.*, 1976). The slowed conduction velocity of the long-fiber system within the cord is consistent with the observation that most of the axons in the fasciculus gracilis at the third cervical segmental level are of Aδ size (Hwang *et al.*, 1975), although peripherally the axons are all of A$\alpha\beta$ size.

The ascending branches of dorsal column afferents form a narrow band that is along the ventrolateral margin of the dorsal column at the level of entry over a dorsal root but that shifts dorsomedially as the fibers ascend; fibers entering more rostral dorsal roots then assume the ventrolateral position (Walker and Weaver, 1942). The fibers of the long dorsal column system terminate in the dorsal column nuclei (Fig. 6.3). The dorsal column nuclei include the nucleus gracilis (of Goll), the nucleus cuneatus (of Burdach), and the lateral (external, accessory) cuneate nucleus (of Clarke–Monakow or of Monakow). In some animals there is also a midline nucleus (of Bischoff). The dorsal column–medial lemniscus sensory pathway relays in the gracile and cuneate nuclei, but not in the lateral cuneate nucleus, which projects

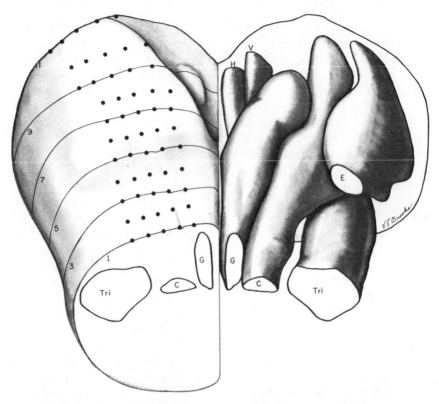

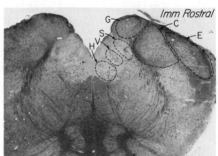

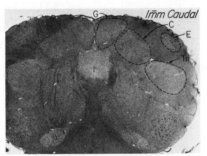

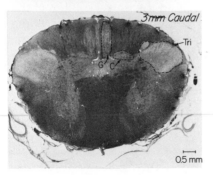

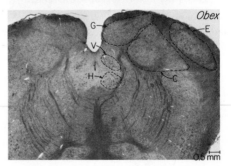

to the cerebellum (Ferraro and Barrera, 1935a,b). However, there is now evidence for a thalamic projection from the lateral cuneate nucleus of the monkey, but not of the cat (Boivie *et al.*, 1975). There are also some neurons in the rostral part of the nucleus gracilis of the cat that receive synaptic excitation from fibers from the hind limb ascending in the fasciculus gracilis and that project to the cerebellum (Gordon and Seed, 1961; Holmqvist *et al.*, 1963; Gordon and Horrobin, 1967). These latter cells may be in a part of the lateral cuneate nucleus (Hand, 1966), although that nucleus is generally regarded as a cerebellar relay for fibers representing the forelimb and rostral body.

The fasciculus gracilis and the fasciculus cuneatus end in the nucleus gracilis and nucleus cuneatus, respectively (Ferraro and Barrera, 1935b; Walker and Weaver, 1942; Chang and Ruch, 1947a; Glees and Soler, 1951; Shriver *et al.*, 1968; Carpenter *et al.*, 1968). The fasciculus gracilis of the monkey consists of the ascending branches of afferents entering the spinal cord over dorsal roots from the eighth (Walker and Weaver, 1942; Carpenter *et al.*, 1968) thoracic segment and caudally, whereas the fasciculus cuneatus is made up of similar fibers entering the cord over the seventh thoracic segment and the more rostral segments (Shriver *et al.*, 1968). A few fibers from segments as low as L1 in the monkey (Carpenter *et al.*, 1968) and L5 or even lower in the cat (Rustioni and Macchi, 1968) project to the nucleus cuneatus. Where there is a nucleus of Bischoff, it may receive input from the tail (Kappers *et al.*, 1936).

Only a fraction—22–23% in the cat, according to Glees and Soler (1951)—of the fibers ascending in the fasciculus gracilis actually reach the medulla. Many of the fibers end in the gray matter of the cord (Walker and Weaver, 1942). At segmental levels, dorsal root fibers terminate in various parts of the spinal gray matter, including the dorsal horn, intermediate region and ventral horn (Sprague and Ha, 1964; Sterling and Kuypers, 1967; Shriver *et al.*, 1968; Carpenter *et al.*, 1968; Réthelyi and Szentágothai, 1973). Ascending fibers of the fasciculus gracilis end in the nucleus dorsalis or column of Clarke (Liu, 1956; Carpenter *et al.*, 1968; Réthelyi and Szentágothai, 1973). Comparable fibers in the fasciculus cuneatus end in the lateral cuneate nucleus (Ranson *et al.*, 1932; Liu, 1956; Shriver *et al.*, 1968). The dorsal columns

←

Fig. 6.3. The drawing at the top shows a three-dimensional reconstruction of the dorsal column nuclei and adjacent nuclei. The cross-sections below were taken at the indicated levels with reference to the obex. Abbreviations: G = nucleus gracilis, C = nucleus cuneatus, Tri = spinal nucleus of the trigeminal, E = external cuneate nucleus, H = hypoglossal nucleus, V = dorsal nucleus of the vagus, S = solitary nucleus. (From Biedenbach, 1972.)

also contain the descending branches of the primary afferent fibers (Sprague and Ha, 1964; Sterling and Kuypers, 1967; Shriver *et al.*, 1968; Carpenter *et al.*, 1968; Réthelyi and Szentágothai, 1973). In addition to the branches of primary afferent fibers, the dorsal columns contain axons belonging to propriospinal neurons (see review by Nathan and Smith, 1959), second-order ascending tract fibers (Uddenberg, 1968b; Rustioni, 1973, 1974; Angaut-Petit, 1975a,b), and several descending pathways (Erulkar *et al.*, 1966; Kerr, 1968), including in some species such as the rat the corticospinal tract (Ramon y Cajal, 1909; Ranson, 1913a; Valverde, 1966). Recently, fibers descending in the dorsal column have been shown to originate in cells of the dorsal column nuclei (Dart, 1971; Kuypers and Maisky, 1975; Burton and Loewy, 1977; Bromberg and Towe, 1977).

The fasciculus gracilis conveys sensory information from the lower extremity and caudal body, while the fasciculus cuneatus contains a representation of the upper extremity and rostral body. Visceral afferents of the splanchic nerve terminate in the ventrolateral part of the gracile nucleus and in the gray matter between the gracile and cuneate nucleus, the same area serving also as the trunk representation (Rigamonti and Hancock, 1974).

A finer-grained topographic organization can also be demonstrated within each of the tracts. The organization of the fibers within the caudal parts of the dorsal column tracts is dermatomal, while that within the rostralmost part, at least of the fasciculus gracilis, is somatotopic. The organization of the neurons within the dorsal column nuclei is somatotopic. The distinction between a dermatomal and a somatotopic organization is illustrated in Fig. 6.4. The primary afferent fibers from a given area of skin, such as from one of the digits of the forepaw, may enter the spinal cord over any of several dorsal roots, and a given dorsal root may innervate a considerable expanse of skin, including that over several digits. For instance, in the raccoon, a model preparation for investigations of tactile innervation, Pubols *et al.*, (1965) found that the fourth digit of the forepaw is supplied by afferents in dorsal roots C7 to T2. Furthermore, a single dorsal root, C8, supplies the skin over all of the digits of the forepaw. Thus, recordings from axons within one of the relevant dorsal roots will demonstrate a dermatomal organization. When the receptive fields of individual axons are mapped, neighboring axons could have receptive fields anywhere within the dermatome (e.g., on any of the digits, if the root is C8). A given body part will not be mapped, and adjacent fibers can have disconnected receptive fields. Pubols *et al.* (1965) point out that the afferent fibers must resort themselves en route to the dorsal column nuclei, since microelectrode recordings here reveal a somatotopic

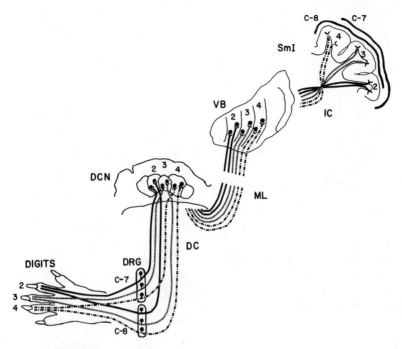

Fig. 6.4. Diagram showing how fiber resorting accounts for a change from a dermatomal to a somatotopic organization in the dorsal column pathway. Abbreviations: DRG = dorsal root ganglion, DC = dorsal column, DCN = dorsal column nuclei, ML = medial lemniscus, VB = ventrobasal complex of thalamus, IC = internal capsule, SmI = sensorimotor area I. (From Pubols *et al.*, 1965.)

organization (Johnson *et al.*, 1968). All the neurons in a certain zone within the nucleus cuneatus will have receptive fields on the fourth digit, and no receptive fields on the fourth digit are found for neurons outside this region (Fig. 6.5). Adjacent neurons have connecting and overlapping receptive fields.

The site of fiber resorting in the dorsal column pathway was investigated in the squirrel monkey by Whitsel *et al.* (1970). At the lumbar level, the fasciculus gracilis had a dermatomal organization, whereas in the cervical cord it had a somatotopic organization. A similar study of the fasciculus cuneatus of the raccoon (Pubols and Pubols, 1973) showed an incomplete resorting of fibers between lower and upper cervical levels. Apparently, the final resorting in the fasciculus cuneatus is done at the level of the nucleus cuneatus.

Because of the fiber resorting, it is understandable that the pattern of degeneration within the dorsal columns following dorsal rhizotomy is complex. The patterns of degeneration have been described both for

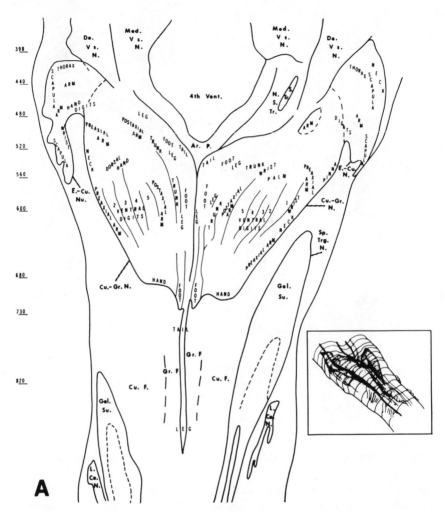

Fig. 6.5. (A) Somatotopic organization of the dorsal column nuclei of the raccoon. The drawing was made from the horizontal section through the widest extent of the dorsal column nuclei shown in (B). Abbreviations: Cu. F., Gr. F., Cu.-Gr. N. = cuneate and gracile fasciculi and nuclei; E.-Cu. Nu. = external cuneate nucleus; Gel. Su. = substantia gelatinosa; L. Ce. N. = lateral cervical nucleus; Sp. Trg. N. = spinal nucleus of the trigeminal; Ar. P. = area postrema; N. and Tr. S. = nucleus and tractus solitarius; De. and Med. Vs. N. = descending and medial vestibular nuclei. (From J. I. Johnson et al., 1968.)

the fasciculus gracilis and for the fasciculus cuneatus (Walker and Weaver, 1942; Carpenter et al., 1968; Shriver et al., 1968) as a sequence of ventromedially oriented bands for successive dorsal roots, but with overlap of the fibers of adjacent dorsal roots. The amount of overlap increases at more rostral levels (Whitsel et al., 1970).

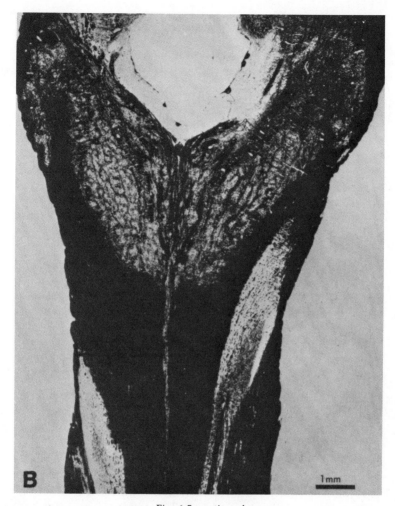

Fig. 6.5 continued.

The pattern of termination of the fasciculus gracilis and the fasciculus cuneatus within the dorsal column nuclei has been described by many investigators (Ferraro and Barrera, 1935b; Walker and Weaver, 1942; Glees and Soler, 1951; Hand, 1966; Shriver et al., 1968; Carpenter et al., 1968; Rustioni and Macchi, 1968; Keller and Hand, 1970; Basbaum and Hand, 1973). Although it has been claimed that the lumbosacral fibers end in the caudal part of the nucleus gracilis and that the thoracic fibers end in the rostral part (Ferraro and Barrera, 1935b; Walker and Weaver, 1942), workers using modern stains for studying degeneration nearer terminals than was possible with the Marchi technique disagree with this (e.g., Hand, 1966). Instead, it ap-

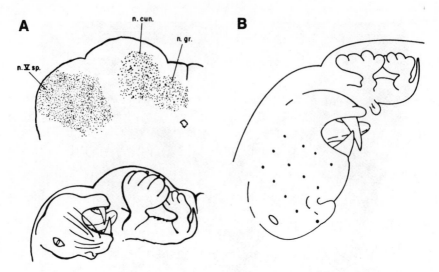

Fig. 6.6. (A) *(top)* The dorsal column nuclei of the cat (n. cun. = nucleus cuneatus; n. gr. = nucleus gracilis) and the spinal nucleus of the trigeminal, pars caudalis (n. V sp.). *(bottom)* A "feliculus," showing the somatotopic organization of the somatosensory nuclei of the caudal medulla. (From Kruger *et al.*, 1961.) (B) A similar somatotopic arrangement for the rat, although in this animal the representation of the face is proportionately larger. (From Nord, 1967.)

pears that projections from any given dorsal root end at all rostrocaudal levels of the dorsal column nuclei. However, the overlap of dermatomal projections is greater in the rostral than in more caudal levels of the dorsal column nuclei (Hand, 1966; Rustioni and Macchi, 1968).

The somatotopic organization mentioned above has been described for a number of species (Fig. 6.6) (Kruger *et al.*, 1961; Nord, 1967; J. I. Johnson *et al.*, 1968; Woudenberg, 1970; Hamilton and Johnson, 1973; Millar and Basbaum, 1975). The caudal part of the body is represented medially and the rostral part laterally. The distal extremities are represented dorsally and the proximal parts of the body ventrally. Essentially the same somatotopic map can be demonstrated at various rostrocaudal levels of the dorsal column nuclei, as might be predicted from the anatomy of the projections. The manner of termination of the ascending fibers of the dorsal column in the dorsal column nuclei was first described by Ramon y Cajal (1909), and additional detail was added by others (Glees and Soler, 1951; Valverde, 1966; Gulley, 1973). The dorsal column divides into several bundles, which project ventrally into the dorsal column nuclei (Fig. 6.7), where the axons branch and end among the cells of the nuclei. A given axon may give off several collaterals as it ascends along the dorsal aspect of its nucleus of termination (Figs. 6.7 and 6.8) (Ramon y Cajal, 1909; Gulley, 1973). A given axon tends to remain in a parasagittal plane in the caudal and middle parts of the dorsal column nuclei, so the same somatotopic information is distributed longitudinally over a considerable distance. In the rostralmost part of the dorsal column nuclei, the precision of the projection is lost, since here individual afferent axons may bend transversely in either direction (Fig. 6.8) (Gulley, 1973). There are also a few axons that cross the midline to terminate in the contralateral dorsal column nuclei (Hand, 1966; Rustioni and Macchi, 1968). However, the bulk of the afferent projection to the dorsal column nuclei is suited to transmit somatotopic information in a highly orderly fashion.

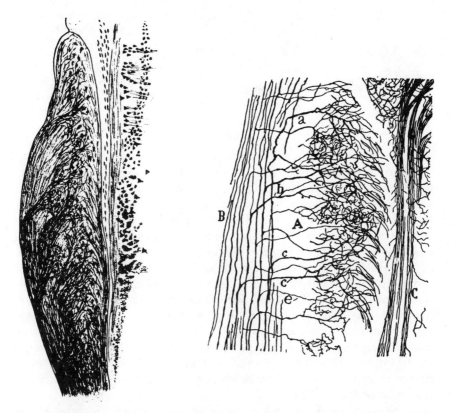

Fig. 6.7. (left) A sagittal section through the nucleus gracilis and the termination of the fasciculus gracilis. (From Glees and Soler, 1951.)   (right) A sagittal section through the cuneate fasciculus (B) and nucleus (A) showing collaterals of the afferents entering the nucleus. (From Ramon y Cajal, 1909.)

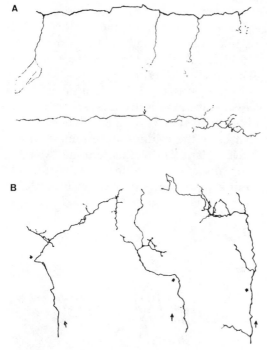

Fig. 6.8. The dorsal column axons in A are in a sagittal section of Golgi-stained material from rat. The upper fiber in A was in the caudal part of the nucleus gracilis and is shown giving off a series of four collaterals. The lower axon in A is in the rostral part of the nucleus gracilis and is shown terminating. The three dorsal column axons in B are in horizontal sections of the nucleus gracilis. The level of the obex is indicated by the asterisks. Above this level, the fibers bend and terminate. (Gulley, 1973.)

Ramon y Cajal (1909) (Fig. 6.9) recognized three types of neurons in the dorsal column nuclei: (1) neurons with short, bushy dendrites located in cell "islands" or nests; (2) neurons with long dendrites located around the margins of the nuclei; and (3) stellate, fusiform, or triangular neurons with radiating dendrites placed between the cell nests or ventrally in the nuclei. Recent studies using the horseradish peroxidase labeling technique have shown that most of the cells that project to the thalamus are in the cell nests, although some of the multipolar neurons also label following injections of horseradish peroxidase into the thalamus (Fig. 6.10) (Albe-Fessard et al., 1975; Berkley, 1975; Blomqvist and Westman, 1975; Cheek et al., 1975). Some of the marginal and multipolar cells project into the spinal cord through the dorsal column (Fig. 6.10) (Burton and Loewy, 1977), and other multipolar cells project to the cerebellum or to the inferior olive (Cheek et al., 1975; Berkley, 1975).

The dorsal column nuclei have several cytoarchitectural zones (Ramon y Cajal, 1909; Taber, 1961; Kuypers and Tuerck, 1964; Hand, 1966; Keller and Hand, 1970; Biedenbach, 1972; Basbaum and Hand, 1973). Experimenters using cats and monkeys (Fig. 6.11) subdivide the nuclei into a rostral, a middle, and a caudal zone (Hand, 1966; Bieden-bach, 1972). Biedenbach (1972) distinguishes five cell types in the monkey cuneate nucleus. The most common cell is the "round" cell, which is synonymous with the "cluster" or "nest" cells of others (Fig. 6.9) (Ramon y Cajal, 1909; Kuypers and Tuerk, 1964; Hand, 1966; Kel-ler and Hand, 1970). The dendrites of these cells are short and bushy (Kuypers and Tuerk, 1964), giving the cells the idiodendritic pattern (Ramón-Moliner and Nauta, 1966) typical of sensory relay neurons. The "round" cells occur most abundantly in the middle zone of the dorsal column nuclei and are grouped in clusters or nests. They in-clude a large portion of the neurons that project to the thalamus. "Large" cells make up a minor fraction of the population of cuneate neurons. They range in size up to 60 μm and are relatively abundant in the rostral zone of the nucleus. "Small" cells, having a typical diam-eter of about 10 μm, are scattered throughout the three zones, al-though there are proportionately more caudally. "Spindle" and "po-lygonal" cells are the other categories. Some of the "polygonal" cells have diameters of up to 50 μm. The "polygonal" cells are the most common type in the caudal zone of the cuneate nucleus. "Spindle" cells are also proportionately abundant caudally. The dendrites of the "spindle" and "polygonal" cells are long and sparsely branching, and

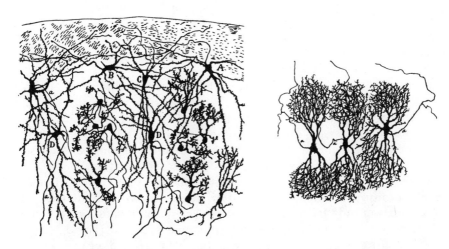

Fig. 6.9. Drawing on the left is of a transverse section through the cuneate nucleus of a kitten (Golgi stain). A–C are marginal neurons (note the axons projecting into the dorsal column). The neurons labeled D are large multipolar cells (*"cellules de cloisons"*). The smaller neurons that are arranged in clusters, E, are the round stellate cells of the cell nests. The last two cell types project into the medial lemniscus. A view of a cell nest from human fetal material is shown at the right. (From Ramon y Cajal, 1909.)

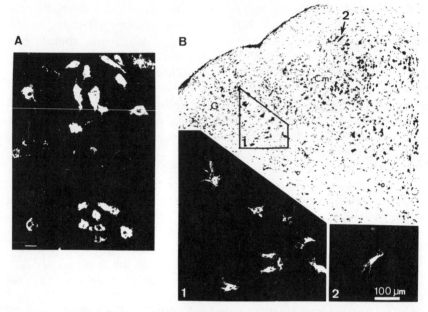

Fig. 6.10. (A) Dark-field plot showing several cell nests in the cuneate nucleus of the cat labeled following injection of horseradish peroxidase into the contralateral thalamus. (From Cheek *et al.*, 1975.) (B) Dark-field photos of neurons in the dorsal column nuclei of the cat were labeled by horseradish peroxidase injected into the spinal cord; the bright-field photo shows the positions of cells in the nuclei. (From Burton and Loewy, 1977.)

hence can be described as isodendritic (Ramón-Moliner and Nauta, 1966), like reticular neurons. The total number of neurons in the monkey cuneate nucleus is approximately 48,000 (Biedenbach, 1972).

When dorsal roots are cut and the primary afferent fibers allowed to degenerate, altered terminals are found in all three zones of the dorsal column nuclei, although the density of degeneration is greatest among the cell clusters of the middle zone (Hand, 1966). Different roots produce different amounts of degeneration; the density of degeneration reflects the density of peripheral innervation of a given root, rather than the size of the dermatome supplied (Hand, 1966). Degenerating afferent terminals can be demonstrated near neurons that project to the thalamus and also near neurons that do not project to the thalamus (Blomqvist and Westman, 1975).

The cytoarchitectural arrangement of the cuneate nucleus in the rat appears somewhat simpler than that in the cat and monkey. Basbaum and Hand (1973) found that the rat cuneate nucleus could be subdivided into a caudal zone and a rostral zone. The caudal zone consisted of a single population of "round" cells arranged in "slabs" or "bricks" oriented dorsoventrally and from side to side. The slablike arrangements could be seen just in horizontal or sagittal, but not in transverse, sections. The rostral part of the cuneate nucleus was composed of "round," "spindle-shaped," and "multipolar" cells arranged in a dispersed fashion. When individual dorsal roots were sectioned, degenerating terminal fields were found to occupy vertically oriented bands in the caudal part of the nucleus at levels corresponding to the

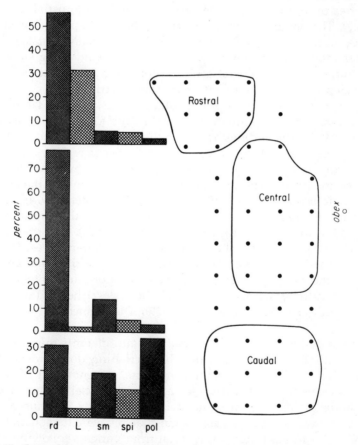

Fig. 6.11. Cytoarchitecture of the cuneate nucleus of the monkey. The outlines of the rostral, central, and caudal parts of the cuneate nucleus are shown at the right. The dots correspond to the sites indicated in Fig. 6.3. The histograms indicate the proportions of different cell types in the three zones of the nucleus. Abbreviations: rd = round, L = large, sm = small, spi = spindle, pol = polygonal. (From Biedenbach, 1972.)

cellular slabs. The cranialmost roots distributed ventrolaterally and the caudalmost dorsomedially. In the rostral region, the degeneration was diffuse, rather than focal, and the topographic arrangement, while present, showed more overlap than in the caudal part of the nucleus.

The Golgi picture of the rat nucleus gracilis is complementary to the description just given of the rat cuneate nucleus. The dendrites of the neurons of the caudal part of the gracile nucleus form dendritic "columns" which are vertically oriented (Gulley, 1973). Dorsal column afferent collaterals project vertically within the nucleus and appear to contact the dendrite columns. A single afferent may give off collaterals to a series of four to six columns arranged in a caudorostral sequence (Fig. 6.8). The dendrites of the neurons in the rostral part of the gracile nucleus, on the other hand, are oriented longitudinally. Dorsal column afferents may terminate in a horizontal arborization along such dendrites, but often the afferents bend abruptly in a transverse plane and end on dendrites of an adjacent "somatotopic strip."

The synaptic endings of dorsal column fibers are often large, up to 7 μm in diameter and more than 30 μm^2 in surface area (Rozsos, 1958; Walberg, 1965). The endings appear at the light microscopic level to be on dendrites and on cell bodies in the cell cluster region, but mostly on dendrites in the rostral zone (Hand, 1966). However, axodendritic synapses are much more common than axosomatic ones at the electron microscopic level (Walberg, 1965; Rustioni and Sotelo, 1974). Axoaxonal synapses are found upon the large terminals of the dorsal column afferents (Walberg, 1965; Rustioni and Sotelo, 1974). The presynaptic elements of these axoaxonal complexes contain flattened vesicles (Fig. 6.12); they also form synapses with the same dendrites that are contacted by the primary afferent terminals (Rustioni and Sotelo, 1974). Dendrodendritic synapses have recently been described in the cuneate nucleus of the monkey (Wen *et al.*, 1977). Their functional role is unknown.

The large terminals of the dorsal column afferents might suggest the possibility that deafferentation by sectioning dorsal roots or the dorsal columns would lead to transneuronal degeneration of cells in the dorsal column nuclei. The dorsal column nuclei do not develop when limbs are removed from neonatal opossums (J. I. Johnson *et al.*, 1972). However, no true transneuronal changes were demonstrated by Loewy (1973) in adult human material from patients following spinal cord transections due to accidental trauma. Some atrophy could be seen in neurons of the gracile nucleus of monkeys after experimental sectioning of the dorsal column.

The dorsal column nuclei project to the contralateral diencephalon by way of the internal arcuate fibers and the medial lemniscus (Fig.

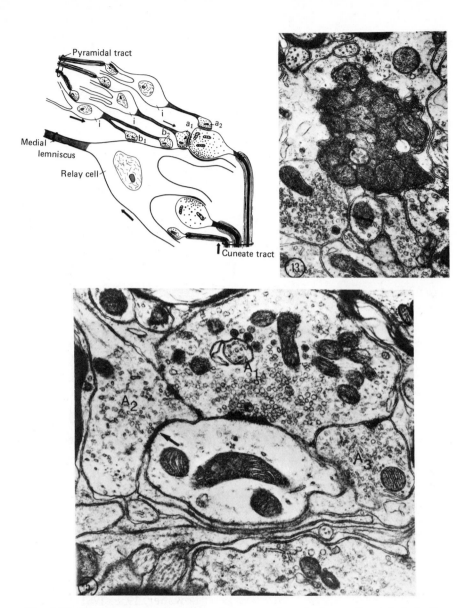

Fig. 6.12. *(top left)* An interpretation of the arrangement of synaptic contacts in the cuneate nucleus for afferents in the fasciculus cuneatus and also for fibers descending in the pyramidal tract. The cuneate terminals make axodendritic contacts with cuneothalamic relay cells. The pyramidal tract fibers terminate on interneurons, which in turn form axoaxonic synapses with the afferent endings and also axodendritic endings on the cuneothalamic relay cells. (From Walberg, 1965.) *(top right)* Electron micrograph showing a degenerating bouton 48 hours after dorsal rhizotomy. *(bottom)* Electron micrograph at the bottom showing the type of bouton, A1, which originates from a dorsal column afferent and synapses with a dendrite. A1 is also postsynaptic to A2 and A3 in an axoaxonic complex. A2 in addition synapses with the dendrite. Note that A1 contains spherical synaptic vesicles, while A2 and A3 contain flattened vesicles. (From Rustioni and Sotelo, 1974.)

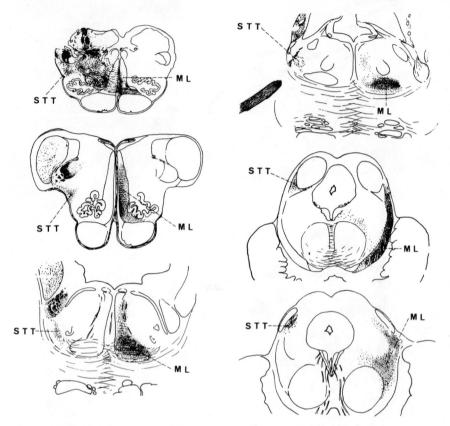

Fig. 6.13. Degeneration ascending through a human brainstem following lesions that damaged the spinothalamic tract and the dorsal column nuclei on the left. A Marchi stain demonstrates the course of the left spinothalamic tract and the right medial lemniscus. (From Rasmussen and Peyton, 1948.)

6.13) (Mott, 1895; Ranson and Ingram, 1932; W. E. L. Clark, 1936; Rasmussen and Peyton, 1948; Matzke, 1951; Bowsher, 1958, 1961; Clezy *et al.*, 1961; Hand and Liu, 1966; Lund and Webster, 1967a; Ralston, 1969; Boivie, 1971a; Jane and Schroeder, 1971; Schroeder and Jane, 1971; Hazlett *et al.*, 1972; Rockel *et al.*, 1972; Jones and Burton, 1974; Blomqvist and Westman, 1975; Groenewegen *et al.*, 1975; Berkley, 1975; Cheek *et al.*, 1975; Hand and van Winkle, 1977). The nuclei of termination in the cat [following the Rinvik (1968) terminology] include the ventral posterior lateral nucleus (VPL), the posterior nuclear group (PO$_m$) and also the zona incerta (Fig. 6.14) (Boivie, 1971a). The projection to the VPL nucleus is somatotopic, with the nucleus gracilis

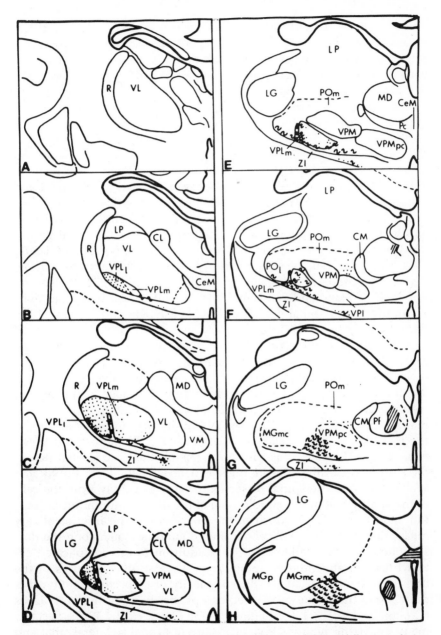

Fig. 6.14. Pattern of terminal degeneration in the thalamus of the cat following a lesion of the contralateral gracile nucleus. Fibers of passage are represented by wavy lines, while terminal fields are shown by dots. Abbreviations: VPL_l and VPL_m = lateral and medial segments of the ventral posterior lateral nucleus of the thalamus, PO_m = medial part of the posterior nuclear complex, ZI = zona incerta. (From Boivie, 1971a.)

projecting to VPL_l and the nucleus cuneatus to VPL_m (Boivie, 1971a; Groenewegen et al., 1975). The projections show a complete inversion (Fig. 6.15): the dorsal cuneate projects to the ventral VPL_m, the ventral cuneate to the dorsal VPL_m, the lateral part of cuneate to medial VPL_m, and medial cuneate to lateral VPL_m (Hand and van Winkle, 1977).

The dorsal column nuclei also project to other parts of the central nervous system than the diencephalon. There are projections to the dorsal and medial accessory olivary nuclei (Hand and Liu, 1966; Morest, 1967; Ebbesson, 1968; Jane and Schroeder, 1971; Schroeder and Jane, 1971; Hazlett et al., 1972; Walsh and Ebner, 1973; Berkley, 1975; Boesten and Voogd, 1975; Groenewegen et al., 1975; Hand and van Winkle, 1977) and to the cerebellum (Gordon and Seed, 1961; Gordon and Horrobin, 1967; Cooke et al., 1971; Cheek et al., 1975; Rinvik and Walberg, 1975; Johansson and Silfvenius, 1977c). Rostral projections reach a number of nuclei of the midbrain (Kuypers and Tuerk, 1964; Hand and Liu, 1966; Lund and Webster, 1967a; Jane and Schroeder, 1971; Schroeder and Jane, 1971; Hazlett et al., 1972; Walsh and Ebner, 1973; Hand and van Winkle, 1977), and descending projections distribute to the spinal cord (Dart, 1971; Kuypers and Maisky, 1975; Burton and Loewy, 1977).

The different projections of the dorsal column nuclei can be associated in some cases with different cytoarchitectural regions. The thalamic projection originates from cells distributed over much of the longitudinal extent of the nuclei, including the most rostral region, where they are less concentrated (Berkley, 1975; Blomqvist and Westman, 1975; Cheek et al., 1975). The largest density of cells projecting to the thalamus is in the cell nests (Berkley, 1975; Blomqvist and Westman, 1975). The cells projecting to the cerebellum are located just in the rostral part of the cuneate nucleus (Cheek et al., 1975: Rinvik and Walberg, 1975). The spinal projection originates chiefly from the cells of the ventral half of the middle zone of the dorsal column nuclei (Burton and Loewy, 1977). Much of the projection to the inferior olivary nucleus comes from small cells scattered longitudinally along the dorsal column nuclei (Berkley, 1975). In addition to the complicated cytoarchitecture and multiple projections, several other features of the dorsal column nuclei add to the complexity of their connectivity. It is quite likely that some of the neurons project to more than one locus (Gordon and Seed, 1961; Berkley, 1975; Cheek et al., 1975). Second, many projecting neurons give off recurrent axonal collaterals that end within the dorsal column nucleus and presumably affect the activity of adjacent neurons; third, there are interneurons within the dorsal column nuclei (Gulley, 1973; Blomqvist and Westman, 1976); these are rare in the rodent, according to Valverde (1966).

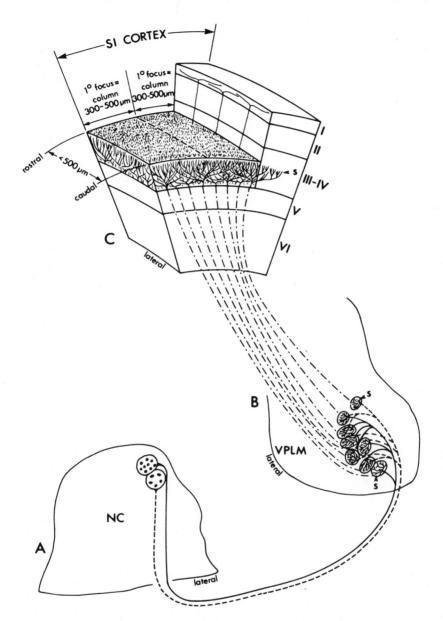

Fig. 6.15. Diagram showing the inversion of topographic relationships between the cuneate nucleus and VPL. Neurons in the dorsolateral part of the cuneate nucleus connect with neurons in the ventromedial VPL. In addition, the possible relationships between clusters of cuneate and VPL neurons and cortical columns is shown. (From Hand and van Winkle, 1977.)

An intriguing suggestion has been made by Hand and van Winkle (1977) that the cell cluster region is the source of afferent connections to cell clusters within the VPL nucleus of the thalamus, and that the VPL clusters are in turn connected with functional columns in the sensory cerebral cortex (Fig. 6.15).

In summary, the dorsal column pathway is the long system of fibers of the dorsal columns. The short and intermediate systems serve other purposes, providing information to segmental levels and to such pathways as the dorsal spinocerebellar tract. The dorsal column pathway is subdivided into a fasciculus gracilis, which ends in the nucleus gracilis, and a fasciculus cuneatus, which ends in the nucleus cuneatus. Fibers of the fasciculus cuneatus also terminate in the lateral cuneate nucleus, which relays chiefly to the cerebellum. The fasciculus and nucleus gracilis convey information concerning the hind limb and caudal body (a Bischoff's nucleus may transmit information about the tail, depending upon species), while the fasciculus and nucleus cuneatus are concerned with a representation of the forelimb and rostral body. The dorsal columns have a dermatomal organization caudally, but through fiber resorting they acquire a somatotopic organization by the time their fibers terminate in the dorsal column nuclei. A given afferent fiber will send off collaterals that terminate within a parasagittal plane along the length of a dorsal column nucleus. This accounts for the observation that the somatotopic map appears to be similar at all levels of the nuclei. However, the afferent terminals are less precise in the rostral part of the dorsal column nuclei. The cytoarchitecture of the dorsal column nuclei reflects a highly ordered caudal and middle region and a less ordered rostral zone. The terminals of the dorsal column afferents are large and contain spherical vesicles. Their removal, at least in adult primates, produces only slight evidence for transneuronal changes. The output from the dorsal column nuclei includes a highly organized projection to the contralateral VPL nucleus of the thalamus. There are also connections to the PO_m and zona incerta in the diencephalon, various mesencephalic nuclei, parts of the inferior olivary nuclei, the cerebellum, and the spinal cord. There is evidence that different projections originate in part from different cytoarchitectural regions of the dorsal column nuclei, although the pattern of organization is complex.

COMPOSITION OF DORSAL COLUMNS

Although all of the afferents entering the spinal cord over the dorsal roots are contained in the dorsal column or in the dorsolateral fasciculus of Lissauer in the same and adjacent segments (Carpenter *et al.*, 1968), only a fraction of the primary afferents ascends the fasciculus gracilis all the way to the medulla. Glees and Soler (1951) found that only 22–23% of the fibers in the lumbosacral dorsal roots of the cat reach the upper cervical cord, and they state that the fiber population of the fasciculus cuneatus becomes even more attenuated en route to the nucleus cuneatus.

The best evidence concerning the functional categories of axons within the dorsal funiculus comes from single-unit recordings in experiments utilizing natural stimulation of receptors. Yamamoto *et al.* (1956) investigated the response characteristics of axons in the dorsal column at an upper cervical level in cats. Rapidly adapting tactile responses were the most common responses observed. These were produced by hair movement or by tactile stimulation of the pads. Other units showed slowly adapting responses to pushing, pulling, or pinching the skin. Units were also observed that were discharged by moving joints or by applying pressure to joint capsules, tendons, or muscle. Some of these units supplied the chest wall and discharged with respiration. [Similar units were found in the human dorsal column by Puletti and Blomquist (1967).] Finally, slowly adapting discharges from units activated by distention of the urinary bladder were found. The numbers of various classes of units are given in Table 6.1. There was a topographic localization, with units from the bladder located along the paramedian, superficial part of the fasciculus gracilis, the hind limb and lower body in the fasciculus gracilis, the upper body and forelimb in the fasciculus cuneatus. At the first cervical level, the fasciculus gracilis was found to migrate ventrally and to be surrounded by the fasciculus cuneatus. The observation of visceral afferents within the dorsal columns is in agreement with the findings of others using electrical stimulation (Amassian, 1951; Aidar *et al.*, 1952). The fasciculus gracilis contained more tactile than proprioceptive fibers, whereas the opposite was true of the fasciculus cuneatus.

Werner and Whitsel (1967) have shown that the fasciculus gracillis of the squirrel monkey also has a topographic organization. At the lumbar level, axons carrying information from cutaneous receptors were intermingled with those carrying information from deep receptors (Werner and Whitsel, 1967). The proportions of axons from cutaneous and deep receptors varied according to the locations of the receptors in the hind limb; there were more fibers representing the skin than the deep tissues of the distal extremity, while there were more from deep than superficial tissues of the proximal extremity (Werner and Whitsel, 1967; Whitsel *et al.*, 1969). This presumably reflects the density of innervation of the skin and deep structures of the distal versus the proximal limb. The organization of the fasciculus gracilis at an upper cervical level was rearranged as compared to that at the lumbar level (see previous section), and the proportion of afferents from the skin was much greater than from deep structures of the hind limb (Whitsel et al., 1969, 1970). The Whitsel group failed to find any axons that responded to joint bending or that were slowly adapting in the cervical fasciculus gracilis of the squirrel monkey (Whitsel et al., 1969). Presumably, many of the afferents from deep structures leave the fasciculus gracilis to terminate in Clarke's column and other nuclei of origin of ascending tracts, and/or in segmental nuclei. The fasciculus cuneatus at an upper cervical level contained large numbers of afferents from deep structures of the forelimb, as well as from the skin (Whitsel et al., 1969), but it is possible that at least some of these were destined for the lateral cuneate rather than for the main cuneate nucleus.

Several studies provide detailed information about the types of receptors whose axons project from the hind limb up the dorsal columns to the upper cervical cord of the cat. Brown (1968) restricted his survey to dorsal column fibers connected with cutaneous receptors, although he often found units that were activated by joint movement. The types and numbers of axons found by A. G. Brown (1968) are summarized in Fig. 6.16 and in Table 6.1. The most common units supplied hair follicles. Some of the afferents were from receptors having the properties of Pacinian corpuscles. A number of other kinds of rapidly adapting receptors were also represented. In addition, both type I and type II touch units were present. The most striking negative finding was the absence of afferents having peripheral conduction velocities in the Aδ range—Type D hair-follicle units and nociceptors.

Petit and Burgess (1968) recorded in the periphery from primary afferents that could be antidromically activated by stimulation of the dorsal columns at a high cervical level. They obtained similar results to those of Brown in that the most common receptor types in the fasciculus gracilis by their classification included G1 and G2 hair-follicle units. They also found numerous "field" receptors, which can be activated by the movement of hair or skin (Burgess et al., 1968). In addition, Petit and Burgess (1968) encountered several type II slowly adapting units, and they described Pacinian corpuscle-like units in the fasciculus gracilis; the latter were stated by Horch et al. (1976) to be misidentified intermediate hair units. The dorsal column sample did not include any nociceptors, but Petit and Burgess did find a few D hair-follicle units (in the plantar nerve, but not in the sural, posterior femoral cutaneous, or superficial peroneal nerves) that projected to the medulla. Unlike Brown, they did not record the activity of any type I

TABLE 6.1. Types of Afferents in the Dorsal Columns

| | Number | | | | | | |
| | Fasciculus gracilis | | | | Fasciculus cuneatus | | |
Afferent type	Yamamoto et al., 1956	A. G. Brown, 1968	Petit and Burgess, 1968	Burgess and Clark, 1969a	Uddenberg, 1968a	Pubols and Pubols, 1973[a]	Bromberg and Whitehorn, 1974
Cutaneous receptors							
Hair-follicle units	276	—	—	—	—	—	—
Type T (tylotrich)	—	42	—	—	—	—	—
Type G (guard hair)	—	48	—	—	79	—	—
G_1	—	—	54	—	—	—	3
G_2	—	—	28	—	—	—	14
Type D (down hair)	—	0	1	—	0	—	1
Field	—	—	38	—	—	—	14
Pacinian corpuscle and rapidly adapting pad	19	11	9[b]	—	4	40	—
Type I slowly adapting	42[d]	11[c]	0	—	—	202	3
Type II slowly adapting	—	7	29	—	30	71[d]	8
Nociceptors	—	0	0	—	0	—	0
Other	129	11	18	—	16	—	6
Deep receptors							
Muscle							
Group I	—	—	—	—	71	—	—
Group II?[e]	—	—	—	—	16	—	—
Joints							
Rapidly adapting	—	—	—	40	—	—	—
Slowly adapting	—	—	—	0	—	—	—
Visceral receptors							
Bladder distention	13	—	—	—	—	—	—

[a] Glabrous skin only. [b] Misidentified intermediate hair units, according to Horch et al. (1976). [c] May have been second-order dorsal column units (Angaut-Petit, 1975b). [d] Identification uncertain. [e] Thresholds to electrical stimulation above 1.5 times threshold of largest afferents.

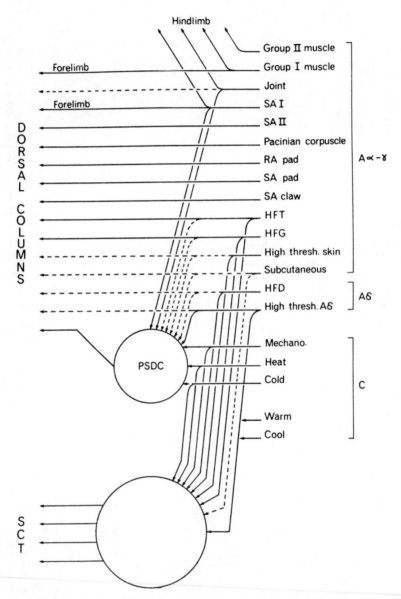

Fig. 6.16. Receptor types represented in the dorsal column and spinocervical tract. The second-order dorsal column pathway is shown, as well as the primary afferent projection (PSDC = postsynpatic dorsal column path). (From A. G. Brown, 1973.)

slowly adapting units (Fig. 6.2). Since touch domes can activate second-order dorsal column neurons (see below), it has been suggested that Brown recorded type I activity from second-order axons rather than from ascending collaterals of primary afferents (Angaut-Petit, 1975b).

Uddenberg (1968a) did not subdivide the receptor types represented in the fasciculus cuneatus as finely as did A. G. Brown (1968) and Petit and Burgess (1968) for the fasciculus gracilis. He found hair-follicle units, touch units, and Pacinian corpuscle-like units. In addition, Uddenberg (1968a) found large numbers of muscle afferents, most of which had a low threshold to electrical stimulation and so were classified as group I. The hair units were located superficially in the dorsal column; muscle units were in an intermediate position; and touch units were deep (and hard to excite by surface electrodes).

Pubols and Pubols (1973) investigated the afferent fiber types to be found in the fasciculus cuneatus of the raccoon. They limited their sample to the afferents supplying the glabrous skin, although they did observe activity in axons from hairy skin and joints. The classes of receptors represented in the fasciculus cuneatus included Pacinian corpuscles, rapidly adapting (RA) receptors, and two kinds of slowly adapting receptors (Table 6.1). There were proportionately many more rapidly adapting receptors than slowly adapting ones in the dorsal column as compared with peripheral nerve or dorsal root. It was not clear what the relationship was between the two slowly adapting receptor types found and the type I and type II receptors of other species, but one of the receptor types in the raccoon did fulfill most of the criteria generally used for identification of type I receptors.

Bromberg and Whitehorn (1974) examined the receptor types projecting in the fasciculus cuneatus of the cat (see Table 6.1). Although their sample was small (56 units), they did find that three of four type I units identified in recordings from the superficial radial nerve projected all the way to the medulla.

Evidently, the fasciculus cuneatus differs from the fasciculus gracilis not only in containing large numbers of group I muscle afferents but also type I slowly adapting cutaneous mechanorecptors. Some of the slowly adapting afferents, at least from muscle, no doubt end in the lateral cuneate nucleus, but many must terminate in the cuneate nucleus, judging from the response properties of some cuneate neurons (see below). It would be interesting to know if slowly adapting joint afferents from forelimb joints project up the fasciculus cuneatus, since only rapidly adapting joint afferents project in the fasciculus gracilis (Burgess and Clark, 1969a).

In summary, not all receptors are represented in the population of dorsal column axons that project directly to the brainstem. The largest proportion of the cutaneous afferents that project arise from rapidly adapting receptors, especially hair-follicle receptors. However, some slowly adapting tactile receptors also have ascending collaterals in the dorsal column (type II but not type I in the fasciculus gracilis; both in the fasciculus cuneatus). Rapidly, but not slowly, adapting joint afferents are present as well as muscle afferents. Visceral afferents, including some responding to bladder distention, and proprioceptive afferents with a respiratory rhythm have also been found. Receptors that are poorly, if at all, represented include those with axons that have a peripheral conduction velocity in the $A\delta$ range (type D hair-follicle units, nociceptors) and receptors with unmyelinated axons (C mechanoreceptors, nociceptors, thermoreceptors).

SECOND-ORDER DORSAL COLUMN PATHWAY

In addition to the branches of primary afferent fibers, the dorsal columns contain second-order axons of ascending tract cells (Uddenberg, 1968a,b; Petit, 1972; Pubols and Pubols, 1973; Rustioni, 1973, 1974; Angaut-Petit, 1975a,b). Uddenberg (1968b) found that most of the second-order units in his experiments on the forelimb could be activated following electrical stimulation of more than one peripheral nerve. Natural stimulation revealed a convergence of several receptor types onto these cells. All of the units could be activated by hair movement, and these responses were rapidly adapting. Pressure on the skin evoked slowly adapting responses, which were probably related to the activation of touch receptors. The discharges of the second-order dorsal column units were increased by pinching the skin or by intense stimulation of deep receptors of the forelimb. The cells of origin of the forelimb pathway (Fig. 6.17) are in the cervical enlargement, chiefly in lamina IV (Rustioni and Kaufman, 1977).

A comparable pathway from the hind limb has also been described (Petit, 1972; Rustioni, 1973; Angaut-Petit, 1975a,b). When the lumbar dorsal column was cut in an animal with chronic dorsal rhizotomies, fresh degeneration could be followed into the nucleus gracilis, the rostral part of the cuneate nucleus, and nucleus z (Rustioni, 1973). Thus, second-order dorsal column fibers terminate in part in the dorsal column nuclei. The specific regions of termination are somewhat different from those of the primary afferents (Rustioni, 1973) but similar to the area of termination of the projection from the cerebral cortex (Kuypers and Tuerk, 1964). A similar description applies to the

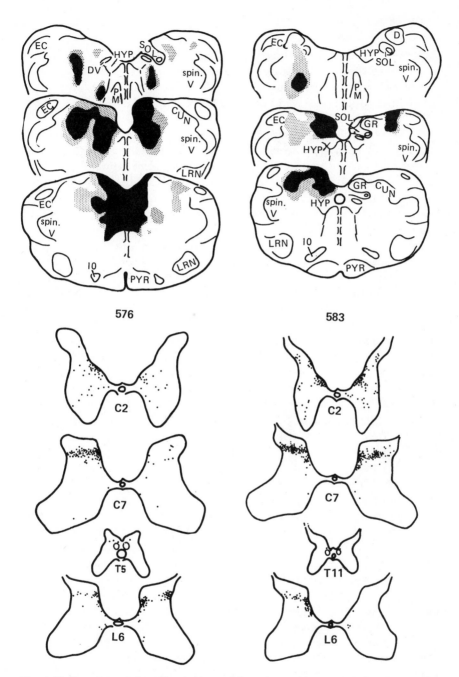

Fig. 6.17. Locations of the cells of origin of the second-order dorsal column pathway. The injection sites in the medulla for horseradish peroxidase labeling are shown above for two experiments. The locations of labeled neurons at several levels of the spinal cord are plotted below. (From Rustioni and Kaufman, 1977.)

second-order fibers from the cervical cord, which end in the rostral part and base of the cuneate nucleus (Rustioni, 1974). The cells of origin of the hindlimb pathway (Fig. 6.17) are largely in lamina IV and in the medial part of laminae V–VI of the lumbosacral enlargement (Rustioni and Kaufman, 1977).

The activity of the second-order dorsal column fibers from the lumbosacral cord has been studied by Angaut-Petit (1975a,b). The units were excited synaptically following electrical stimulation of the sciatic nerve or natural stimulation of the hind limb. The axons could be antidromically activated by stimulation of the cervical dorsal column, and the conduction velocities of the axons were determined (range 16–71 m/s). The axons lay within the thoracic dorsal column at a depth between that of primary afferents from skin and that of proprioceptive afferents. The cells could be classified according to their responses to natural stimulation. Some (16%) were activated just by weak mechanical stimuli, such as hair movement or tapping. A few (6%) were excited just by noxious mechanical stimuli. Most (77%) received a convergent input from sensitive mechanoreceptors and nociceptors. These were activated by hair movement in a rapidly adapting fashion and by maintained tactile stimulation in a slowly adapting fashion. The latter response could often be produced by stimulation of tactile domes. An additional response was obtained by pinching a fold of skin with forceps or by heating the skin to 45°C or more (Fig. 6.18). A firing rate as high as 350 impulses per second could result from a noxious heat stimulus. The receptive fields of these cells were fairly small when on the distal part of the limb (a few square millimeters), but could be large when proximal (up to 20 or 30 cm^2). No inhibitory receptive fields were found.

It has been questioned whether the second-order fibers of the dorsal column actually arise from the cord or from the cells that project down from the dorsal column nuclei into the dorsal columns (Burton and Loewy, 1977). However, Angaut-Petit (1975b) recorded comparable activity in cats with transected spinal cords, so at least some of her units arose from neurons located within the spinal cord. Furthermore, her collision tests were consistent with rostrally projecting and not caudally projecting units (Angaut-Petit, 1975a). Finally, the anatomic demonstration of a second-order projection through the dorsal column to the dorsal column nuclei (Rustioni, 1973, 1974) and of the cells of origin of this pathway in the spinal cord dorsal horn (Rustioni and Kaufman, 1977) is in agreement with the interpretation that the units studied by Uddenberg and by Angaut-Petit project rostrally. A study is needed of the response properties of the dorsal column nucleus cells that do project caudally into the cord. Preliminary evidence indicates

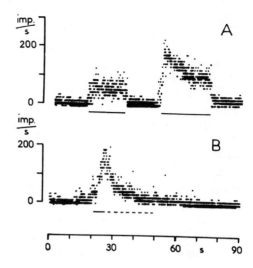

Fig. 6.18. Responses of a unit in the second-order dorsal column pathway (A) to noxious mechanical stimuli and (B) to noxious radiant heat. (From Angaut-Petit, 1975b.)

that many of these cells also project to the thalamus and show responses like those of other relay cells (Bromberg and Towe, 1977).

DORSOLATERAL FASCICULUS PATHWAY TO DORSAL COLUMN NUCLEI

Another pathway that must be considered in studies of the dorsal column nuclei ascends in the dorsal part of the lateral column (Gordon and Grant, 1972; Tomasulo and Emmers, 1972; Hazlett *et al.*, 1972; Dart and Gordon, 1973; Rustioni, 1973, 1974; Rustioni and Molenaar, 1975; Nijensohn and Kerr, 1975). Terminals have been demonstrated in the dorsal column nuclei in the same regions in which the second-order dorsal column pathway ends (Rustioni, 1973, 1974). Most of the cells of origin seem to lie rostral to L5, since lesions at L4 or L5 result in only a sparse amount of degeneration in the nucleus gracilis (Gordon and Grant, 1972; Rustioni, 1973). The suggestion that these fibers may be collaterals of the spinocervical tract (Tomasulo and Emmers, 1972) is made less attractive by these anatomic findings, since cells of origin of the spinocervical tract are abundant in the lumbosacral enlargement (Bryan *et al.*, 1973). Initially, it was thought that the fibers are not branches of the dorsal spinocerebellar tract or other spinocerebellar tracts, since no actions on cells of the dorsal column nuclei could be demonstrated following stimulation within the cerebellum (Dart and Gordon, 1970). However, recent evidence indicates that cells in the rostral part of the cuneate nucleus can in fact be activated by stimulation within the cerebellum via collaterals of the dorsal spinocerebellar tract (Johansson and Silfvenius, 1977c). The physiological effects of the dorsolateral fasciculus pathway to the dorsal column nuclei include activation of neurons that relay into the medial lemniscus, as well as of "interneurons" (Dart and Gordon, 1973). Some of these "interneurons" (so identified because they were not antidromically activated from the medial lemniscus) may very well project to the cerebellum, since cells of this type have now also been shown to receive excitatory drive from the dorsolateral fasciculus path (Johansson and Silfvenius, 1977c). The responses of some dorsal column neurons that relay to the thalamus had normal responses to natural stimuli even after the dorsal columns had been sectioned (Dart and Gordon, 1973). This observation indicates that it cannot be assumed that transection of the dorsal columns prevents the participation of the dorsal column nuclei in somesthesis.

In summary, besides the primary afferent fibers, the dorsal columns contain second-order afferent fibers arising from cells in the dorsal horn of the cervical and lumbosacral enlargements. These units typically receive a convergent input from several types of peripheral receptors, including sensitive mechanoreceptors and also nociceptors. Another second-order pathway ascends to the dorsal column nuclei through the dorsolateral fasciculus. These axons appear to arise from a region of the spinal cord above the lumbosacral enlargement, perhaps from Clarke's column. These fibers presumably account for the observation that some dorsal column neurons respond to natural stimuli in a normal fashion, even though the dorsal columns are transected.

RESPONSE PROPERTIES OF DORSAL COLUMN NEURONS TO ELECTRICAL STIMULATION OF PERIPHERAL NERVES

The properties of the relay neurons of the dorsal column nuclei will be considered in some detail, even though they belong to the brainstem rather than the spinal cord, since these cells are in the same position in the dorsal column–medial lemniscus pathway as the cells of origin of the spinocervical and spinothalamic tracts and the second-order dorsal column pathway.

Although studies of sensory pathways using electrical stimulation of peripheral nerves are not as pertinent to sensory experience as are investigations employing natural forms of stimulation, nevertheless, such work has value, especially for an understanding of synaptic mechanisms.

Stimulation of peripheral nerves or of the dorsal columns results in a sequence of field potentials that can be recorded from the dorsal column nuclei (Fig. 6.19). For example, in recordings from the dorsal surface of the cuneate nucleus following stimulation of cutaneous nerves of the forelimb, there is seen an initial spikelike potential, then

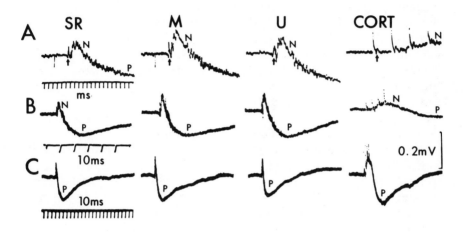

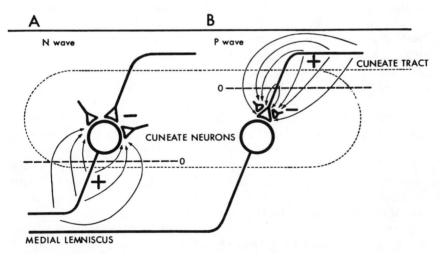

Fig. 6.19. Field potentials recorded from the surface of the cuneate nucleus of the cat. Structures stimulated included the superficial radial (SR), median (M), and ulnar (U) nerves and the sensorimotor cortex (CORT). The negative (N) and positive (P) field potentials are shown on progressively slower time bases in A–C. The diagram at the bottom shows the pattern of current distribution that might account for the field potentials. (From Andersen *et al.*, 1964b.)

slow negative and positive waves (Therman, 1941; Andersen *et al.*, 1964b). The spike potential is due to the arrival of the afferent volley in the fastest fibers of the fasciculus cuneatus, while the N wave is due to a combination of the afferent volley in slower afferents, the summed excitatory postsynaptic currents generated in neurons of the cuneate nucleus following synaptic transmission, and action potentials of cuneate neurons triggered by the excitatory postsynaptic potentials (Andersen *et al.*, 1964b, 1972a; Andres-Trelles *et al.*, 1976). The P wave is considered to be due to the depolarization of the terminals of primary afferents ending in the cuneate nucleus (primary afferent depolarization, PAD) resulting from activation of an interneuronal pathway ending with axoaxonal synapses on the primary afferent endings (Andersen *et al.*, 1964c,d; Walberg, 1965; Rustioni and Sotelo, 1974). PAD would produce presynaptic inhibition of transmission through the dorsal column nuclei (J. C. Eccles, 1964; Schmidt, 1971).

Sometimes the size of the N wave recorded from the surface of the dorsal column nuclei is used as a measure of the output of the nuclei in response to a stimulus applied to a peripheral nerve or to the dorsal column. However, this can be deceptive (Andersen *et al.*, 1972a). The true output is the discharge of relay cells, not the sum of the synaptic potentials and discharges of a mixed population of neurons. A better measure of the output of the dorsal column nuclei (to the thalamus, at least) is the size of the medial lemniscus volley (Andersen *et al.*, 1970, 1972a,b; Bromberg *et al.*, 1975). However, even this approach has limitations, especially if peripheral nerves are stimulated to provide the input, since the potential recorded from the medial lemniscus is composed not only of activity in a diverse set of dorsal column neurons (A. G. Brown *et al.*, 1974), but it may also be contaminated by activity in axons ascending from the lateral cervical nucleus (Carli *et al.*, 1967a) and potentially even the spinothalamic tract. In addition, there is the added complication of the dorsal column reflex (see below). Nevertheless, this technique has proved quite valuable for sorting out the relative contributions of pre- and postsynaptic inhibition in the dorsal column nuclei in experiments in which the stimulus is applied directly in the nuclei. Such stimulation results in a directly evoked response in dorsal column neurons that serves as a test of the excitability of these neurons (excitability reduced during postsynaptic but not presynaptic inhibition) followed by a relayed volley (reduced by either pre- or postsynaptic inhibition).

Krnjević and Morris (1976) examined the input–output curve of the cuneate nucleus by stimulating the dorsal column and recording the antidromically conducted volley in afferents from a peripheral nerve (input) and the relayed volley in the medial lemniscus (output).

The input–output curve was a power function with a very steep rise, indicating a high safety factor for transmission.

Many studies of single-unit responses within the dorsal column nuclei have failed to distinguish between the neurons that relay information to the thalamus and those that serve as interneurons. The relay neurons are identifiable on the basis of antidromic discharges following stimulation within the contralateral medial lemniscus (Fig. 6.20A) (Amassian and DeVito, 1957; Gordon and Seed, 1961; Gordon and Jukes, 1964a; Andersen et al., 1964d; Gordon and Horrobin, 1967; Rosén, 1969b). The collision test (Paintal, 1959; Bishop et al., 1962; Darian-Smith et al., 1963; see discussion of limitations of this technique in Fuller and Schlag, 1976) has been used in some of the studies to help distinguish between orthodromic and antidromic activation (e.g., Gordon and Jukes, 1964a; Rosén, 1969b). Interneurons are not discharged antidromically; however, since the entire medial lemniscus may not be activated by an electrical stimulus, some relay cells will not be discharged antidromically and thus will be misclassified (Gordon and Seed, 1961; Andersen et al., 1964d). Furthermore, some of the neurons not antidromically activated from the medial lemniscus are nevertheless relay neurons to other brain areas. The description to follow of the response properties of neurons in the dorsal column nuclei will emphasize work on identified relay cells. However, consideration will also be given to the behavior of unidentified cells, since many of these are in fact relay cells, and the interneurons are thought to modify the activity of the relay neurons.

The excitatory effects of electrically evoked volleys upon single neurons of the cuneate nucleus of the cat were examined by Amassian and DeVito (1957). In addition to monosynaptic excitation, they observed repetitive discharges, which they attributed to interconnections within the nucleus through axon collaterals. However, Andersen et al., (1964a) found that the excitatory postsynaptic potentials (EPSPs) produced by the afferent volley ascending from peripheral nerve stimulation were large enough to account for a repetitive discharge in the cuneate neurons. Amassian and DeVito (1957) observed that some cuneate neurons could in fact be discharged by a very small afferent volley, representing as little as 0.3% (fewer than eight fibers) of the dorsal column fibers arising from Aβ afferents. Andersen et al. (1964a) agreed that the intracellularly recorded EPSPs produced by single afferents were quite large and that summation of only a few would be needed to cause a discharge. Amassian and Giblin (1974) showed that cuneate neurons could discharge virtually every time that a single afferent discharged, suggesting a complete synaptic security of a single afferent onto a single relay cell. Such powerful excitatory effects may

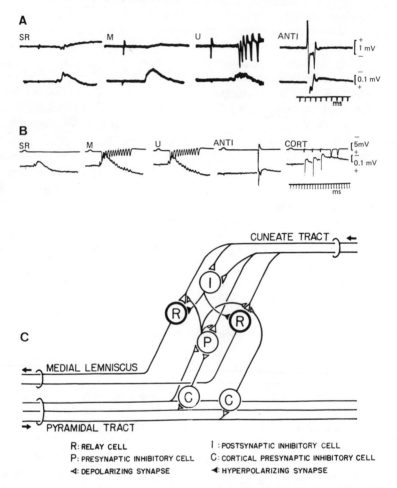

A

SR   M   U   ANTI $\begin{bmatrix} + \\ 1\,mV \\ - \end{bmatrix}$

$\begin{bmatrix} - \\ 0.1\,mV \\ + \end{bmatrix}$

ms

B

SR   M   U   ANTI   CORT $\begin{bmatrix} - \\ 5mV \\ + \end{bmatrix}$

$\begin{bmatrix} - \\ 0.1\,mV \\ + \end{bmatrix}$

ms

CUNEATE TRACT

I

R   R

C   P

MEDIAL LEMNISCUS

C   C

PYRAMIDAL TRACT

R: RELAY CELL   I : POSTSYNAPTIC INHIBITORY CELL
P: PRESYNAPTIC INHIBITORY CELL   C: CORTICAL PRESYNAPTIC INHIBITORY CELL
◁: DEPOLARIZING SYNAPSE   ◀: HYPERPOLARIZING SYNAPSE

Fig. 6.20. (A) Records made from a cuneothalamic relay cell (upper traces) and the dorsal surface of the cuneate nucleus (lower traces). The neuron was activated orthodromically by stimulation of the ulnar nerve (U), but not of the superficial radial (SR) or median (M) nerves. Identification was provided by antidromic invasion of an action potential (ANTI) following stimulation of the contralateral medial lemniscus.   (B) Activity of an interneuron that was excited by stimulation of either the median or ulnar nerves or of the sensorimotor cortex (CORT), but that was not antidromically activated from the medial lemniscus.   (C) A possible circuit that accounts for convergence of excitatory input from peripheral nerves and the sensorimotor cortex onto cuneate interneurons, which then produce presynaptic inhibition of excitatory pathways to cuneothalamic relay neurons. A postsynaptic inhibitory pathway through a different interneuron is also shown. (From Andersen *et al.*, 1964c.)

reflect the large sizes of the synapses made by dorsal column afferents upon neurons of the dorsal column nuclei (Rozsos, 1958; Walberg, 1965, 1966). However, the tendency for dorsal column neurons to discharge repetitively is not due entirely to their synaptic input, since the cells also tend to discharge in doublets or short bursts when activated by the iontophoretic application of drugs like glutamate (Galindo *et al.*, 1968). The repetitive discharge is not the result of an excitatory feedback through recurrent collaterals of the axons of relay cells, since antidromic activation by stimulation within the medial lemniscus does not result in a repetitive discharge (Gordon and Seed, 1961). [Note, however, that some relay cells and interneurons of the cuneate nucleus are synaptically activated following stimulation of the medial lemniscus (Blum *et al.*, 1975).] The tendency toward a repetitive discharge appears to be an intrinsic property of the cells of the dorsal column nuclei (Galindo *et al.*, 1968), possibly due to retriggering of the initial segment by a dendritic spike (Calvin and Loeser, 1975). The latencies of the initial spikes of the neurons of the gracile nucleus show a dispersion in time, which can be accounted for by the dispersion in arrival times of the afferent impulses ascending through the fasciculus gracilis (Whitehorn *et al.*, 1972). This observation does not rule out, however, relayed activity through second-order dorsal column neurons. It simply makes it unlikely that long interneuronal pathways are important for eliciting the initial discharges of gracile neurons.

There is increasing pharmacological evidence that the synaptic transmitter substance used by primary afferents at their excitatory synapses upon neurons of the dorsal column nuclei is glutamic acid (Steiner and Meyer, 1966; Galindo *et al.*, 1967; Duggan and Johnston, 1970; J. L. Johnson and Aprison, 1970; Haldeman and McLennan, 1972; J. L. Johnson, 1972; Davies and Watkins, 1973; Roberts *et al.*, 1973; Roberts, 1974).

Inhibition of spontaneous or evoked activity in the dorsal column nuclei following peripheral stimulation has been reported frequently (Therman, 1941; Amassian, 1952; Gordon and Paine, 1960; Gordon and Jukes, 1964a; Andersen *et al.*, 1964a, 1970, 1972b; Jabbur and Banna, 1968, 1970; Biedenbach *et al.*, 1971; Davidson and Smith, 1972; Silvey *et al.*, 1974; Bromberg *et al.*, 1975). Part of the inhibition in the cat can be ascribed to a postsynaptic inhibitory action, since inhibitory postsynaptic potentials (IPSPs) have been recorded intracellularly from dorsal column neurons, and the excitability of dorsal column neurons to direct electrical stimulation decreases during inhibition (Andersen *et al.*, 1964a, 1970; Schwartzkroin *et al.*, 1974b). The duration of most of the IPSPs observed was only about 15–20 ms, yet the time course of inhibition of dorsal column neurons often exceeds

100–200 ms. The prolonged inhibition can be attributed in part to occasional long-lasting IPSPs, but also in part to presynaptic inhibition (Andersen *et al.*, 1964a, 1970, 1972b; Jabbur and Banna, 1968; 1970; Bromberg *et al.*, 1975). In the frog, there is no evidence for postsynaptic inhibition, but rather just the presynaptic variety (Silvey *et al.*, 1974).

A number of lines of evidence suggest the importance of presynaptic inhibition in the dorsal column nuclei. The responses of dorsal column neurons to electrically evoked afferent volleys are often complicated by the occurrence of a "dorsal column reflex" (Hursh, 1940; Therman, 1941; Andersen *et al.*, 1964c). The "dorsal column reflex" is a discharge in the afferent fibers of the dorsal column and is equivalent to the "dorsal root reflex" (Toennies, 1938; J. C. Eccles *et al.*, 1961; J. C. Eccles, 1964), which is due to PAD. The dorsal column reflex can be generated either at the segmental level or at the level of the dorsal column nuclei (Andersen *et al.*, 1964c). Excitability testing shows that the afferent terminals within the dorsal column nuclei are depolarized as a result of activity evoked by other afferents ascending in the dorsal column (Wall, 1958; Andersen *et al.*, 1964a,c, 1970, 1972b; Jabbur and Banna, 1968, 1970; Silvey *et al.*, 1974; Bromberg *et al.*, 1975). The depolarization results in a negative field potential within the dorsal column nuclei near the terminals made by the dorsal column afferents but a positive field potential at the dorsal surface of the medulla (Fig. 6.15) (Therman, 1941; Andersen *et al.*, 1974a; Silvey *et al.*, 1974).

Putnam and Whitehorn (1973) investigated the organization of the PAD system in the gracile nucleus to see if PAD in rapidly adapting receptor terminals was generated primarily by rapidly adapting afferents and PAD in slowly adapting afferent terminals by slowly adapting afferents, as in the cord (Jänig *et al.*, 1968b). There was no evidence of this. Instead, PAD was produced in the afferent endings of G1 and G2 hair-follicle receptors, field receptors, and type II slowly adapting receptors by the same form of natural stimulation—hair movement by puffs of air but not steady indentation of the skin. They concluded that the receptors responsible for the PAD were G2 and/or G1 hair-follicle afferents. However, in view of the evidence of Bystrzycka *et al.* (1977) that second-order neurons of the cuneate nucleus are inhibited by Pacinian corpuscles, which are so sensitive that they can be activated by hair movement, the receptors responsible for PAD in afferents to the dorsal column nuclei need reevaluation.

PAD is thought to be produced by axoaxonal synapses (Walberg, 1965; Rustioni and Sotelo, 1974) made upon afferent terminals within the dorsal column nuclei by the synaptic endings of local interneurons or of neurons located outside the dorsal column nuclei (Andersen *et al.*, 1964d; Jabbur and Banna, 1968). The interneurons are discharged by excitation from dorsal column afferents, and PAD results, leading to presynaptic inhibition (J. C. Eccles, 1964; Schmidt, 1971). It should be noted that the same boutons that form axoaxonal contacts in the cat dorsal column nuclei also make axodendritic synapses (Rustioni and Sotelo, 1974). It is therefore likely that pre- and postsynaptic inhibition often occur together in this species.

An effort was made by Andersen *et al.* (1964d) to identify the interneurons that might be responsible for inhibition in the cuneate nucleus. Since stimulation of the cerebral cortex also results in PAD (Andersen *et al.*, 1964b), one criterion for identification of the interneurons was a convergent excitation from both peripheral nerve and corticofugal volleys (Fig. 6.20B). Andersen *et al.* (1972b) used the technique of cooling the cuneate nucleus to alter the inhibitory activity as a way to assist in the identification of the interneurons. Cooling enhances and prolongs PAD in the cuneate nucleus (Andersen *et al.*, 1962b). However, postsynaptic inhibition was not changed. When the discharges of interneurons were recorded, it was found that in half the cases cooling depressed the activity, but in the other half of the cells, cooling caused a prolongation of their burst discharges. The same interneurons displayed a poor ability to follow repetitive stimulation, with a curtailed discharge at stimulus rates of 10/per second or greater, a stimulus rate that severely reduces PAD. It seems likely that these interneurons are involved in generating PAD.

Another investigation in which an attempt was made to identify the interneurons responsible for PAD in the cuneate nucleus was that of Bromberg *et al.* (1975) and Blum *et al.* (1975). They observed that PAD can occur with either of two time courses—relatively fast or relatively slow. The faster form of PAD reached its peak in 25 ms and was due to stimulation just of a nerve of the ipsilateral forelimb. The slow PAD peaked later and was smaller in amount. The slow PAD could be evoked by stimulation of the contralateral sensorimotor cortex or of a nerve in the contralateral forelimb. Similar differences in time course of PAD could be recognized when the excitability of single afferents was tested. The PAD was paralleled in time course by a reduction in the synaptically transmitted volley recorded from the medial lemniscus, so it was concluded that the PAD was producing presynaptic inhibition. When interneuronal responses were evaluated, it was found that some interneurons were excited just by stimulation of a peripheral nerve in the ipsilateral forelimb (nonconvergent interneurons), while other interneurons were excited by nerves of more than one limb and by corticofugal volleys (convergent interneurons). When the authors computed synthetic PAD curves based on the latencies of the spikes in the discharges of the whole population of inter-neurons (allowing for synaptic delay), they found that the curve constructed based on the nonconvergent neurons resembled closely the fast PAD and that from the convergent neurons resembled the slow PAD.

Pharmacologic evidence suggests that both pre- and postsynaptic inhibition in the dorsal column nuclei may be mediated by γ-aminobutyric acid (GABA) (Galindo et al., 1967; Banna and Jabbur, 1969, 1971; Davidson and Southwick, 1971; Banna et al., 1972; Davies and Watkins, 1973; Kelly and Renaud, 1973a,b,c; Roberts, 1974; Hill et al., 1976; Andres-Trelles et al., 1976; however, cf. E. S. Boyd et al., 1966). However, an alternative possibility that has not as yet been ruled out is that PAD may be produced by an extracellular accumulation of potassium released by activated neruons (Vyklický et al., 1972, 1975, 1976; Krnjević and Morris, 1974; Kříž et al., 1974, 1975; Syková et al., 1976; however, cf. Bruggencate et al., 1974; Somjen and Lothman, 1974; Lothman and Somjen, 1975).

Recurrent inhibition of cuneothalamic relay neurons has been described following stimulation of the medial lemniscus (Davidson and Smith, 1972). The inhibition is probably in part presynaptic, since PAD is produced concurrently. Interneurons of the cuneate nucleus may be activated by recurrent volleys as well as by input following stimulation of ipsilateral and contralateral peripheral nerves (Davidson and Smith, 1972). It is possible that these interneurons form a final common pathway for PAD in the cuneate nucleus.

In summary, peripheral nerve volleys evoked by electrical stimuli produce excitation and then inhibition in the dorsal column nuclei. The excitation of neurons that relay to the thalamus can be so powerful that a postsynaptic cell can be synaptically driven by one or a few afferent fibers. Neurons in the dorsal column nuclei have a tendency to discharge in doublets or in short bursts; this seems to be an intrinsic property of the cells, perhaps attributable to retriggering by dendritic spikes. The excitatory synaptic transmitter released by dorsal column pathway afferents may be glutamate. Both presynaptic and postsynaptic inhibition occur in the dorsal column nuclei, but presynaptic inhibition seems the more important. Presynaptic inhibition is associated with primary afferent depolarization (PAD), which can be demonstrated by the production of a dorsal column reflex (like a dorsal root reflex), by excitability testing, and by the distribution of the associated field potentials. PAD is thought to be due to interneuronal activity and mediated by axoaxonal synapses. Interneurons of the requisite characteristics have been described. Some evidence suggests that the presynaptic inhibitory transmitter is GABA. However, a role for K^+ has not been ruled out.

RESPONSE PROPERTIES OF DORSAL COLUMN NEURONS TO NATURAL STIMULATION

According to Gordon and Paine (1960), most of the cells in the nucleus gracilis of the cat respond to mechanical stimultion of hair or of the skin, whereas only some 10% respond to stimulation of deep tissues, including joints. Receptive field sizes varied from less than 0.5 cm² to the entire hind limb and lower half of the ipsilateral trunk. Cells with large receptive fields tended to be concentrated in the rostral part of the nucleus, while cells with the smallest receptive fields were in the middle of the nucleus; cells in the caudal part of the nucleus had intermediate-sized receptive fields. Cells that were most likely to show surround inhibition were found to lie in the central zone of the nucleus. Only some of the cells in the rostral part of the nucleus could be activated antidromically, whereas 80–90% of those in the middle zone were discharged antidromically from the contralateral medial lemniscus (Gordon and Paine, 1960). Anatomic studies also suggest that the relay cells of the dorsal column nuclei are concentrated in the middle zone of the nuclei, with fewer cells in the rostral and caudal zones projecting into the medial lemniscus (Kuypers and Tuerk, 1964; Berkley, 1975; Blomqvist and Westman, 1975). A few of the cells in the rostral dorsal column nuclei project to the cerebellum (Gordon and Horrobin, 1967; Cooke et al., 1971; Cheek et al., 1975; Rinvik and Walberg, 1975; Johansson and Silfvenius, 1977c).

Kruger et al. (1961) subdivided units within the dorsal column nuclei of the cat according to the forms of natural stimulation that would activate them. The classes and numbers of units studied are listed in Table 6.2. Most of the neurons were activated by hair movement or by tactile stimulation of the skin. Pressure units may have been activated at least in some cases by subcutaneous receptors. Joint units responded to small changes in joint angle but not to cutaneous stimulation or to manipulation of muscle. The hair units were usually rapidly adapting, whereas touch, pressure, and joint units could be rapidly or slowly adapting. Different classes of cells were found to be intermingled. There was a distinct somatotopic organization in the transverse plane at all levels of the nuclei, but not along the anteroposterior axis of the nuclei. The tail was represented medially and the shoulders laterally; the distal limbs were dorsal and the trunk ventral (Fig. 6.6). The somatotopic organization was similar to that described by Kuhn (1949) and by F. H. Johnson (1952). All the receptive fields were ipsilateral. Receptive field size varied with the position of the field; the smallest fields were on the distal parts of the limbs, while the largest were on the trunk. No relationship was found between receptive field size and rostral–caudal position within the nuclei. No at-

TABLE 6.2. Response Properties of Neurons in Dorsal Column Nuclei and Axons of Medial Lemniscus

	Kruger et al., 1961	Perl et al., 1962	Gordon and Jukes, 1964a	A. G. Brown et al., 1974	Angaut-Petit, 1975b	Rosén, 1969b
Cutaneous						
Hair movement	207	111	209	—	56	—
Type T (tylotrich units)	—	—	—	15	—	—
Touch	189	—	—	—	36	—
Pad-sensitive	—	—	7	4	—	—
Touch–temperature	—	68	—	—	—	—
Type I slowly adapting	—	—	—	2	—	—
Type II slowly adapting	—	—	—	3	—	—
Claw-sensitive	—	—	15	2	—	—
Vibration	—	41	22	—	—	—
Pressure	132	—	—	—	—	—
Convergent						
Hair-multiple types	—	—	—	5	—	—
Hair and pad-sensitive	—	—	19	12	—	—
Hair and touch–pressure	—	—	8	9	—	—
Touch–pressure	—	—	70	—	—	—
Hair–touch–pressure–nociceptive	—	—	—	—	42	—
Subcutaneous	—	—	6	—	—	—
Other	—	—	22	30	—	—
Deep						
Joint movement	72	Few	—	—	—	—
Pressure on deep structures	—	Few	Some	42	—	—
Group I muscle afferents	—	—	—	—	—	105
Groups I and II muscle afferents	—	—	—	—	—	46

tempt was made to identify the neurons by antidromic activation, but the population of cells that was sampled extended throughout the dorsal column nuclei and no doubt included many relay neurons.

Yamamoto and Miyajima (1961) found proprioceptive units within the dorsal column nuclei; there were proportionately more in the cuneate nucleus than in the gracile nucleus. Some of the proprioceptive units had a respiratory rhythm. Slowly adapting pressure units and rapidly adapting hair- and pad-sensitive units were also observed.

An effort was also made by Perl et al. (1962) to relate the discharge properties of neurons of the cat nucleus gracilis to the responsible receptors. They found that they could subdivide the units activated by cutaneous and just subcutaneous stimuli into three groups. The first class was activated by hair movement. Care had to be taken to distinguish these from units activated by vibration. The hair units were rapidly adapting and were discharged when hair was bent and again when it was allowed to straighten. Receptive field size varied from 10 mm^2 to over 2000 mm^2. Receptive fields were smallest distally on the limb and larger more proximally. Surround inhibition of hair-activated units could be demonstrated. A second class of cells was activated by tactile stimulation of the skin and also by cooling. The responses to touch were slowly adapting. Receptive field sizes were larger than for hair-activated units, ranging from 228–28,900 mm^2. Surround inhibition could not be demonstrated; instead, electrical stimulation of the skin surrounding the receptive field often produced excitation. The third class of gracile cell was activated by vibratory stimulation (cf. Amassian and DeVito, 1957), following 100–300 Hz stimuli. These units sometimes fired with each cardiac cycle. The receptors for them appeared to be within the abdominal cavity. It was suggested that the receptors involved were Pacinian corpuscles. A few units were also observed to discharge in response to joint bending or to the application of pressure to deep tissues of the foot.

The responses of units within the gracile nucleus of the rat were investigated by McComas (1963), who applied brief mechanical pulses to the pads of the hind foot. Cells within the rostral, middle, and caudal parts of the nucleus were compared with respect to receptive field size, threshold, latency, and ability to respond to repeated stimulation at a high frequency. The rostral cells had high thresholds, large receptive fields, long latencies, and poor following to repetitive stimulation, in contrast to the cells in the middle and caudal regions of the nucleus gracilis. Furthermore, the cells in the middle of the nucleus could often be inhibited by stimulation of the skin adjacent to the excitatory receptive field, while such inhibition was less commonly seen for cells in the rostral region.

The most elaborate classification of the response properties of neurons in the dorsal column nuclei is that of Gordon and Jukes (1964a) and A. G. Brown et al. (1974). Gordon and Jukes (1964a) concentrated their attention on cells of the nucleus gracilis in the cat receiving different kinds of input from cutaneous receptors. The largest class of cells (Table 6.2) responded to hair movement. Most of them had a rapidly adapting response, although a few were slowly adapting. The receptive field size depended upon the position of the cell within the rostrocaudal extent of the nucleus and with the location of the receptive field on the limb. The smallest fields belonged to cells in the middle part of the nucleus and were on the distal extremity. A second class of cell was unaffected by hair movement but responded to gentle tactile stimulation of the skin. Both rapidly and slowly adapting responses were seen. The cells were in the middle part of the nucleus, and their receptive fields were small. The third class of cells responded both to hair movement and tactile stimulation of the skin. Most were rapidly adapting, although some were slowly adapting. Most of these cells were in the rostral part of the nucleus gracilis, but some were in the middle part. Receptive field sizes varied from 1 to 50 cm². A fourth class of cell responded to claw movement or stimulation of a small area at the base of a claw. The responses were slowly adapting. Almost all of these cells were in the middle part of the nucleus. A fifth class of cells responded to light touch or pressure and were slowly adapting. The cells were located throughout the nucleus, but within the middle part they tended to be deep. The receptive fields were generally large, but the cells in the middle zone of the nucleus had somewhat smaller receptive fields than did the rostrally located cells. The sixth class of cells responded both to hair movement and to touch and pressure. The responses to hair movement were rapidly adapting, while those to touch and pressure were slowly adapting. Such cells were found throughout the nucleus, and the receptive fields for pressure were large. A seventh class of cells were activated by subcutaneous receptors. Both rapidly and slowly adapting responses were seen. The cells were in the middle part of the nucleus, but the receptive fields were large (5–30 cm²). The eighth class included cells that were sensitive to vibration. The cells were discharged by a 100-Hz tuning fork applied to the skin or to bone. The cells were in the middle zone of the nucleus, and they were probably activated by Pacinian corpuscles. Some of the receptors appeared to lie within the abdominal cavity. However, several of these were excited not only by vibration but also by hair movement or tactile stimulation on the hind limb. The remaining cells in the study either gave inconsistent responses or were difficult to excite by the stimuli employed.

Inhibition was often demonstrated for hair-sensitive units, pad-sensitive touch units, claw-sensitive units, and subcutaneous units. Hair units were more commonly inhibited if they were in the middle than in the rostral part of the nucleus. The touch–pressure cells were not inhibited. Antidromic activation was possible for at least some cells of each category, so all classes project into the contralateral medial lemniscus. Most of the antidromically activated cells were in the middle part of the nucleus. However, touch–pressure cells within the middle part of the nucleus were antidromically fired in only 31% of cases.

Gordon and Jukes concluded that the nucleus gracilis has a dual organization. Hair-sensitive, pad-sensitive, pad-and-hair-sensitive, claw-sensitive, and subcutaneous units have small receptive fields, are located in the middle zone of the nucleus, are subject to surround inhibition, are somatotopically organized, and project into the contralateral medial lemniscus. Other hair-sensitive, pad-and-hair-sensitive, and touch–pressure units have large receptive fields, are located in the rostral nucleus gracilis or deep in the middle part, are not subject to surround inhibition (but rather to facilitation), are not somatotopically organized, and often do not project into the contralateral medial lemniscus.

The receptive properties of axons of the cat medial lemniscus have been described by A. G. Brown *et al.* (1974). These authors felt that most of their units were the axons of neurons of the dorsal column nuclei. By recording from the medial lemniscus, they avoided pulsatory movements, which plague microelectrode experiments on the lower medulla, and they also avoided inadvertent damage to the cells studied. Another advantage was that the recordings were restricted to thalamic relay neurons, although there is uncertainty about what proportion actually arose from the dorsal column nuclei and what from the lateral cervical nucleus or belonged to the spinothalamic tract.

A total of ten categories of medial lemniscus axons was distinguished by the receptor types that activated them, and there was another class of unidentified cells. The first class was composed of units fired by movement of tylotrich hairs (Figs. 6.21 and 6.22). Their responses were rapidly adapting, and the receptive fields were small, often only a few square millimeters. Surround inhibition was easily demonstrated. The second class of unit responded with a rapidly adapting discharge to tactile stimulation of one or more foot pads. Inhibition could often be shown. The third class responded to movements of a claw or pressure on the skin adjacent to the claw (Fig. 6.21). Inhibition of these units was seen. The fourth class of unit was excited by a group of touch corpuscles (type I slowly adapting receptors) (Figs. 6.21 and 6.22). Inhibition was found. The fifth class was activated by stimulation of a single spot with a regular, slowly adapting discharge. The receptor was probably a type II ending. No inhibition was seen. The sixth category could be activated by all of the types of hairs within its receptive field, and the responses were rapidly adapting. Inhibition could be produced. The seventh class were activated by hair movement and by pad stimulation. The responses were entirely rapidly adapting for some of the cells, but there was an additional slowly adapting component in some. Inhibition could usually be demonstrated. The eighth class could be activated by hair movement and by maintained skin displacement. The response to hair movement was rapidly adapting. The slowly adapting component could have a low

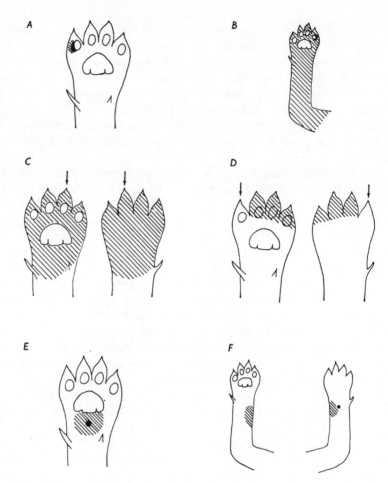

Fig. 6.21. Excitatory (filled areas) and inhibitory (hatched areas) receptive fields of neurons projecting into the medial lemniscus. The receptors for the fields in A and B were tylotrich hair-follicle receptors. The arrows in C and D show locations of fields of units responsive to claw movements. The receptors in E and F were type I slowly adapting receptors. (From A. G. Brown *et al.*, 1974.)

threshold (a touch corpuscle was responsible in one case) or a high threshold. Inhibition was seen in three or five units. A ninth category was activated by hair movement with a rapidly adapting response, but there was no slowly adapting response. The hairs involved were not identified, but some appeared to discharge like type G afferents. The tenth category was activated by joint movement or by stimulation of deep receptors. The responses were slowly adapting. The axons of these units were more commonly found in the ventromedial part of the medial lemniscus.

Angaut-Petit (1975b), in her study of the second-order dorsal column system, also recorded the responses of neurons in the nucleus gracilis that had properties like those of the second-order fibers. Most of the cells she examined were in the deep part of the middle of the nucleus gracilis. No attempt was made to demonstrate if the cells projected into the medial lemniscus. The cells received a convergent input from sensitive mechanoreceptors (rapidly adapting response to hair movement, slowly adapting response to maintained touch) and from mechanical and thermal nociceptors. Similar units could be found after all the spinal cord except the dorsal columns had been transected,

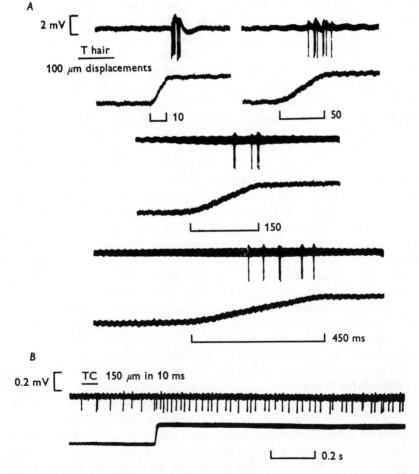

Fig. 6.22. (A) Responses of a unit in the medial lemniscus to ramp displacements of a tylotrich hair at different velocities. (B) Responses of another unit to indentation of a touch corpuscle. (From A. G. Brown *et al.*, 1974.)

suggesting that the responses were due, at least in part, to the second-order fibers of the dorsal column.

The projections of forelimb group I muscle afferents to the cuneate nucleus have been demonstrated in experiments utilizing electrical stimulation of muscle afferents (Rosén, 1967, 1969a,b). Relay cells were identified by antidromic activation from the contralateral medial lemniscus (Rosén, 1969b). Over half of the cuneate neurons discharged by group I axons could be activated antidromically in this fashion. The fact that group I afferents were the effective ones was judged by grading the stimulus intensity from threshold to a strength just sufficient to fire the cell. Stimulus intensities below 1.5 times threshold for the most excitable afferents were considered to belong to group I when a muscle nerve was stimulated. Most of the cells were activated by group I fibers of only a single muscle nerve, but some received a convergent input from several muscle nerves. Many of the cells also received an excitatory input from group II fibers (but not from group III). There was sometimes a weak input from a cutaneous nerve, but natural stimulation of the skin failed to produce any discharge of such cells. Electrical stimulation of cutaneous and high-threshold muscle afferents produced an inhibition. "Interneurons" had similar properties, except that they were generally fired by cortical stimulation, whereas the cells relaying to the thalamus were rarely fired by corticofugal volleys but were instead inhibited. The cells that received Group I input were preferentially distributed deep within the cuneate nucleus below most of the cells having cutaneous inputs. No group I projections were found to cells in the rostral part of the cuneate nucleus (Rosén, 1969a), and no similar projections are known to the gracile nucleus. However, recently, Johansson and Silfvenius (1977c) have found neurons in the rostral cuneate nucleus that receive a Group I input. The projections are by second-order fibers in the dorsolateral fasciculus. This path is not part of the spinocervical tract, but rather is the spinomedullothalamic pathway, which relays in nucleus z (Landgren and Silfvenius, 1971), as will be discussed in Chapter 7. Some of the "interneurons" of the rostral cuneate nucleus receiving a Group I input project to the cerebellum (Johansson and Silfvenius, 1977c).

The group I projections to the cuneate nucleus have been further investigated using natural forms of stimulation, as well as by electrical stimuli (Rosén and Sjölund, 1973a,b). All of the cuneothalamic relay neurons studied were activated by group Ia muscle spindle afferents, but not by group Ib Golgi tendon organ afferents (Rosén and Sjölund, 1973a). This was shown by a low threshold to passive stretch of muscle, by a pause during twitch contraction, by excitation during longitudinal vibration of muscle (50 μm amplitude) and by activation following administration of succinylcholine. Several interneurons were activated by Golgi tendon organ afferents, but most were excited by Ia afferents. Most of the cuneothalamic relay cells and interneurons examined received an excitatory input from just a single muscle, although some were excited by afferents of several muscles, almost always synergistic ones (Rosén and Sjölund, 1973b). Few cells were inhibited, even by muscles antagonistic to those producing excitation.

The responses to neurons in the gracile nucleus to bending the knee joint were studied by Williams et al. (1973). The hind limb was denervated except for the medial and posterior articular nerves. The units studied were all relatively rapidly adapting and signaled either velocity or acceleration in changes of joint angle. The lack of slowly adapting neurons signaling position is consistent with the evidence that slowly adapting afferents from the knee joint do not project all the way up the fasciculus gracilis (Burgess and Clark, 1969a).

Amassian and Giblin (1974) were able to demonstrate that single slowly adapting afferents could determine the periodicity of the discharges of tactile and proprioceptive neurons of the cuneate nucleus. The cells studied were shown to project to the thalamus by antidromic activation from the medial lemniscus. The discharge pattern of a given neuron reflected both the period of discharge of a single afferent and the mixture of inputs from several afferents. A differently coded output would be expected for an input from a population of slowly adapting afferents excited, for example, by a rough surface as compared with a smooth surface. Such differences in coding might contribute to the discriminative ability of a population of dorsal column neurons known not to be subject to afferent inhibition (Perl et al., 1962; Gordon and Jukes, 1964a).

A different approach to the classification of neurons within the cuneate nucleus was attempted by Blum et al. (1975). In addition to identifying the cells by their reactions to natural stumuli applied to the skin and to stimulation of the medial lemniscus, these workers divided the cells in two other ways. Using both natural and electrical stimulation, they could distinguish two subsets of cells. One subset was characterized by an ability to follow rapidly repeated stimuli ("strong" synaptic connection), while the other had a poor ability to do so ("weak" connection). Another subdivision was according to whether a given cell was activated from just the ipsilateral forelimb or whether it received a convergent input from more than one limb. Figure 6.23 summarizes their conclusions. Cuneothalamic relay cells might have strong or weak synaptic drive. Interneurons might have strong or weak input, and they might be nonconvergent or convergent. It should be noted that excitatory inputs from other regions of

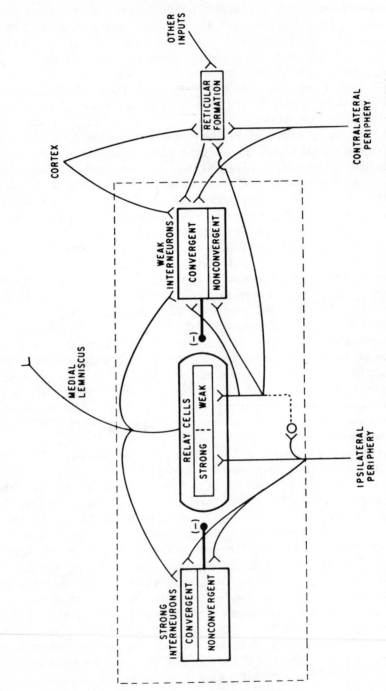

Fig. 6.23. Scheme showing some of the neural circuits of the dorsal column nuclei. (From Blum *et al.*, 1975.)

the brain, such as the cerebral cortex, reticular formation, or cerebellum, activate the convergent interneurons (either directly or indirectly through the reticular formation).

Recently, Bystrzycka *et al.* (1977) reexamined the excitatory and inhibitory responses of neurons of the cuneate nucleus using unanesthetized, decerebrate cats. They employed carefully controlled natural stimuli to activate particular afferent types selectively. The cells were subdivided into slowly and rapidly adapting classes by their responses to step indentations of the skin. The rapidly adapting cells were further divided into those that were most sensitive to vibratory stimuli in the frequency range of 20–50 Hz and those that were best fired by vibrations of 200–300 Hz. The thresholds for the latter were often of the order of 1–2 μm of displacement, and the receptive fields were very large. It was suggested that the cells responsive to 300 Hz stimulation have a specific input from Pacinian corpuscles. Hair movement also activates these cells, but this kind of stimulus will excite Pacinian corpuscles as well as hair-follicle receptors. All three kinds of neuron could be inhibited by Pacinian corpuscle input and probably not by other inputs. Some previous workers who did not find inhibition of slowly adapting neurons of the dorsal column nuclei used barbiturate anesthesia, which may have interfered with the inhibition. The findings of Bystrzycka *et al.* (1977) are consistent with the evidence (McIntyre, 1962; McIntyre *et al.*, 1967; Silfvenius, 1970) for a strong projection of Pacinian corpuscle afferents through the dorsal column–medial lemniscus system to the cerebral cortex.

The effects of partial or complete deafferentation of the lumbosacral enlargement by dorsal rhizotomy have been investigated on the receptive field properties of neurons of the gracile nucleus (Dostrovsky *et al.*, 1976; Millar *et al.*, 1976). When all but one of the dorsal roots are cut, a large number of cells unresponsive to stimulation of the skin are found, as expected. However, in addition, a number of cells with receptive fields on the trunk or with split receptive fields (e.g., one on the limb and one on the trunk) appear. The findings are similar whether the roots are cut acutely or chronically, but exaggerated in chronic animals (Millar *et al.*, 1976). When all the dorsal roots of the lumbosacral enlargement were cut, there were again many more cells than normal responsive to receptive fields on the trunk, especially the abdomen. Another change was a greatly expanded inhibitory field. Similar changes occurred whether the deafferentation was acute or chronic. A cold block could be used to show the reversible appearance of an abdominal receptive field for cells normally responsive to receptive fields just on the limb. The best explanation for these findings seems to be that dorsal column neurons have ineffective synapses from afferents that are disinhibited when the normal input is removed.

In summary, the response properties of neurons in the dorsal column nuclei that relay to the thalamus reflect two distinctive patterns of organization. There are cells that appear to transmit information from one or a few specific receptor types, and there are cells that receive a convergent input from a variety of receptor types. Among the specific relay cells, activity originating from such receptors as type T (tylotrich hair), rapidly adapting pad receptors, type I and type II slowly adapting receptors, vibration receptors (presumably Pacinian corpuscles), and claw receptors can be recognized. In addition, there are cells that respond specifically to input from group I muscle afferents (presumably from primary endings of muscle spindles). By contrast, some of the relay neurons in the dorsal column nuclei receive convergent inputs form hair, tactile and pressure receptors, and nociceptors. There are also interneurons within the dorsal column nuclei. These may also receive rather specific input, or they may receive a convergent input. The convergent input to interneurons may come from receptors of several extremities and from a number of regions of the brain. One difficulty in the experiments on neurons of the dorsal column nuclei is the possibility that some cells labeled "interneurons" are likely to be misidentified relay neurons, either because of failure to backfire them from the medial lemniscus or because the axon projected to some region that was not stimulated (e.g., cerebellum, inferior olive, or spinal cord).

DESCENDING CONTROL OF DORSAL COLUMN NUCLEI

Hagbarth and Kerr (1954) showed that stimulation within the reticular formation inhibits activity ascending in the lateral and ventral funiculi of the spinal cord and also through the dorsal column nuclei. Similar effects were produced by stimulation of the sensorimotor cortex, SII, the anterior part of the cingulate gyrus, and the anterior cerebellar vermis. The depression of transmission through the dorsal column nuclei has also been shown by the reduction in evoked potentials following stimulation of the reticular formation, the cerebral cortex, or the pyramidal tract (Hernández-Peón *et al.*, 1956; Guzmán-Flores *et al.*, 1962; Magni *et al.*, 1959).

Reticular formation stimulation results in PAD of afferents ascending to the dorsal column nuclei (Cesa-Bianchi *et al.*, 1968). Inhibition of dorsal column thalamic relay neurons can be demonstrated at the single-unit level, while interneurons in the cuneate nucleus are excited by comparable stimuli (Cesa-Bianchi and Sotgiu, 1969). Thus, the inhibitory effects of the reticular formation may be mediated by interneurons located in the dorsal column nuclei. The most effective part of the reticular formation appears to be the nucleus gigantocellularis, which is the nucleus of origin of a direct projection to the dorsal column nuclei (Fig. 6.24) (Sotgiu and Margnelli, 1976; Sotgiu and Marini, 1977). Stimulation of the cerebellar nuclei and of the nonspecific nuclei of the thalamus results in PAD of afferents to the cuneate nucleus (Sotgiu and Cesa-Bianchi, 1970), inhibition of many cuneothalamic relay cells, and excitation often followed by inhibition of cuneate interneurons (Sotgiu and Cesa-Bianchi, 1972). Cuneate neurons, especially cuneothalamic relay neurons, are also inhibited by stimulation of the caudate nucleus (Jabbur et al., 1977). Presumably, many of these inhibitory actions are transmitted by way of the reticular formation and from there the inhibition may be mediated via inhibitory interneurons in the dorsal column nuclei (Sotgiu and Cesa-Bianchi, 1972).

The projection pathway from the cerebral cortex to the dorsal column nuclei is well established (e.g., Chambers and Liu, 1957; Walberg, 1957; Kuypers, 1958; Kuypers and Tuerk, 1964; Levitt et al., 1964; Valverde, 1966; Shriver and Noback, 1967; McComas and Wilson, 1968; Gordon and Miller, 1969; Martin et al., 1971; Weisberg and Rustioni, 1976, 1977). The projection originates in cats from the sensory cortex, partly from cells in cytoarchitectonic area 3a and partly from cells of areas 4, 3b, 1, 2, and SII (Gordon and Miller, 1969; Weisberg and Rustioni, 1976) and in monkeys (Fig. 6.25) also from the supplemental motor and supplemental sensory areas (Weisberg and Rustioni, 1977). The projection to the nucleus gracilis comes from the medial part of the sensorimotor cortex and that to the nucleus cuneatus from the lateral part, suggesting a somatotopic arrangement comparable to that of the ascending pathways (Kuypers, 1958; Levitt et al., 1964; however, cf. Walberg, 1957). The region of termination of the cortical projection is largely in the rostral and ventral portions of the dorsal column nuclei (Fig. 6.26), rather than in the cell cluster zone (Kuypers and Tuerk, 1964). Presumably, the cortical inhibitory actions are brought about by way of interneurons.

Recordings from neurons within the dorsal column nuclei show that cortical stimulation results in the excitation of some neurons and inhibition of others (Towe and Jabbur, 1961; Jabbur and Towe, 1961; Levitt et al., 1964). The excitation is chiefly of interneurons (Fig. 6.20), while the inhibition is most prominently seen in cuneothalamic relay cells (Gordon and Jukes, 1964b; Andersen et al., 1964d). However,

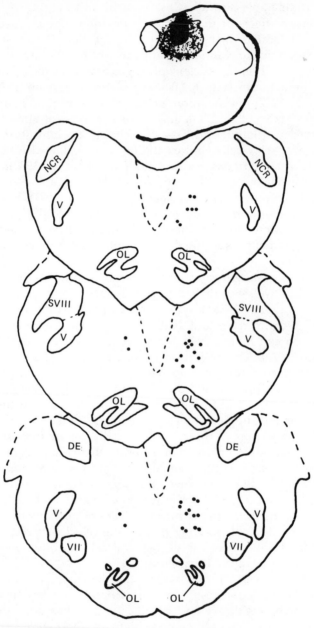

Fig. 6.24. Reticular formation neurons that project to the dorsal column nuclei. The site of an injection of horseradish peroxidase into the dorsal column nuclei is shown at the top, and the distribution of retrogradely labeled neurons in the nucleus reticularis gigantocellularis is shown in the other drawings of brainstem sections. (From Sotgiu and Marini, 1977.)

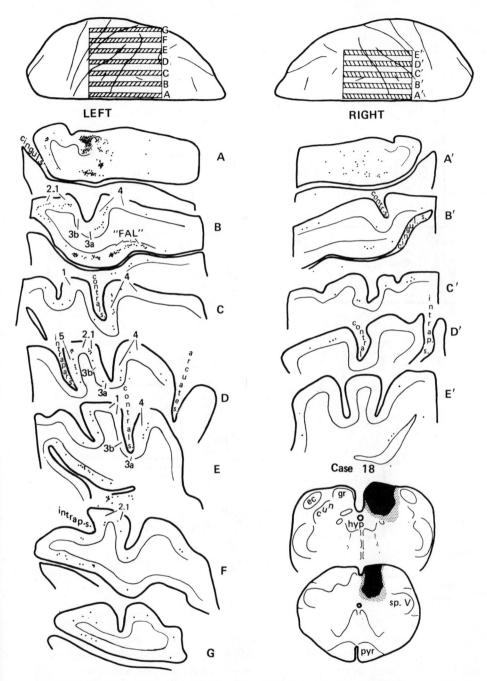

Fig. 6.25. Neurons of the sensorimotor cortex that project to the dorsal column nuclei were labeled by horseradish peroxidase. The injection site is shown at the bottom on the right. Sagittal sections were made through the monkey brain at the levels indicated above. Cytoarchitectonic areas in the cortex are indicated. (From Weisberg and Rustioni, 1977.)

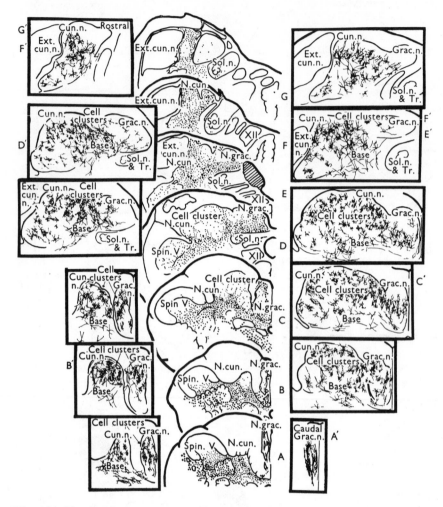

Fig. 6.26. The distribution of terminal degeneration in the dorsal column nuclei following a lesion of the sensorimotor cortex is shown in the column of drawings at the center. The cytoarchitecture of the dorsal column nuclei is shown by the flanking columns of drawings of Golgi-stained material. (From Kuypers and Tuerk, 1964.)

both excitation and inhibition were commonly seen in individual neurons by Winter (1965). The inhibition is presumably in part presynaptic, since cortical volleys produced PAD in the afferents to the dorsal column nuclei (Fig. 6.19) (Andersen *et al.*, 1964b,c). The excitatory action is mediated primarily by way of the pyramids, whereas inhibition can still be obtained after the pyramids are sectioned at the level of the trapezoid body (Jabbur and Towe, 1961; Levitt *et al.*, 1964). The inhibition of dorsal column cells that relay to the thalamus would presumably be in part mediated by interneurons that are directly excited by pyramidal tract fibers and in part by neurons in the reticular formation that are activated by pyramidal fibers.

A projection has been described anatomically from the red nucleus to the rostral cuneate nucleus and also to the gracile nucleus (Edwards, 1972), but there do not appear to be any physiological studies of this pathway.

The functional significance of the various efferent pathways to the dorsal column nuclei is conjectural. The inhibitory actions common to many of the inputs are thought to explain the changes in transmission through the dorsal column nuclei that occur (1) as a result of polysensory stimulation (lights, clicks) (Atweh *et al.*, 1974); (2) during sleep (Carli *et al.*, 1967a,b,c; Favale *et al.*, 1965; Ghelarducci *et al.*, 1970); (3) during voluntary movement (Coquery *et al.*, 1971; O'Keefe and Gaffan, 1971; Ghez and Lenzi, 1971; Ghez and Pisa, 1972; Coulter, 1974; Dyhre-Poulsen, 1975); and (4) during seizures experimentally induced in the sensory cortex (Schwartzkroin *et al.*, 1974a,b). The feedback during movement could sum with peripheral feedback (Evarts, 1971), or it could substitute for peripheral feedback in its absence (Taub and Berman, 1968). The inhibitory feedback might serve as a kind of "corollary discharge" by counteracting that part of the sensory input predicted from a voluntary movement, yet allowing information not due simply to the movement to be transmitted (Holst, 1954; Teuber, 1960). Alternatively, the inhibition might serve to interfere with input that might disturb preprogrammed ballistic movements (Dyhre-Poulsen, 1975). More studies are needed to determine the role of centrifugal control of the dorsal column nuclei during exploratory movements, preferably in a primate.

In summary, the dorsal column nuclei are under the control of afferent pathways of the brain, as are other sensory systems. The best-studied efferent systems that act on the dorsal column nuclei are the reticular formation, especially the nucleus reticularis gigantocellularis, and the sensorimotor cortex. Stimulation of either structure produces PAD in the dorsal column nuclei and inhibition of neuronal activity. Cortical stimulation excites some neurons in the dorsal column nuclei; these may be inhibitory interneurons. The role of efferent control systems is not entirely clear, but such control might (1) serve to sum with or substitute for peripheral feedback, (2) serve as a corollary discharge, or (3) prevent the disruption of motor programs by peripheral feedback.

CONCLUSIONS

1. The dorsal column pathway is present in amphibia, reptiles, and birds, as well as in mammals.

2. In the human embryo, the dorsal column pathway begins to be recognizable at 8–9 weeks, as the dorsal root ganglia and dorsal column nuclei differentiate and the dorsal columns form.

3. The dorsal columns are comprised of short, intermediate, and long systems of fibers. The short system operates segmentally. The intermediate system has effects segmentally but also at the level of Clarke's column. The long system from the lumbosacral cord appears to have connections at the segmental level, at the cervical enlargement, and in the dorsal column nuclei. Less than 25% of dorsal column fibers belong to the long system.

4. The long-fiber system of the dorsal column forms most of the spinal portion of the dorsal column (dorsal column–medial lemniscus) pathway.

5. The dorsal column pathway includes the fasciculus gracilis, containing ascending branches of afferents supplying the lower body and hind limb, and the fasciculus cuneatus, which contains afferents from the upper body and forelimb.

6. The fasciculus gracilis synapses in the nucleus gracilis, and the fasciculus cuneatus synapses in the nucleus cuneatus.

7. The dorsal column axons have a topographic organization. At caudal levels, the organization is dermatomal, while at the level of the dorsal column nuclei, the pattern is somatotopic due to fiber resorting.

8. Dorsal column axons terminate at all rostrocaudal levels of the dorsal column nuclei. As a result, the dorsal column nuclei have a somatotopic organization that is roughly comparable at all rostrocaudal levels.

9. The dorsal column nuclei have several cytoarchitectonic zones. In the cat and monkey, these are rostral, middle, and caudal; in the rat, they are rostral and caudal.

10. When three cytoarchitectonic zones are recognized, the middle zone is the one richest in neurons projecting to the contralateral thalamus. Where only two zones are found, the caudal zone contains the larger concentration of cells that relay to the thalamus.

11. Dorsal column axonal terminals are often large, axodendritic boutons. They contain spherical synaptic vesicles, and they often participate in axoaxonic complexes as postsynaptic elements.

12. Transection of the dorsal columns in adult primates results in only minimal evidence of transneuronal degeneration in the dorsal column nuclei.

13. The dorsal column nuclei project via the medial lemniscus to the contralateral diencephalon, with terminals in the ventral posterior lateral nucleus (VPL), the medial part of the posterior nuclear complex, and the zona incerta. The projection to VPL is somatotopic.

14. Other projections of the dorsal column nuclei are to parts of the inferior olivary complex, the cerebellum, the midbrain, and the spinal cord.

15. Recordings from axons of primary afferents that project to the level of the medulla, as shown by antidromic activation, show that the receptor types represented in the fasciculus gracilis include G_1 and G_2 hair-follicle receptors, field receptors, type II slowly adapting receptors, Pacinian corpuscles, and rapidly adapting joint receptors. The fasciculus cuneatus includes also type I slowly adapting receptor and group I muscle receptor afferents.

16. The axons of second-order sensory neurons are also present in the dorsal columns. Some of these receive a convergent input from mechanoreceptors and nociceptors, while others respond just to mechanoreceptors or just to nociceptors.

17. The dorsal column nuclei receive synaptic connections from second-order fibers ascending in the dorsolateral fasciculus, in addition to inputs from the dorsal columns. The dorsolateral pathway accounts for the failure of a transection of the dorsal column to change the response properties of some neurons of the dorsal column nuclei.

18. Field potentials can be recorded from the dorsal column nuclei in response to electrical stimulation of peripheral nerves. A negative (N) wave at the dorsal surface of the medulla reflects excitatory processes in the dorsal column nuclei, while a positive (P) wave is associated with primary afferent depolarization and presynaptic inhibition.

19. Neurons of the dorsal column nuclei have a tendency to respond to a variety of stimuli with a short burst discharge. This tendency appears to reflect in part the membrane properties of these cells.

20. Cells of the dorsal column nuclei that relay information to the thalamus can be identified by antidromic activation from the contralateral medial lemniscus. However, not all cells that fail to respond antidromically to such stimuli are interneurons, since the stimulus may not discharge all of the axons of the cells that relay to the thalamus and since some cells in the dorsal column nuclei relay information to other sites in the central nervous system than the thalamus.

21. The excitatory synaptic transmitter released by primary afferent fibers in the dorsal column nuclei may be glutamic acid.

22. Short-lasting inhibition in the dorsal column nuclei may be due to inhibitory postsynaptic potentials (IPSPs) and long-lasting in-

hibition to presynaptic inhibition. However, occasional prolonged IPSPs have been observed, so this distinction is not absolute.

23. Primary afferent depolarization (PAD) in the dorsal column nuclei due to stimulation of cutaneous receptors does not seem to have the specificity observed in the lumbosacral spinal cord.

24. PAD in the dorsal column nuclei may be produced by axoaxonal synapses formed between interneuronal terminals and primary afferent terminals. The same interneuronal terminals also form axodendritic synapses, suggesting that pre- and postsynaptic inhibition may occur simultaneously.

25. Presumed interneurons in the dorsal column nuclei can be excited by stimulation of peripheral nerves and of the sensorimotor cortex. Some of these interneurons are thought to be responsible for PAD.

26. Pre- and postsynaptic inhibition in the dorsal column nuclei may be mediated by γ-aminobutyric acid. Alternatively, PAD may result from an extracellular accumulation of potassium ions.

27. Responses of cells in the dorsal column nuclei to natural forms of stimulation indicate that the most prominent input is from the skin. The cells with the smallest excitatory receptive fields tend to lie in the middle zone; the same is true for cells that are most likely to have surround inhibitory receptive fields. Furthermore, cells in the middle zone are the most likely to show antidromic invasion when stimuli are applied to the contralateral medial lemniscus.

28. The somatotopic relations of the dorsal column nuclei are the following: the tail is represented medially, the shoulders laterally, the distal limbs dorsally and the trunk ventrally.

29. Receptive fields are smallest when distal on a limb and largest when proximal.

30. Many dorsal column neurons are excited by hair movement; these have surround inhibition. Other neurons respond to touch and lack surround inhibition. Still others can be discharged by vibration at rates of 100–300 Hz. A few can be activated by deep receptors.

31. Cells in the rostral part of the dorsal column nuclei differ from those in the middle zone in having larger receptive fields, higher thresholds, longer latencies, and poorer ability to follow repetitive stimuli; surround inhibition is also less common for rostral cells.

32. Other details about the responses of dorsal column neurons to natural stimuli include the observation that both rapidly and slowly adapting responses are seen; some neurons respond to claw movement or pressure at the base of a claw; convergence of input from hair, touch, and pressure receptors can be demonstrated for some neurons;

for vibration-sensitive cells, the receptors are often located in the abdomen (presumably Pacinian corpuscles).

33. The dorsal column nuclei can be considered to have a dual organization. Some of the neurons are responsive in a selective way to particular receptor types; their receptive fields tend to be small and are somatotopically organized; there is often surround inhibition; the cells are generally in the middle zone, and they can be antidromically activated from the medial lemniscus. Other dorsal column neurons receive a convergent input from several receptor types; they have large receptive fields that are not clearly somatotopic; there is no surround inhibition; these cells are located in the rostral zone or deep in the middle zone, and they often do not project into the medial lemniscus.

34. Cuneate neurons that are activated by group I muscle afferents are located deep to the cells that have cutaneous inputs. Many of the cells project to the contralateral thalamus. The relay neurons are excited by group Ia muscle spindle afferents, although some interneurons can be activated by group Ib fibers from Golgi tendon organs.

35. Gracile neurons that respond to knee joint afferents signal either velocity or acceleration but not position.

36. The discharge periodicity of the slowly adapting responses of cuneate neurons to tactile or proprioceptive input can be modified by the activity of a single afferent.

37. Inhibition of dorsal column neurons with either rapidly or slowly adapting responses to cutaneous stimulation can be produced by Pacinian corpuscles.

38. Partial denervation results in the immediate appearance of proximal or split receptive fields that could not be detected prior to denervation. Inhibitory fields also increase. This suggests that there are normally ineffective synapses that are disinhibited following denervation.

39. The dorsal column nuclei are subject to descending control from the reticular formation, from a number of other brain sites via the reticular formation, and from the sensorimotor cerebral cortex. The control is generally inhibitory, although corticofugal volleys often excite dorsal column neurons. The latter may, however, be interneurons that in turn inhibit relay cells.

40. Descending control may account for changes in transmission through the dorsal column nuclei as a result of polysensory stimulation, during sleep and during voluntary movements. The control may be considered feedback that can sum with or substitute for peripheral feedback. It may represent a corollary discharge. Or the inhibition may prevent disruption of motor programs.

7 Sensory Pathways in the Dorsolateral Fasciculus

The two major sensory pathways that are located in the dorsolateral fasciculus are the spinocervicothalamic and the spinomedullothalamic pathways. There is also a second-order projection to the dorsal column nuclei (see Chapter 6).

THE SPINOCERVICOTHALAMIC PATHWAY

A previously unrecognized sensory pathway in the spinal cord was described by Morin in 1955. This is the spinocervicothalamic pathway. The cells of origin of the path are in the gray matter of the dorsal horn. Axons from these cells project up the dorsal part of the ipsilateral lateral column and synapse on cells of the lateral cervical nucleus. This part of the pathway is referred to as the spinocervical tract. Cells of the spinocervical tract receive afferent input over the dorsal roots from sensory receptors of the ipsilateral body, and the sensory information is transmitted to the lateral cervical nucleus of the same side of the cord at C1–C2. The cells of the lateral cervical nucleus project through the medial lemniscus to the contralateral thalamus as the cervicothalamic tract (Fig. 7.1).

Phylogeny

The most distinctive component of the spinocervicothalamic pathway in neuroanatomic material is the lateral cervical nucleus. This nucleus can be recognized in the upper cervical spinal cord in a number of mammalian species (including the cat, dog, sheep, seal,

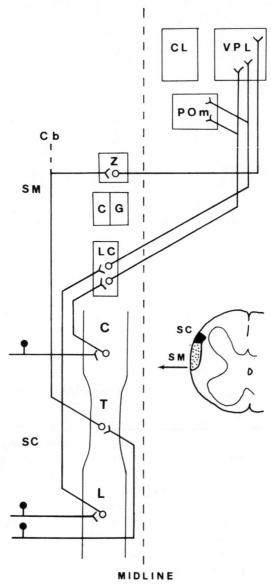

Fig. 7.1. Sensory pathways of the dorsolateral fasciculus. The organization of the spinocervical and spinomedullothalamic pathways is shown. Primary afferent fibers end upon cells of the dorsal horn in the cervical (C) and lumbar (L) enlargements. The second-order neurons project through the spinocervical tract (SC) to the lateral cervical nucleus. The axons of third order cells decussate and project through the medial lemniscus to the medial part of the posterior nuclear complex (PO_m) and the ventral posterior lateral (VPL) nucleus of the thalamus. Other primary afferent fibers ascend in the dorsal column to the thoracic cord (T), where they synapse upon cells in Clarke's column (and also on cells caudal to Clarke's column), which in turn project in the spinomedullary tract (SM) to nucleus z. Some of these axons also project to the cerebellum (Cb). Nucleus z projects contralaterally to the VPL and adjacent parts of the ventral lateral nucleus. The transverse section of the spinal cord indicates the locations of the spinocervical and spinomedullary pathways.

whale, raccoon, and monkey) (Rexed, 1951, 1954; Brodal and Rexed, 1953; Gardner and Morin, 1957; Ha and Morin, 1964; Ha et al., 1965; Kitai et al., 1965; Mizuno et al., 1967; Kircher and Ha, 1968; Shriver et al., 1968; Ha, 1971). The lateral cervical nucleus is larger in the raccoon and dog than in the cat (Ha et al., 1965; Kitai et al., 1965). A column of cells just ventral to the dorsal horn and extending the entire length of the spinal cord has been described in several species (rat, guinea pig, rabbit, ferret, and hedgehog). It has been suggested that this column is equivalent to the lateral cervical nucleus (Gwyn and Waldron, 1968, 1969; Waldron, 1969), but no evidence was advanced that the cell column has a thalamic projection.

The presence of a lateral cervical nucleus in man is controversial. None was seen by several investigators (Rexed, 1951; Brodal and Rexed, 1953; Gardner and Morin, 1957; Seki, 1962). However, others have observed a lateral cervical nucleus in at least some human spinal cords (Ha and Morin, 1964; Kircher and Ha, 1968; Truex et al., 1965). Possibly the nucleus is not distinctly separate from the dorsal horn in some specimens. The total number of cells in the lateral cervical nucleus of the two sides combined from the medulla through C1 (presumably not the entire extent of the nucleus) in one human cord was 5173 (Truex et al., 1965). This is a somewhat smaller number of cells than has been reported for a similar extent of the nucleus in the cat (2800–2950 for one side) (Morin and Catalano, 1955), but it can be concluded that the nuclei are of roughly comparable size in the cat and human.

Degenerating ascending tract fibers to the human lateral cervical nucleus were abundant in a cord examined by Kircher and Ha (1968) from a victim of a diving accident. The ascending degeneration observed by Nathan and Smith (1955) following cordotomy at a high cervical level in human patients may have been due to interruption of the cervicothalamic projection.

Anatomy of the Spinocervical Tract and the Lateral Cervical Nucleus

The locations of the cells of origin of the spinocervical tract have been mapped (Fig. 7.2A–C) in electrophysiological experiments in the cat and monkey (Hongo et al., 1968; Bryan et al., 1973, 1974; A. G. Brown et al., 1976; Cervero et al., 1977a). Most of the cells were in Rexed's laminae IV and V (Rexed, 1952, 1954), although some appeared to be in laminae VI–VIII (Bryan et al., 1973, 1974); note, however, that not all of the cells were checked for a projection above C1, and so some of the neurons may have projected to a level rostral to the lateral cervical nucleus. There may also be some spinocervical tract

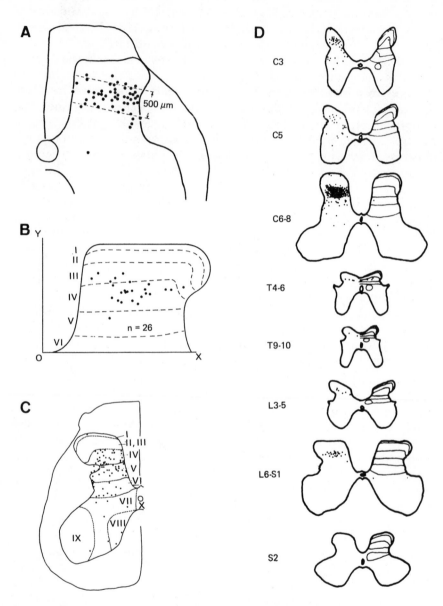

Fig. 7.2. The locations of neurons of the spinocervical tract determined by different techniques. Extracellular recordings were used for A (cat) and C (monkey), with histological reconstruction of the recording points. Intracellular dye injections (procion yellow) were employed for B (cat). Horseradish peroxidase was injected into the lateral cervical nucleus in the experiment of D (cat). (A and B from Brown *et al.*, 1976; C from Bryan *et al.*, 1974; D from Craig, 1976.)

cells in lamina I (Bryan *et al.*, 1974; Cervero *et al.*, 1977a). The locations of spinocervical tract cells have also been studied in experiments in which the neurons were labeled intracellularly with procion yellow (Fig. 7.3) (Bryan *et al.*, 1973; Jankowska, 1975; A. G. Brown *et al.*, 1976). The proportions of cells located in lamina IV are higher when this technique is used than with extracellular reconstructions of microelectrode positions. Possibly extracellular recordings reflect dendritic, as well as somatic, activity, and so the recording sites are more

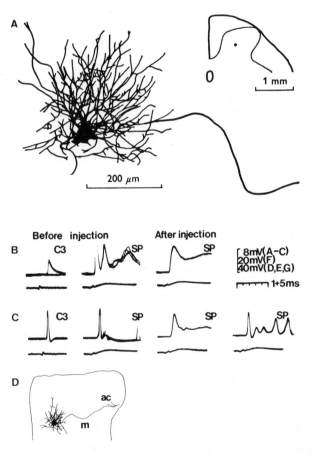

Fig. 7.3. Drawing in A shows the dendritic tree and the initial part of the axon of a spinocervical tract neuron that was labeled by an intracellular injection of procion yellow. (From Brown *et al.*, 1976.) The recordings in (B and C) are from two different spinocervical tract neurons before and after the intracellular injection of horseradish peroxidase. The drawing in D shows the dendritic tree and initial axon of the cell from which the records in B were made. (From Jankowska *et al.*, 1976.)

scattered. Alternatively, if spinocervical tract cells in lamina IV are larger than those elsewhere, intracellular recordings may be from a sample biased toward larger cells. However, a recent study of Craig (1976), using retrograde labeling of spinocervical tract cells by injections of horseradish peroxidase into the lateral cervical nucleus of cats and dogs, showed that spinocervical tract cells in the lumbar enlargement are predominantly in lamina IV (Fig. 7.2D). In the cervical cord, some labeled cells were also found in laminae I and V–VII. Almost all of the cells were ipsilateral to injection. Assuming that the horseradish peroxidase labeled a fair sample of the cells of origin of the spinocervical tract, it appears that the lumbar projection, at least, arises from lamina IV.

Spinocervical tract cells marked with procion yellow display a variety of different dendritic patterns, although in general the bulk of the dendrites of these cells project dorsally (A. G. Brown et al., 1976). The dendritic pattern can rarely be correlated with other morphological or functional characteristics of the cells.

Another approach to marking spinocervical tract cells (Fig. 7.3) is with intracellular injections of horseradish peroxidase (Jankowska et al., 1976; Snow et al., 1976). This technique has the advantage that it allows an ultrastructural as well as a light microscopic analysis. It appears that axons and axon collaterals can be followed more readily in cells marked with horseradish peroxidase than with procion yellow.

It has been suggested that some of the axons of spinocervical tract cross the spinal cord and ascend the contralateral side (Brodal and Rexed, 1953; Ha and Liu, 1966). This possibility does not necessarily conflict with many of the electrophysiological mapping studies, since the contralateral gray matter was not searched systematically for cells antidromically discharged following stimulation of the spinocervical tract. However, it is not in agreement with the distribution of receptive fields of neurons in the lateral cervical nucleus, which are ipsilateral (Rexed and Ström, 1952; Morin et al., 1963; Kitai et al., 1965; Ha et al., 1965; Horrobin, 1966; however, Gordon and Jukes, 1963, and Oswaldo-Cruz and Kidd, 1964, reported some contralateral receptive fields for cells of the lateral cervical nucleus). Furthermore, only a few contralateral cells were labeled by horseradish peroxidase injections into the lateral cervical nucleus (Craig, 1976).

Cells in the nucleus proprius have been shown to project axons into the dorsolateral column (Ramon y Cajal, 1909). The axons of the spinocervical tract ascend in the dorsal part of the lateral funiculus (Brodal and Rexed, 1953; Lundberg and Oscarsson, 1961; Grant, 1962; Loewy, 1974; Nijensohn and Kerr, 1975), presumably from such neurons. The fibers of the spinocervical tract are said to be of two

types, coarse and fine (Ramon y Cajal, 1909; Westman, 1968a). However, Loewy (1974) found an essentially unimodal distribution of axon
diameters in the area of white matter occupied by the spinocervical
tract. A large fraction of the fibers were small (less than 5 μm), but
others were large (up to 22 μm). Although there was no way to distinguish between spinocervical and propriospinal axons, this size range
does account for the wide range of conduction velocities of spinocervical tract axons—7–90 m/s (Bryan et al., 1973); 12–92 m/s (Cervero et
al., 1977a).

The axons of the spinocervical tract terminate in the lateral cervical nucleus, entering it chiefly from the dorsolateral and lateral sides
(Fig. 7.4) (Ramon y Cajal, 1909; Ha and Liu, 1966; Westman, 1968a).
The fibers entering the nucleus can sometimes be shown to be collaterals of larger fibers (Ha and Liu, 1966; Westman, 1968a). For this
reason, it has been suggested that the spinocervical connections are
made, at least in part, by collaterals of the dorsal and ventral spinocerebellar tracts (Busch, 1961; Ha and Liu, 1963, 1966). Lesions placed
in Clarke's column and in the contralateral region of origin of the ventral spinocerebellar tract result in terminal degeneration within the lateral cervical nucleus (Ha and Liu, 1966). The fact that the afferents to
the lateral cervical nucleus arise at all levels of the cord, including segments above and below Clarke's column (Brodal and Rexed, 1953;
Grant, 1962), argues against the possibility that all of the afferents are
collaterals of the dorsal spinocerebellar tract, as does the fact that the
cells of origin of the spinocervical tract that have so far been investigated do not lie within Clarke's column (e.g., J. C. Eccles et al., 1960;
Hongo et al., 1968; Bryan et al., 1973, 1974; A. G. Brown et al., 1976;
Cervero et al., 1977a). Further evidence against this suggestion is that
stimulation within the cerebellum has no effect upon most cells within
the lateral cervical nucleus (Horrobin, 1966), even though the dorsal
spinocerebellar tract would have been activated antidromically. Furthermore, the bulk of the spinocervical tract appears to end in the lateral cervical nucleus (Beusekom, 1955; Grant, 1962), Finally, cells of
Clarke's column do not label when horseradish peroxidase is injected
into the lateral cervical nucleus (Craig, 1976).

The endings of the axons of the spinocervical tract within the lateral cervical nucleus (Fig. 7.4) include terminal boutons, boutons de
passage (Westman, 1968a), and baskets or calices (Ha and Liu, 1963).
One axon may branch repeatedly to supply terminals over a broad expanse of the nucleus. The coarse fibers have a larger terminal field
than do the fine fibers (Westman, 1968a). The synaptic contacts are
both axodendritic and axosomatic (Ha and Liu, 1963), although the
majority are axodendritic, as shown by the distribution of degenerat-

ing terminals at the electron microscopic level after sectioning the spinocervical tract (Westman, 1969). Most of the synaptic terminals within the lateral cervical nucleus do not degenerate following chronic transection of the spinocervical tract, indicating that most of the synapses within the nucleus come from other sources (Westman, 1969). Likely sources include axon collaterals of the neurons of the lateral cer-

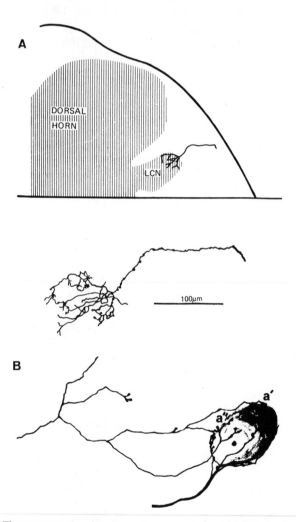

Fig. 7.4. (A) The manner of termination of an axon from the spinocervical tract in the lateral cervical nucleus. (From Westman, 1968a.) (B) Terminations of two different spinocervical tract axons on a cell in the lateral cervical nucleus. (From Ha and Liu, 1963.)

vical nucleus itself, interneurons, descending fibers, and possibly trigeminal afferents (Wall and Taub, 1962; Westman, 1968a, 1969). However, degenerating fibers could not be demonstrated following lesions at the level of the midbrain (Grant and Westman, 1969) or lower medulla (Ha and Liu, 1966), and there is physiological evidence against trigeminal connections (Gordon and Jukes, 1963; Oswaldo-Cruz and Kidd, 1964). No evidence was obtained in the anatomic studies for a somatotopic organization of the spinocervical afferents to the lateral cervical nucleus; the degeneration produced by lesions either at the cervical or at the lumbar level was distributed throughout the nucleus (Brodal and Rexed, 1953).

The lateral cervical nucleus was depicted from Golgi material by Ramon y Cajal (1909), who named it the *noyau du faisceau cérébelleux*. Ranson *et al.*, (1932) thought the nucleus belonged to the reticular formation of the cord and called it the posterior reticular nucleus. It was renamed the lateral cervical nucleus by Rexed and Brodal (1951). The distribution of the nucleus in the cat spinal cord is described in the paper by Rexed and Brodal (1951) and in Rexed's cytoarchitectonic atlas (Rexed, 1954), and it is further depicted (Fig. 7.5) by Ha and Liu (1966) and by Oswaldo-Cruz and Kidd (1964). It lies within the lateral funiculus and is restricted to the first and second cervical segments, with only a slight continuation into the medulla. The nucleus disappears at the level at which the dorsal column nuclei appear and the pyramidal decussation ends. The nucleus tapers in the caudal third of the second cervical segment and disappears by the boundary of the second and third segments. In the rostral part of the first cervical segment, the nucleus connects with the dorsal horn by way of small islands of cells (Fig. 7.5C). At this level, the nucleus lies ventral and lateral to the dorsal horn. It is more easily recognized further caudally, where it is distinctly separated from the dorsal horn and it lies lateral or even dorsolateral to it. In the cat, a total of about 3000 cells are found in C1 through the medulla on each side (Morin and Catalano, 1955).

The cells of the lateral cervical nucleus resemble those of Clarke's column (Rexed and Brodal, 1951; Rexed, 1954). Most of the cells in the cat are medium-sized to large, measuring about 30 μm in transverse section and 30–50 μm in longitudinal section (Westman, 1968b). However, there are small neurons scattered throughout the nucleus (Westman, 1968a,b). Some of these may be interneurons (Westman, 1969). The dendrites are seen in Golgi-stained material to be richly branched and to have spines (Ramon y Cajal, 1909; Ha and Liu, 1966; Westman, 1968a). The axons course ventromedially toward the gray matter, although they may at first travel in other directions, including dorsally,

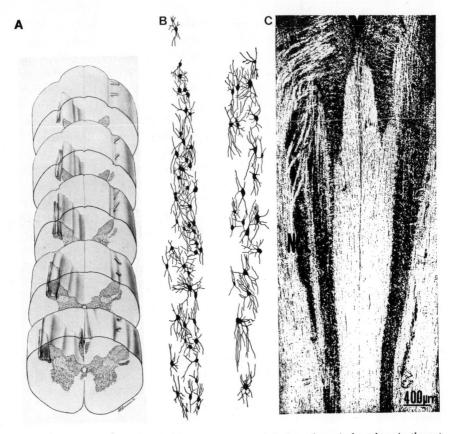

Fig. 7.5. (A) A three-dimensional reconstruction of the lateral cervical nucleus in the cat C1 and C2 spinal cord segments. (From Oswaldo-Cruz and Kidd, 1964.)   (B) The lateral cervical nucleus of the cat bilaterally in a horizontal section in Golgi-stained material.   (C) Similar to B but in a Nissl preparation. This section shows the lateral cervical nucleus (NCL) well just on the left side. (From Ha and Liu, 1966.)

for a short distance. The axons give off collaterals that end with small terminals within the lateral cervical nucleus (Westman, 1968a).

The lateral cervical nucleus was initially considered to be a spino-cerebellar relay nucleus by Rexed and Brodal (1951). This belief was based on the finding of retrograde chromatolysis in neurons of the lateral cervical nucleus in kittens after a cerebellar lesion. However, other workers have failed to produce similar retrograde changes by cerebellar damage (Morin and Catalano, 1955; Morin and Thomas, 1955; Grant et al., 1968). Instead, retrograde changes have been found after lesions of the contralateral medial lemniscus (Morin and Catalano, 1955; Morin and Thomas, 1955; Ha and Liu, 1961; Grant and Westman, 1969). Furthermore, cells of the lateral cervical nucleus of the monkey are labeled following injection of horseradish peroxidase into the contralateral thalamus (Albe-Fessard *et al.*, 1975). Lesions of the lateral cervical nucleus result in anterograde degeneration that can be traced across the spinal cord in the ventral white commissure (Fig. 7.6). The degeneration then passes rostrally in the ventral funiculus to the brainstem; it is found lateral to the inferior olivary nucleus and eventually in the dorsolateral part of the medial lemniscus (Morin and Thomas, 1955; Busch, 1961; Hagg and Ha, 1970; Boivie, 1970; Ha, 1971). If the dorsal spinocerebellar tract is first interrupted chronically and time is given for the degeneration to disappear, lesions of the lateral cervical nucleus fail to produce any degeneration in the cerebellum (Grant *et al.*, 1968). The material of Rexed and Brodal (1951) has been reexamined and found to show the chromatolysis originally described; it is suggested that a vascular change may have resulted in the chromatolysis (Grant *et al.*, 1968). The evidence thus indicates that the lateral cervical nucleus is a relay for sensory information to the thalamus, rather than a cerebellar relay. However, there is some anatomic and physiological evidence that the cervicothalamic projection gives off collaterals to the contralateral inferior olivary nucleus (Morin and Thomas, 1955; Horrobin, 1966; Hagg and Ha, 1970). This suggests that the spinocervicothalamic pathway also serves as a spinoolivocerebellar pathway. However, Mizuno (1966) and Boivie (unpublished work quoted in Boivie and Perl, 1975) do not confirm a significant projection from the lateral cervical nucleus to the inferior olive.

The thalamic nuclei in which the cervicothalamic fibers end have been variously stated to include the lateral part of the ventrolateral nucleus (Morin and Thomas, 1955), the ventrobasal complex (Busch, 1961), or the nucleus ventralis posterolateralis (Landgren *et al.*, 1965; Hagg and Ha, 1970; Ha, 1971). In a thorough study utilizing both the Nauta and the Fink–Heimer stains, Boivie (1970) found that lesions of the cat cervicothalamic tract produced terminal degeneration in the following thalamic nuclei (Fig. 7.7): the lateral and medial parts of the nucleus ventralis posterolateralis (VPL_1 and VPL_m), the medial part of the posterior nuclear complex (PO_m), and the magnocellular part of the medial geniculate nucleus (MG_{mc}). The projection is entirely crossed. A similar pattern of degeneration resulted whether lesions were made in the rostral or the caudal part of the lateral cervical nucleus, indicating that a rostral-to-caudal somatotopic organization like that proposed by Catalano and Lamarche (1957) is unlikely.

At least some of the cells of the thalamus that are activated by cervicothalamic projections receive a convergent input from the dorsal column pathway (Landgren *et al.*, 1965; Andersen *et al.*, 1966). Fur-

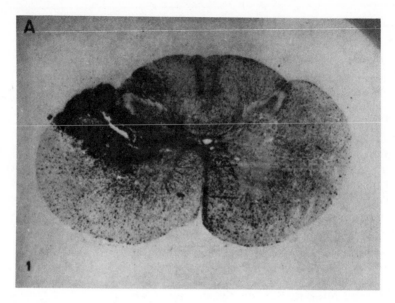

Fig. 7.6. Marchi preparation showing the course of the cervicothalamic pathway. The lesion of the lateral cervical nucleus is shown in A, as is the decussation of the cervicothalamic path (arrows). The ascending fibers of the cervicothalamic pathway are seen in medullary and midbrain levels in B and C. (From Hagg and Ha, 1970.)

thermore, thalamic neurons in the spinocervicothalamic path may project to both the SI and the SII sensory regions of the cerebral cortex (Andersen *et al.*, 1966).

In summary, the cells of origin of the spinocervical tract are concentrated in lamina IV of the spinal cord dorsal horn (although some may be in laminae I and V–VIII). The axons project up the ipsilateral dorsolateral fasciculus to end in the lateral cervical nucleus. The area of termination of a single axon within the nucleus may be large. There is no morphologic evidence of a somatotopic organization of the lateral cervical nucleus. The lateral cervical nucleus is located ventrolateral to the dorsal horn and extends from the caudal medulla through C2. Axons from cells of the lateral cervical nucleus decussate in the ventral white commissure and then ascend in the ventral quadrant to the medulla. They pass lateral to the inferior olivary nucleus and eventually join the dorsolateral part of the medial lemniscus. The cervicothalamic tract ends in several thalamic nuclei, including the medial part of the posterior nuclear complex and the nucleus ventralis posterolateralis.

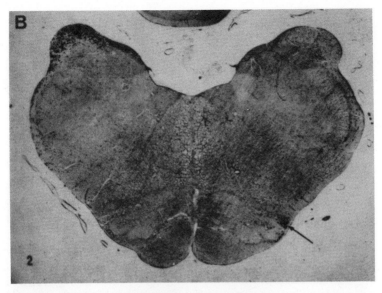

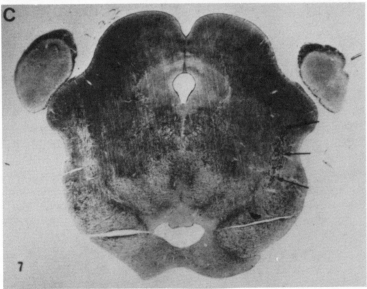

Fig. 7.6 continued.

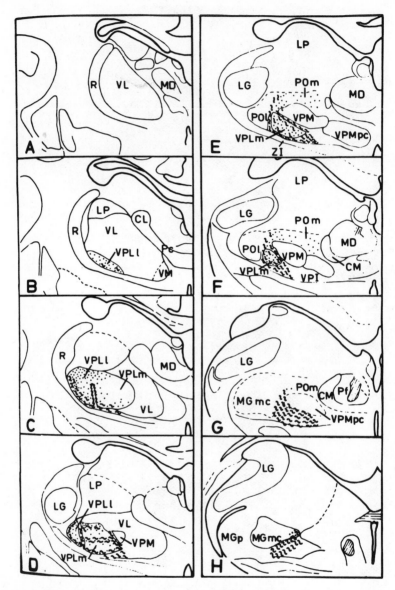

Fig. 7.7. Areas of termination of the cervicothalamic pathway in the cat. Pertinent abbreviations: VPL$_l$ and VPL$_m$ = ventral posterior lateral nucleus, lateral and medial segments; PO$_m$ = posterior complex, medial part. Terminals indicated by dots, fibers of passage by wavy lines. (From Boivie, 1970.)

Responses of Spinocervical Tract Neurons to Electrical Stimulation

Many studies of the activity ascending in the spinocervical tract have involved the recording of evoked potentials, either from the lateral cervical nucleus (Rexed and Ström, 1952) or from the cerebral cortex (e.g., Morin, 1955; Catalano and Lamarche, 1957; Gardner and Morin, 1957; Mark and Steiner, 1958; Norrsell and Wolpow, 1966). The lateral cervical nucleus was shown to generate evoked potentials in response to stimulation of ipsilateral cutaneous nerves, but not muscle nerves, and no activity resulted from stimulation of cutaneous or muscle nerves to the contralateral fore- or hind limb (Rexed and Ström, 1952). The studies utilizing evoked potentials recorded from the cerebral cortex in animals with lesions interrupting other sensory pathways give only indirect evidence about the activity of spinocervical tract cells (see Chapter 5), since the responses also reflect the information processing that occurs within the lateral cervical nucleus and the thalamus. However, it is interesting that the latencies of the evoked potentials due to volleys transmitted via the spinocervicothalamic pathway and recorded from the SI and SII cortex in the cat are actually shorter than the latencies of the evoked potentials due to the dorsal column pathway (Mark and Steiner, 1958; Norrsell and Voorhoeve, 1962; Norrsell and Wolpow, 1966). A criticism of such studies is that lesions of the dorsal column (or of the dorsolateral fasciculus) may be incomplete, even in the face of adequate histological controls, and pathways with very steep input–output relations, such as the dorsal column pathway, may produce large cortical evoked potentials even though only a few fibers are left intact (Whitehorn *et al.*, 1969; Ennever and Towe, 1974). Towe's group could not evoke a substantial cortical potential when they stimulated the dorsolateral fasciculus lateral to a mica plate inserted between the dorsolateral fasciculus and the dorsal column to reduce stimulus spread. However, Andersson and Leissner (1975) were able to evoke a large cortical potential by stimulation of the dorsolateral fasciculus isolated from the dorsal column by a Teflon sheet. They suggested that Towe's group damaged the spinocervical tract or lateral cervical nucleus in their preparations.

J. C. Eccles *et al.* (1960) described several types of interneurons in the lumbosacral enlargement. One class of neuron was excited monosynaptically following electrical stimulation of cutaneous afferents and was also activated antidromically by stimulation of the "ventrolateral" funiculus on the same side. The same neurons were often activated polysynaptically by high-threshold afferents. The tract cells were located at depths of 1.6–2.5 mm from the surface of the cord. It was suggested that these cells might project to the lateral cervical nucleus.

Taub and Bishop (1965) found that axons within the dorsolateral funiculus were activated both antidromically and orthodromically by stimuli applied to the dorsolateral column and to the dorsal column, unless suitable lesions were made. Almost all of the axons found that could be excited monosynaptically by sural nerve stimulation were activated antidromically by stimulation of the dorsolateral column at C4, and 89% responded orthodromically to dorsal column stimulation at C1–C2. Stimulation of the dorsolateral column rostral to C1 in animals without a section of this region of the cord produced antidromic activation of only a few of the axons judged to belong to the spinocervical tract, and the conduction velocities of the axons so discharged slowed considerably at the upper cervical level, suggesting either termination of the fibers or collaterization at the level of the lateral cervical nucleus. The identified spinocervical tract axons were excited by both Aα and Aδ afferent fibers.

Mendell (1966) recorded the activity of axons in the dorsolateral column at caudal L4 or L5. Since this is below Clarke's column, he assumed that the axons belonged to the spinocervical tract. The cells responded monosynaptically to stimulation of large Aβ fibers, and 60% of them were also excited by stimulation of C fibers. There may have been a contribution of excitation from Aδ fibers as well. With repeated stimulation of certain frequencies, the response to C fiber stimulation increased, a phenomenon named "windup." This was apparently due to a facilitation lasting some 2–3 seconds. Natural stimulation showed that spinocervical tract cells that responded to both A and C fiber inputs had a much larger dynamic range of stimulus strengths, which altered the discharge of the cell. The two response types corresponded to the activity seen in two of the pathways of the dorsolateral column described by Lundberg and Oscarsson (1961). Both Wall (1967) and Fetz (1968) found some cells in lamina IV that had a small dynamic range and others that had a wide dynamic range. Convergence of A and C fiber inputs onto spinocervical tract cells was confirmed by Fetz (1968) and by A. G. Brown et al. (1973a,b, 1975).

Intracellular recordings were made from neurons identified as spinocervical tract cells by Hongo et al. (1968) in order to determine if the cells are subject to postsynaptic inhibition. The cells were identified by antidromic invasion from stimulation of the lateral white matter of the cord at a lower thoracic level, monosynaptic activation by large cutaneous afferents, and location of the cell body at 1.1–1.8 mm depth in the cord. Electrical stimulation of cutaneous afferents produced monosynaptic excitatory postsynaptic potentials and disynaptic inhibitory postsynaptic potentials, while high-threshold muscle afferents produced polysynaptic EPSPs. IPSPs were also observed following natural stimulation of the skin, including hair movement, touch of the pad, pressure, and pinch. The inhibitory fields were eccentric, rather than surround, in type. Stimulation of flexion reflex afferents of the ipsilateral and contralateral limb also produced IPSPs, or mixed EPSPs and IPSPs, with a polysynaptic latency. No effects were found when group I muscle afferents were stimulated, and no recurrent IPSPs were observed. In addition to postsynaptic inhibition, it was suggested that presynaptic inhibition could also play a role in limiting the discharges of spinocervical tract neurons. Further evidence for this possibility was obtained by J. C. Eccles *et al.* (1962b), Brown and Kirk (1972), and Brown *et al.* (1973a), who found a long-lasting depression of the activity of spinocervical tract neurons following stimulation of cutaneous nerves.

A. G. Brown *et al.* (1975) employed an anodal blocking technique to demonstrate the effects of C fiber volleys on cat spinocervical tract units in the absence of volleys in A fibers. Of a sample of 52 cells, 29% were excited just by A fibers, while 71% were excited by both A and C fibers. All of the latter but none of the former were activated by pressure as well as by hair movement, suggesting that the C fibers were responsible for the excitation produced by pressure. Noxious heat activated both categories of units; it was proposed that in addition to C fibers, some myelinated fibers must be excited by noxious heat to account for this. Conditioning volleys in A fibers of peripheral nerves or in pathways descending in the cord white matter (dorsolateral fasciculus and also ventral funiculus) produced a prolonged inhibition of the responses of spinocervical tract cells to A or C fibers; however, conditioning volleys in C fibers had no effect on either the response to A or to C fiber volleys. Thus, C fibers either excite spinocervical tract cells or have no effect.

In summary, the spinocervical tract is activated by ipsilateral cutaneous and high-threshold muscle afferents (the flexion reflex afferents) but not by low-threshold muscle afferents or by contralateral afferents. The spectrum of cutaneous afferents that are effective may include Aαβ, Aδ, and C fibers. The C fiber excitation shows windup when stimuli are repeated at intervals less than 3 s. Some ipsi- and contralateral afferents produce inhibitory postsynaptic potentials in spinocervical tract neurons. Inhibition of activity in the spinocervical tract reflects pre- as well as postsynaptic mechanisms, since volleys in A fibers result in a prolonged inhibition that is probably presynaptic. C fibers either excite spinocervical tract cells or have no effect.

Responses of Spinocervical Tract Neurons to Natural Stimulation

Wall (1960) recorded the activity of interneurons within the lumbosacral enlargement of the cat spinal cord (see Chapter 4). The axons of some of the cells were found to lie within the dorsolateral funiculus, and so they may have belonged to the spinocervical tract. The cells had a somatotopic relationship to their peripheral receptive fields. The distal leg was represented medially in the dorsal horn, while the proximal leg was represented laterally. The anterior leg was represented by cells around L4, while the posterior leg and perineum was represented by cells of S2. The receptive fields were oval, with the long axis running down the leg. The cells were most responsive to stimuli applied at a central region of the receptive field, with a gradient of responsiveness out to the periphery. Inhibition was possible with heavy pressure in areas surrounding the excitatory receptive field, but weak stimuli did not produce inhibition. The response to tactile stimulation was rapidly adapting, but the same cells displayed a slowly adapting discharge to pressure and to noxious stimuli.

The activity of tract cells can be recorded from axons within the cord white matter. The experiments of Lundberg and Oscarsson (1961) distinguished between axons of the dorsal spinocerebellar tract and those of the spinocervical and other tracts by observing the effects of stimulation within the cerebellum and of the lateral column below the caudal end of Clarke's column. The axons belonging to the dorsal spinocerebellar tract were directly activated by cerebellar stimulation, but not by stimulation of the lateral column below Clarke's column, whereas the converse was true for axons belonging to the spinocervical or other tracts. The axons presumed to be in the spinocervical tract were excited monosynaptically by cutaneous nerve stimulation but not by muscle nerves. Natural stimulation revealed that all of the axons could be excited by hair movement, and there was no increased excitation with pressure or pinch. The receptive fields were usually small (10 mm^2 for fields on the toes), but they could be large when they were on the proximal limb or on the trunk (up to 20 cm^2). No inhibition of the resting discharge was seen with touch, pressure, or pinch. Two other pathways in the dorsal part of the lateral column were also described by Lundberg and Oscarsson (1961). One was excited by both cutaneous and high-threshold muscle afferents. Effective natural stimuli included both touch and also pressure and pinch. The receptive fields varied from a few square centimeters to much larger. The third pathway was activated after a long latency by flexion reflex afferents of both the ipsilateral and the contralateral side, although the ipsilateral effects were stronger. Such units were distinguished from the ones in the other tracts by their being excited or inhibited by stimulation of the cerebellum and inhibited by descending fibers in the dorsal part of the lateral column. The site of termination of these pathways was not demonstrated. It was suggested that the cells described by J. C. Eccles *et al.* (1960) receiving a convergent input from cutaneous and high-threshold muscle afferents and the neurons studied by Wall (1960) belonged to the second of the three pathways, which Lundberg and Oscarsson did not identify with the spinocervical tract. However, the first two pathways of Lundberg and Oscarsson (1961) were considered to be subdivisions of the spinocervical tract by Lundberg *et al.* (1963).

Responses were recorded from axons of the dorsolateral funiculus by Taub (1964). Although the termination of the axons was unknown, Taub identified the cells as spinocervical on the basis of monosynaptic excitation by cutaneous afferents. The units had the characteristics described by Wall (1960), except that their firing slowed rather than accelerated with heating of the skin. All of the units were discharged by hair movement or by spraying with ethyl chloride, and none were activated by touch on the glabrous skin. The discharges of the units were depressed by strong cutaneous stimuli applied to the ipsi- and contralateral hindlimb. Light brushing outside the excitatory receptive field sometimes slowed the spontaneous activity. Inhibition could also be produced by stimulation of the forelimbs or pinching the nose, pinnae, or tip of the tail. Descending effects will be mentioned in the next section.

A. G. Brown and Franz (1969) studied the effects of specific receptor types upon spinocervical tract neurons (Fig. 7.8). They recorded from axons ascending in the dorsolateral column and identified by antidromic activation from the C3 level. The axons had to fail to respond to stimulation at C1 or to show a reduction in conduction velocity of 50% or more between C3 and C1 to be included in the sample. The three classes of cells identified in spinal cats were: (1) units excited by hair movement alone, (2) units excited by hair movement and by pressure, and (3) units excited by heavy pressure and pinch of skin and/or subcutaneous tissue. The units that were activated just by hair were rapidly adapting and had small receptive fields on the distal limbs (down to 3×2 mm). All three kinds of hairs were effective. Inhibition was found for some units, requiring squeezing. The second class of units showed a rapidly adapting response to hair movement and a slowly adapting response to pressure on the skin. All three hair types were effective. No evidence was found that type I or II slowly adapting receptors were responsible for the responses to pressure. Most of the units could be inhibited, often by squeezing the contralateral ankle.

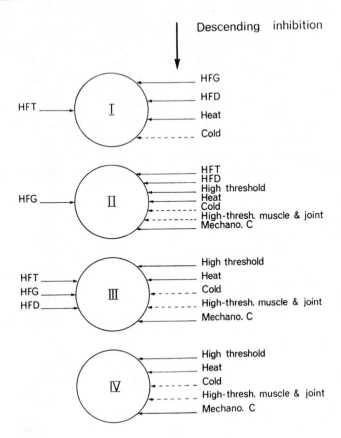

Fig. 7.8. Classification of spinocervical tract neurons according to their responses to peripheral input in the decerebrate cat (left) and in the spinal cat (right). The difference in the responses is attributable to tonic descending inhibitory pathways that are interrupted by spinal transection. The various hair-follicle receptors are abbreviated HFT, HFG, and HFD. (From A. G. Brown, 1973.)

Hair movement, pressure, and squeezing could be effective in inhibiting such units. When an inhibitory receptive field was ipsilateral, it was not of the surround type. The third class of unit was not excited by hair movement but did respond to heavy pressure or pinch with a slowly adapting discharge. The discharge outlasted the stimulus by as long as 30 s. Inhibitory fields were almost always found and resembled those of the second class of units. Anesthetized or decerebrate cats were distinctly different from spinal cats. They had five classes of spinocervical tract neurons: (1) units excited by guard hairs, (2) units excited by tylotrich hairs, (3) units excited by all types of hair, (4) units excited by heavy pressure and pinch of the skin and/or subcutaneous tissue, (5) units not influenced by peripheral stimulation. The guard hair activated units were sometimes also discharged by pressure. Inhibition was not seen, but only two units were adequately tested. Nor was inhibition seen for three of the four tylotrich units. However, almost all of the units activated by all types of hairs could be inhibited, and the inhibitory fields were like those of the units in spinal cats that were excited by hair and pressure. Thermal stimuli excited spinocervical tract cells. The cells began to discharge when the skin was heated to 40–55°C, with the maximum rate occurring at 50–65°C. Some units also discharged when the skin temperature was lowered to below 15–25°C, with a maximum response at 4–18°C. There was no obvious dynamic effect of warming or cooling. Brown and Franz (1970) later showed that mechanical stimulation and heating could have opposite effects on the coefficient of variation in the interspike intervals of spinocervical tract cells without necessarily changing the mean frequency of discharge. Thus, different modalities could be represented in the discharges of a given neuron. The discharge of spinocervical tract cells by pressure or pinch correlated well with a convergence of C fiber input (A. G. Brown et al., 1973a).

The receptive fields of spinocervical tract cells were examined in the cat by Bryan et al. (1973) and in the monkey by Bryan et al. (1974). The cells were identified by antidromic activation from the dorsolateral column at C3 and in many instances by failure of antidromic activation from C1 or rostrally. Most of the cells responded to hair movement or tactile stimulation of the skin. Some responded also to pressure, and a few just to pressure or pinch. A somatotopic relationship was observed between the location of the cells in the dorsal horn and the position of the receptive fields on the limb. The rostrocaudal location of the cells had a dermatomal arrangement (Fig. 7.9). The lateral-to-medial position related to the position of the receptive field on the dorsal versus the ventral surface of the hindlimb. Laterally placed cells had receptive fields on the dorsal surface, while medially placed cells had fields on the ventral surface (Fig. 7.9). A similar scheme has been suggested by Brown and Fuchs (1975) for unidentified interneurons of the cat dorsal horn, although they indicated that the medial-to-lateral organization can be equally well described by a distoproximal gradient, as suggested by Wall (1960), and by a ventrodorsal one, as suggested by Bryan et al. (1973, 1974). The receptive fields in the monkey (Fig. 7.9) were clearly located in some instances on the glabrous skin (Bryan et al., 1974), although comparable receptive fields were not observed in the cat by A. G. Brown and Franz (1969).

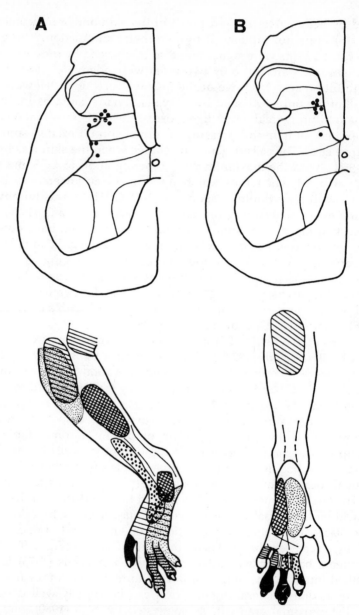

Fig. 7.9. Somatotopic organization of spinocervical tract neurons. The cells in A, which were located in the lateral part of the monkey spinal cord, had receptive fields on the dorsal aspect of the limb, while the cells in B had ventrally placed fields. The receptive fields shown in C were spinocervical tract neurons in the segments indicated. (From Bryan *et al.*, 1974.)

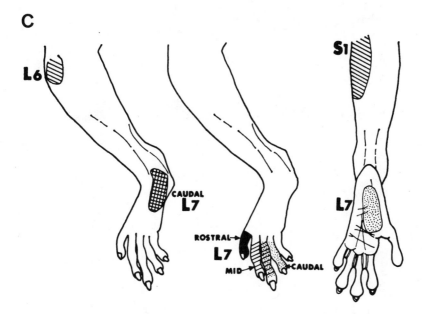

Fig. 7.9 continued.

Cervero *et al.* (1977a) reinvestigated the convergence of nonnoxious and noxious afferent inputs onto spinocervical tract cells in the cat. All but one of their units were excited by nonnoxious stimuli. However, most were also excited by noxious stimuli (Fig. 7.10), and one only by noxious stimuli. Some units were inhibited or both excited and inhibited by noxious input. It was concluded that spinocervical tract neurons might assist in the recognition or discrimination of potentially damaging stimuli, although other pathways might be required to provide information about the specific quality of a noxious stimulus.

Further evidence for a convergence of input from skin and from high-threshold muscle receptors onto spinocervical tract cells has recently been obtained by Kniffki *et al.* (1977). They used intraarterial injections of algesic chemicals (K^+, bradykinin, serotonin) into the circulation of the triceps surae muscles. The agents used had previously been shown to excite group III and IV muscle afferents (Fig. 2.14) but not group I and II fibers (Mense and Schmidt, 1974; Franz and Mense, 1975; Fock and Mense, 1976; Mense, 1977). Thus, spinocervical tract cells are excited by high-threshold muscle afferents using chemicals that in humans produce pain and in animals pain reactions

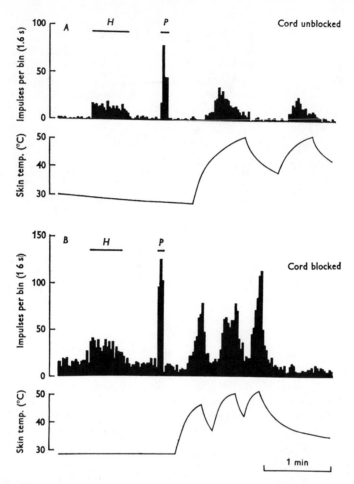

Fig. 7.10. Responses of a spinocervical tract neuron in the spinal cord of the cat. The stimuli were hair movement (H), pinprick (P), and noxious heat. The responses at the top were with the spinal cord intact (animal anesthetized), while those below were after cold block of the cord. (From Cervero *et al.*, 1977a.)

(Burch and DePasquale, 1962; Coffman, 1966; Lim, 1970). This and the other observations mentioned above that show a convergent input to spinocervical tract cells from nociceptors makes the possibility of a role of spinocervical tract cells in nociception an attractive one.

In summary, spinocervical tract cells are best identified by antidromic activation following stimulation of the dorsolateral white matter at C3 or C4 and either by failure of antidromic activation from C1 or by evidence of *a slowed conduction velocity between C3 and C1. Most spinocervical tract cells are excited by hair movement with ipsilateral receptive fields. Receptive field sizes are small distally and large proximally. Inhibition, when seen, is not of the surround type. Some spinocervical tract cells are activated by pressure or pinch, as well as, or instead of, hair movement. Furthermore, many spinocervical cells are discharged by noxious heat and by substantial cooling of the skin. The responses to low-intensity mechanical stimulation can be attributed to monosynaptic excitation by cutaneous $A\alpha\beta$ fibers, while the other responses may be due to activation of $A\delta$ and C fibers. There is also a convergent input from high-threshold muscle receptors onto many spinocervical tract cells. The inhibitions are probably due in part to IPSPs, although presynaptic inhibition may also play a role. There is evidence for a somatotopic organization of the spinocervical tract cells within the dorsal horn. It is possible that the spinocervical tract may play a role in pain mechanisms.*

Descending Control of Spinocervical Tract Neurons

Axons in the dorsolateral column presumably belonging to the spinocervical tract were found by Lundberg and Oscarsson (1961) to respond both to touch and to pressure and pinch and also to high-threshold muscle afferents. Stimulation of a descending pathway in the dorsal half of the lateral column did not change the responsiveness of these units to cutaneous stimulation but interfered with their activation by high-threshold muscle afferents. Stimulation of the sensorimotor cortex had only a weak action (Lundberg *et al.*, 1963). Taub (1964) found that axons presumed to belong to the spinocervical tract could be inhibited by stimulation of cutaneous receptors of the head and also by electrical stimulation of the deep cerebellar nuclei and the brainstem tegmentum. Such supraspinal stimulation could produce a constriction of receptive fields.

Wall (1967) studied the effects of descending pathways on interneurons of laminae IV–VI by comparing their responses before, during, and after reversible block of conduction down the cord by cooling (see Chater 4). Some of the neurons were probably spinocervical tract cells. Units in lamina IV increased their spontaneous discharge rate following spinal block, and many developed a wider dynamic range. However, the receptive fields did not expand. Stimulation of the pyramidal tract had no effect on these cells. Units in lamina V also showed an increased excitability following spinal block, and in addition, their receptive fields expanded. Stimulation of the pyramidal tract excited six of these cells, inhibited twelve others, and had no effect on just one. Units in lamina VI responded to skin stimulation and to joint rotation. Spinal block caused an increase in sensitivity to cutaneous stimulation and in most a reduction in responsiveness to joint movement. Pyramidal tract stimulation excited eleven, inhibited seven, and did not affect one of these cells.

Fetz (1968) examined the effects of pyramidal tract stimulation further, looking at changes in the activity of dorsal horn interneurons, including cells projecting into the dorsolateral column. Most of the latter can be presumed to belong to the spinocervical tract. Units in lamina IV were found to have either a narrow or a wide dynamic range. About two-thirds of the cells were inhibited by pyramidal tract volleys. Some cells were weakly excited and then inhibited, and a few were unaffected. Of sixty cells tested, ten were antidromically fired by stimulation of the dorsolateral column. Many cells in lamina VI failed to respond to joint movement. However, pyramidal tract stimulation was found to affect the response to cutaneous or proprioceptive input in the same way, either by facilitating or inhibiting. About two-thirds of the cells were excited by pyramidal tract stimulation, whereas inhibitory, mixed, or no effects were less common. None of the lamina VI cells projected into the dorsolateral column. Fetz suggests that the inhibitory effects on more dorsally located interneurons are produced by pyramidal tract axons arising from the postcruciate cortex, whereas the excitatory actions on more ventrally located neurons are produced by axons from the precruciate cortex (cf. Nyberg-Hansen and Brodal, 1963).

A. G. Brown (1970, 1971) extended his previous work with Franz showing different responsiveness of spinocervical tract neurons to natural stimuli in the spinal state as compared with the decerebrate or anesthetized state by the use of reversible cold block of the cord. This allowed him to characterize a particular unit in an animal with and without a functional transection of the cord. The units were identified by antidromic activation from C3 and not from C1 (or from C1 with a slowed conduction velocity). They were subdivided into four classes (Fig. 7.8). Type I units were excited by the movement of tylotrichs, but not by pressure or pinch; with blocked conduction of descending pathways, these units could be excited by any type of hair but, again, not by pressure or pinch. Type II units were excited by movement of guard hairs and by pressure or pinch in the decerebrate state; in the spinal state they could be activated by any kind of hair and by pressure. Type III units were the most common and responded with a rapidly adapting discharge to movement of any kind of hair and often also with a slowly adapting discharge to pressure or pinch in the decerebrate state; after cold block of the cord, a similar pattern was seen, but the thresholds were lower and all were excited by pressure or pinch. Type IV units were difficult to excite in the decerebrate animal; in the spinal animal they were activated by pinch. A few units did not fit into any of these categories. The sizes of the receptive fields of most units were unaffected by cold block. Spinalization did not result in the development of inhibitory fields in type I units. Some type III units had no inhibitory field in the decerebrate condition but developed one after spinal block, and inhibition was generally easier to elicit in the spinal state.

The discharges of spinocervical tract cells were shown by A. G. Brown et al. (1973b, 1973c) to be inhibited by stimulation of the dorso-lateral fasciculi, the ventral columns (Figs. 7.11 and 7.12) and the dor-sal columns (above a section at L1). Facilitation was not seen. The inhibitory actions were long lasting, with a maximum at 20–40 ms and a duration of 150–250 ms. It was suggested that the inhibitory effects from stimulation of the dorsolateral and ventromedial white matter were mediated by descending pathways. The action of dorsal column stimulation was thought to be secondary to activation of propriospinal

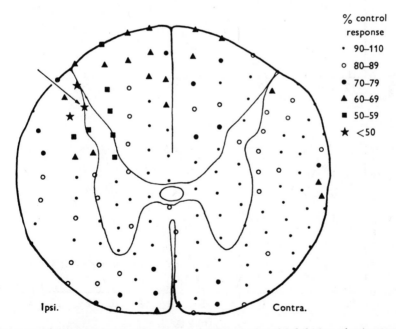

Fig. 7.11. Sites within the spinal cord at C2 that produced inhibition of spinocervical tract neurons. The arrow indicates the only location that when stimulated resulted in antidromic activation. The degree of inhibition is shown by the choice of symbol. (From A. G. Brown et al., 1973.)

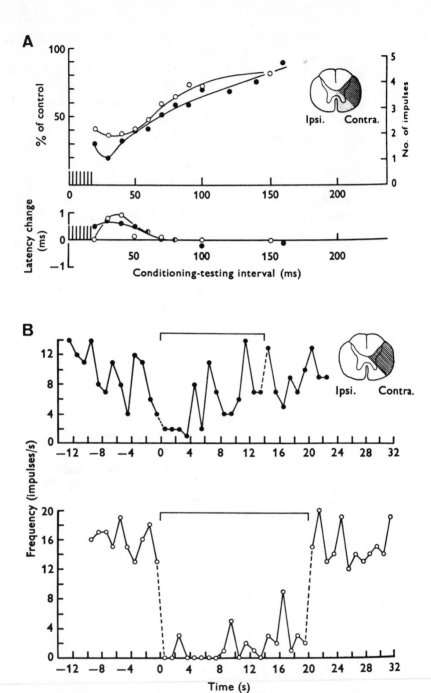

Fig. 7.12. (A) Time course of inhibition of a spinocervical tract cell produced by stimulation of the contralateral dorsolateral fasciculus (filled circles) or ventral funiculus (open circles). (B) Inhibition of spontaneous activity (above) and of the response to noxious mechanical stimulation of a spinocervical tract cell during stimulation of the contralateral dorsolateral fasciculus (below). (From A. G. Brown *et al.*, 1973c.)

neurons. The inhibitory volleys produced P waves recorded from the dorsal surface of the cord; these plus the long time course of the inhibition led to the hypothesis that the inhibitory effects were due to presynaptic inhibition. The pathway mediating the inhibition produced by dorsal column stimulation was investigated further by A. G. Brown and Martin (1973) in animals having an interruption of the dorsal columns at C4. Low-intensity electrical stimulation over the ipsilateral or contralateral dorsal columns or dorsal column nuclei was effective in decerebrate and in decerebrate–decerebellate preparations. However, the inhibition was less after cerebellar removal, suggesting that part of the pathway passes through the cerebellum. The inhibition was eliminated by a transection of the brainstem just above the rostral end of the dorsal column nuclei, indicating that the remainder of the pathway involves the brainstem. It was argued that neurons in the dorsal column nuclei and projecting caudally in the dorsolateral column (Dart, 1971) did not mediate the inhibition, unless the axons of such cells ascend first before descending into the cord.

Stimulation of the SI and SII regions of the cat cerebral cortex was found by A. G. Brown and Short (1974) and A. G. Brown et al. (1977a) to produce a profound inhibition of spinocervical tract cells, as well as cord dorsum P waves. There was also weak excitation of some neurons from areas 5 and 7. The inhibition was abolished by bilateral sectioning of the dorsolateral funiculus and reduced by barbiturate anesthesia. Several different cytoarchitectural areas, including area 4, were shown to be effective by use of microstimulation (A. G. Brown et al., 1977a). The effects of barbiturate presumably account for the negative results of Lundberg et al. (1963) in otherwise similar experiments.

In summary, there is ample evidence that descending pathways, both from the brainstem and from the cerebral cortex, affect the response properties of spinocervical tract neurons. The descending pathways generally inhibit the cells and tend to make the cells more selective in terms of what receptor types activate them. However, some of the descending actions are excitatory in sign. The inhibition may be presynaptic. The important point is that the sensory information signaled by the spinocervical tract is in part determined by pathways descending from the brain. Stimulation of the sensorimotor cortex may be excitatory or inhibitory, whereas unidentified pathways descending in the dorsolateral fasciculi and in the ventral columns produce a long-lasting inhibition.

Responses of Neurons of the Lateral Cervical Nucleus

Morin et al. (1963) recorded the activity of neurons in the lateral cervical nucleus of the cat. Of the 160 cells studied, 125 responded to touch, 27 to pressure, 5 to joint movement, and 3 to touch and pressure. More receptive fields were on the limbs than on the body. The tactile responses were rapidly adapting ones to hair movement. The cells excited by pressure had slowly adapting responses. Several cells required intense stimulation. The units activated by joint movement were sensitive to both rate and the amount of the movement. Receptive field size varied from restricted to very large. The cells with large (more than one segment of a limb or a whole limb) or very large (trunk and two limbs) fields represented 64% of the population.

Kitai *et al.* (1965) obtained somewhat different results in a study of the lateral cervical nucleus of the dog. Some of the cells had a rapidly adapting response to touch and a slowly adapting response to pressure; otherwise, the description of the classes of units resembled that in the cat. However, the proportion of units with restricted receptive fields was high in the dog (86 of 136 neurons), in contrast to the cat (36% of neurons). The lateral cervical nucleus of the raccoon was similar to that of the dog (Ha *et al.*, 1965) in having a large proportion of neurons (about 72%) with restricted receptive fields. Furthermore, none of the units in the raccoon responded to joint movement. Most were responsive to touch, while some were responsive to pressure. It should be noted that receptive fields were found on the glabrous skin.

Oswaldo-Cruz and Kidd (1964) found both similarities and differences in the activity of neurons of the lateral cervical nucleus of the cat when comparing their results with those of Morin *et al.* (1963). Of the 164 neurons studied, 73% were activated by hair movement in a rapidly adapting fashion. Other cells were excited by skin contact or by subcutaneous receptors. The latter were not joint receptors, but instead were often in fascia. A few atypical cells had discontinuous or very large receptive fields. Most receptive fields were relatively restricted, although distal ones were much smaller than proximal ones (Fig. 7.13). Surround inhibition was not detected, although a few cells did have inhibitory receptive fields. No somatotopic organization was noted. Synaptic coupling was secure enough that many cells would follow stimuli repeated at 50 Hz.

Horrobin (1966) also recorded the activity of neurons in the lateral cervical nucleus of the cat. He identified the neurons by antidromic invasion from the contralateral medial lemniscus. About 90% of the cells were activated by tactile stimuli. Of these, most were excited by hair movement, while some were fired by touch or claw receptors. A few cells were activated by noxious stimuli, pressure over a muscle belly, or by convergent inputs (hair movement and pressure). The receptive fields were distributed over the body, with no preference for rostral or caudal regions of the nucleus to respond to stimulation in the rostral

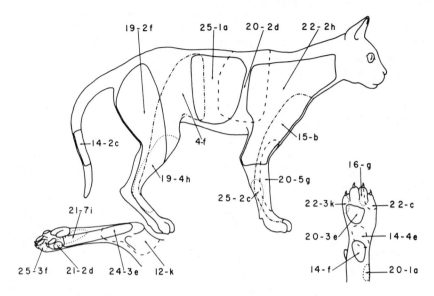

Fig. 7.13. Receptive fields of neurons in the lateral cervical nucleus responsive to hair movement. (From Oswaldo-Cruz and Kidd, 1964.)

or caudal parts of the body. However, forelimb units appeared to be concentrated laterally and hindlimb units medially in the nucleus, although there was overlap. Most of the receptive fields were relatively large, although smaller ones were found on the forelimb than on the hindlimb. The axons within the medial lemniscus seemed to be somatotopically organized: the axons of cells with forelimb receptive fields were dorsolateral and those of cells with hindlimb fields were dorsomedial in the medial lemniscus. Inhibition was demonstrated for only a few cells, and it was not of the surround type. Most of the inhibited cells received a convergent input or responded just to pressure. The cells that responded just to noxious stimuli were excited from all of the ipsilateral body and inhibited from the contralateral side. The inhibitory receptive fields were either contralateral or on the other limb of the same side. Stimulation within the cerebellum did not antidromically activate any of the cells, confirming the finding that the lateral cervical nucleus does not project to the cerebellum (Grant *et al.*, 1968). Only two cells were activated synaptically following cerebellar stimulation. It was concluded that the afferents to the lateral cervical nucleus are not collaterals of spinocerebellar tracts. Evidence was found that collaterals from the cervicothalamic tract terminate in the inferior olivary nucleus, since some lateral cervical nucleus cells could be antidromically fired by stimulation within the contralateral inferior olivary nucleus; all such neurons were also antidromically activated from the contralateral medial lemniscus.

Inhibition of neurons in the lateral cervical nucleus was examined further by Fedina *et al.* (1968). They obtained evidence for both post-synaptic inhibition of cells in the lateral cervical nucleus and presynaptic inhibition of the input over the spinocervical tract. The inhibitory actions were from a wide area of the body and seemed to depend heavily upon transmission through pathways in the ventrolateral columns. Inhibition could be produced by natural or electrical stimulation of cutaneous afferents, as well as by electrical stimulation of high-threshold muscle afferents.

In summary, the cells of the lateral cervical nucleus respond as might be predicted, given a convergent input to them from several spinocervical tract axons. The majority of lateral cervical nucleus cells are activated by tactile stimuli, but some respond to pressure or to stimulation of subcutaneous receptors. Receptive fields tend to be relatively small if distal or large if proximal. A few receptive fields are very large. Inhibition, when observed, is not of the surround type. Inhibition can be attributed both to pre- and postsynaptic inhibition within the lateral cervical nucleus, as well as to inhibition at the level of spinocervical tract neurons.

THE SPINOMEDULLOTHALAMIC PATHWAY

Recent work has shown that group I afferents from hindlimb muscles provide information to the cerebral cortex over a previously unrecognized pathway, the spinomedullothalamic path (Fig. 7.1). The group I afferents synapse on spinal neurons at the level of Clarke's column and also caudal to Clarke's column. Axons of these cells ascend in the dorsolateral fasciculus and end within a cell group once considered part of the vestibular complex called nucleus z. The cells of nucleus z project contralaterally by way of the medial lemniscus to the thalamus, terminating in parts of the ventral posterior lateral nucleus and its boundary with the ventral lateral nucleus. The thalamic cells in turn project to the sensorimotor cortex. The pathway is specific to the hindlimbs; group I afferents from the forelimbs utilize the dorsal column pathway.

Phylogeny

Most of the work on the spinomedullothalamic pathway has been done in cats. However, a nucleus comparable to the cat nucleus z has been described in human material (Sadjadpour and Brodal, 1968), suggesting that there may be a similar pathway in man. There is also a nucleus z in the monkey, and it receives a synaptic input from fibers in the dorsolateral fasciculus (Nijensohn and Kerr, 1975).

Morphology of the Spinomedullothalamic Pathway

A pathway from the spinal cord to nucleus z (Fig. 7.14) was first recognized by Pompeiano and Brodal (1957). Previous authors had considered these fibers to be spinovestibular projections, since they accompany ascending axons to the vestibular complex proper. Although nucleus z was listed among the nuclei of the vestibular complex by Brodal and Pompeiano (1957), this was because of topographic rather than functional relations. Since nucleus z receives no vestibular afferents (Walberg et al., 1958) and projects to the thalamus (Grant et al., 1973), it is proper to consider it a part of the somatosensory system rather than the vestibular system.

The cells of origin of the spinomedullothalamic pathway appear to be located at least in part below the level of Clarke's column, since ample ascending degeneration can be seen in nucleus z following midlumbar lesions (Pompeiano and Brodal, 1957; however, cf. Landgren and Silfvenius, 1971). Recordings have revealed the presence of cells at L5 and L6 in the medial base of the dorsal horn and intermediate region (Fig. 7.15) that respond to group I muscle afferent volleys and that project rostrally at least to C1 (Aoyama et al., 1973). At least some of these cells project to the cerebellum and may be considered a component of the dorsal spinocerebellar tract. However, these and/or cells of Clarke's column appear to give off axon collaterals that end in nucleus z (Johansson and Silfvenius, 1977a), and so the cells observed by Aoyama et al. (1973) may correspond to a part of the origin of the spinomedullothalamic pathway. Against this possibility is the observation that these cells receive a convergent input from several muscles (see below), unlike nucleus z cells, which are generally activated by just one muscle (Johansson and Silfvenius, 1977a).

The ascending pathway to nucleus z is chiefly through the dorsal part of the lateral funiculus (Pompeiano and Brodal, 1957; Busch, 1961; Landgren and Silfvenius, 1971; Rustioni, 1973; Nijensohn and Kerr, 1975), although some second-order fibers of the dorsal column end in nucleus z (Rustioni, 1973). In addition, Hand (1966) found that a few primary afferents reach nucleus z (see also Johansson and Silfvenius, 1977a; however, cf. Pompeiano and Brodal 1957; Landgren and Silfvenius, 1971).

The axons of neurons of nucleus z project to the contralateral thalamus by way of the medial lemniscus, and they terminate in the rostral part of the ventral posterior lateral nucleus (lateral segment) and in the ventral lateral nucleus (Grant *et al.*, 1973). Projections from this part of the thalamus ascend to the cerebral cortex, accounting for the group I activity from hindlimb muscle nerves that can be recorded in the sensorimotor areas (Landgren *et al.*, 1967; Landgren and Silfvenius, 1971). Presumably, the spinomedullothalamic pathway is also responsible for conveying hindlimb group I afferent input to the sensory cortex of primates (e.g., Hore *et al.*, 1976), although this possibility does not seem to have been investigated yet.

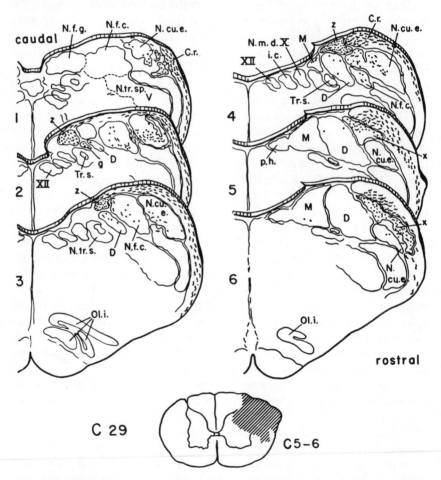

Fig. 7.14. Terminal degeneration in nucleus z of the cat following dorsolateral cordotomy. (From Pompeiano and Brodal, 1957.)

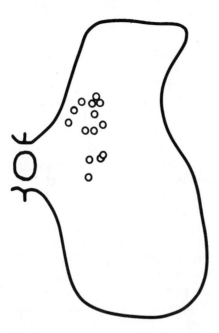

Fig. 7.15. Locations of cells in the segment of the cat spinal cord responding to group I muscle afferent volleys. (From Aoyama et al., 1973.)

Responses of Spinal Neurons That May or Do Project to Nucleus z

The cells investigated by Aoyama et al. (1973) generated monosynaptic excitatory postsynaptic potentials (EPSPs) following electrical stimulation of group I fibers of hindlimb muscle nerves. Responses to graded stimulus strengths suggested that both group Ia and group Ib fibers contributed to the EPSPs. Some cells were excited by volleys in only one muscle nerve, but most could be activated by input from more than one nerve. Furthermore, a few of the cells had a convergent input from skin or joint afferents. The conduction velocities of the ascending axons ranged from 27 to 114 m/s.

Recordings were made by Magherini et al. (1974, 1975) from the axons of some ascending tract cells at the level of nucleus z. The axons had a conduction velocity of about 100 m/s. They responded monosynaptically to sinusoidal stretch of hindlimb muscle at amplitudes of stretch that selectively excite group Ia muscle spindle afferents. The responses of some units increased as the stimulus recruited secondary endings, indicating a convergence of group Ia and group II afferents on some tract cells.

Responses of Neurons in Nucleus z

Landgren and Silfvenius (1971) found that volleys in group I afferents of hindlimb muscles evoked by electrical stimulation activated cells in nucleus z. Group II afferents contributed an additional excitation of some cells. There was also a convergent input in some cases from cutaneous afferents. The muscle input was powerful, since many cells could follow repetitive stimulation at rates of 150–200 Hz. Most cells were activated by stimulation of just one muscle nerve, some by just cutaneous input, and some both by muscle and cutaneous volleys. Some of the neurons were antidromically activated following stimulation in the contralateral medial lemniscus.

Magherini *et al.* (1974, 1975) utilized sinusoidal stretch of hindlimb muscles to test the effects of group Ia and group II muscle afferents upon cells in nucleus z. Such stimuli excited nucleus z cells or produced excitation followed by inhibition. The latencies of discharges indicated that at least in some instances there was a disynaptic connection between primary afferents and cells of nucleus z. Alterations in the amplitudes of the stretch stimuli showed that most units were excited by group Ia afferents, although some were in addition activated by group II fibers (in a few cases by group II alone). Dynamic but not static stretch also excited the neurons. Only two of the twelve units tested were antidromically activated from the contralateral medial lemniscus.

The question of whether the input to the neurons of nucleus z is at least in part by way of collaterals of the dorsal spinocerebellar tract was recently investigated by Johansson and Silfvenius (1977a). They stimulated within the cerebellum and looked for responses of neurons in nucleus z, especially in cells proven to project to the thalamus by antidromic activation. Most of the nucleus z cells were excited by cerebellar stimulation, and a collision test indicated that the excitation in at least half the cases was transmitted via the dorsal spinocerebellar tract. Johansson and Silfvenius (1977b) also studied cells in nucleus z that were not antidromically activated from stimulation of the medial lemniscus. The responses were often like those of relay cells, but many of these neurons were excited by cutaneous afferents or by low-threshold joint afferents. It is likely that many of these cells actually project to the thalamus but that technical factors prevented the demonstration of antidromic activation. The ones excited by joint afferents may account for the information that reaches the cerebral cortex from joint afferents via the dorsolateral fasciculus (Clark *et al.*, 1973). Cells of the dorsal spinocerebellar tract have been described that are activated by joint afferents (Lindström and Takata, 1972; Kuno *et al.*, 1973).

Descending Control of the Spinomedullothalamic Pathway

Virtually nothing is known about a possible descending control of the spinomedullothalamic tract. Johansson and Silfvenius (1977a) observed a synaptic excitation of some nucleus z units following stimulation in the contralateral diencephalon. Otherwise this issue does not seem to have been investigated. Since the dorsal spinocerebellar tract is under the control of the pyramidal tract (cf. Hongo and Okada, 1967; Hongo *et al.*, 1967), it can be predicted that stimulation of the pyramidal tract should also affect transmission through the spinomedullothalamic tract.

In summary, the cells of origin of the spinomedullothalamic tract may include neurons of Clarke's column and also dorsal horn neurons at levels of the cord caudal to Clarke's column. The pathway ascends in the dorsolateral fasciculus to end in nucleus z. From here, the pathway continues to the contralateral VPL and VL nuclei of the thalamus and thence to the sensorimotor cortex. The spinomedullary tract cells and cells of nucleus z are activated by group Ia and sometimes also group II muscle afferents. Some cells have convergent inputs, although most are activated by afferents of just a single muscle. It is possible that low-threshold joint afferents also utilize this pathway.

CONCLUSIONS

1. Judging from the presence of a lateral cervical nucleus, the spinocervicothalamic pathway is present in a variety of mammals, including monkeys and probably man. Some mammals have a cell column beginning in the usual location of the lateral cervical nucleus but extending the length of the spinal cord. It is not known if this column projects to the thalamus.

2. The cells of origin of the spinocervical tract are concentrated in lamina IV of the dorsal horn. There may in addition be such cells in laminae I and V–VIII.

3. The spinocervical tract ascends ipsilaterally in the dorsolateral fasciculus.

4. The spinocervical tract terminates in the lateral cervical nucleus. The tract does not appear to consist of collaterals of the dorsal spinocerebellar tract, as has sometimes been proposed.

5. The majority of the terminals of the spinocervical tract are axodendritic. Cells of the lateral cervical nucleus receive numerous synapses from other sources in addition to the spinocervical tract.

6. The lateral cervical nucleus extends from the caudal medulla to the caudal margin of C2. In the cat, there are at least 3000 cells on each side.

7. The lateral cervical nucleus does not project to the cerebellum, as was originally proposed. A possible projection to the contralateral inferior olivary nucleus is controversial. The main projection is to the contralateral thalamus by way of the medial lemniscus. The particular nuclei of termination include the ventral posterior lateral (VPL), medial part of the posterior (PO_m), and the magnocellular medial geniculate nuclei.

8. Spinocervical tract neurons respond to electrical and natural stimuli in much the same way as do other dorsal horn interneurons. Some of the cells are activated just by innocuous mechanical stimuli, while others are in addition excited by pressure and pinch.

9. Some spinocervical tract cells are excited just by A fibers, while others are excited by both A and C fibers. The A fibers in the case of the latter type of cell would include $A\delta$ as well as $A\alpha\beta$ fibers. The responses to C fiber volleys show "windup," a progressive increase in responses with stimuli repeated at intervals less than 3 s.

10. Spinocervical tract cells can have peripheral inhibitory receptive fields, but these fields are not arranged in a surround fashion.

11. Intracellular recordings reveal that spinocervical tract cells generate monosynaptic EPSPs in response to volleys in cutaneous nerves and polysynaptic EPSPs following high-threshold muscle afferent volleys. Cutaneous volleys also evoke disynaptic IPSPs. Mechanical stimuli applied to the skin can produce IPSPs in spinocervical tract cells.

12. It is likely that presynaptic inhibition plays a significant role in limiting the responses of spinocervical tract cells to peripheral inputs.

13. The specificity of the inputs to spinocervical tract cells depends upon the integrity of pathways descending from the brain. In intact anesthetized cats or in decerebrate cats, spinocervical neurons can be found that respond just to guard or to tylotrich hairs, as well as others that have a convergent input. In spinalized animals, units activated by hair did not respond to just one type of hair, but rather to all types.

14. Spinocervical tract cells are often responsive to intense thermal stimuli, including noxious heat and intense cold.

15. Spinocervical tract cells have a somatotopic organization like that of other dorsal horn interneurons.

16. Many spinocervical tract cells can be activated following the intraarterial injection of algesic chemicals into the circulation of skeletal muscle.

17. It is likely that spinocervical tract cells play a role in pain mechanisms.

18. Pyramidal tract volleys often inhibit spinocervical tract cells. Inhibition or sometimes a weak facilitation results from stimulation of the sensorimotor cortex.

19. Other descending inhibitory pathways descend in the dorsolateral fasciculi and in the ventral funiculi. The dorsolateral path is probably involved in determining the receptive field selectivity mentioned in statement 13. There is also an inhibitory pathway that includes an ascending limb in the dorsal column and a relay both in the cerebellum and in the caudal medulla.

20. Neurons in the lateral cervical nucleus commonly respond to tactile stimuli, although some respond to convergent inputs or to joint movement. Receptive fields can be very large, but sometimes they are restricted. Inhibitory receptive fields, when present, are not of the surround type.

21. Both presynaptic and postsynaptic inhibition are found at the level of the lateral cervical nucleus.

22. Nucleus z, a brainstem nucleus that was originally described as part of the vestibular complex has now been shown to project to the contralateral thalamus and is a somatosensory relay.

23. The spinomedullothalamic pathway originates from cells in the cord gray matter. Some of the cells are probably in Clarke's column, but others are at levels caudal to Clarke's column.

24. The spinomedullary pathway ascends in the dorsolateral fasciculus to end in nucleus z. At least part of this projection is formed by collaterals of axons of the dorsal spinocerebellar tract.

25. Nucleus z projects via the medial lemniscus to the contralateral thalamus. The terminals are in the rostral part of VPL and the adjacent ventral lateral (VL) nucleus.

26. Neurons in nucleus z respond to group I muscle afferent volleys and sometimes also to group II muscle afferents. There may be a cutaneous input to some cells. Sinusoidal stretch of muscle shows that the group I effects on cells of nucleus z are due in part to an input from group Ia muscle spindle afferents.

8 Sensory Pathways in the Ventral Quadrant

This chapter will be concerned with several pathways in the ventral quadrant of the spinal cord—the spinothalamic, spinoreticular, and spinotectal tracts.

THE SPINOTHALAMIC TRACT

The spinothalamic tract in primates originates largely from neurons in the dorsal horn of the spinal cord. The axon of a given spinothalamic tract cell decussates in the same or in a nearby segment and ascends in the ventrolateral white matter to the thalamus (Fig. 8.1). Associated with the spinothalamic tract are other pathways, several of which are often regarded as forming with the spinothalamic tract a system of direct and indirect projections to the thalamus. The indirect pathways include the spinoreticular (Fig. 8.1) and the spinotectal tracts. These will be discussed separately. The spinothalamic tract is often subdivided into a lateral and a ventral spinothalamic tract. The lateral spinothalamic tract is traditionally considered to carry pain and temperature information, while the ventral spinothalamic tract is supposed to convey tactile and pressure data to the brain. It is not evident at this time whether or not such a subdivision is warranted.

Phylogeny of the Spinothalamic Tract

Although Gowers (1878) suggested that pain and temperature sensation is transmitted by fibers in the ventrolateral white matter, Edinger (1889, 1890) is generally regarded as the first to suggest a

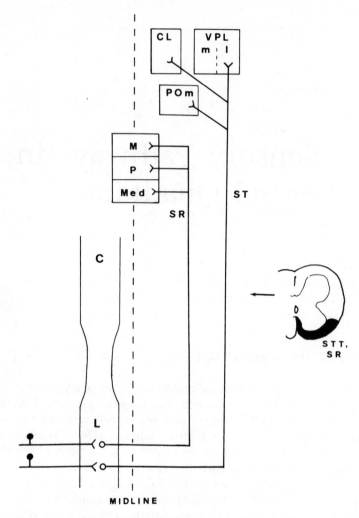

Fig. 8.1. The spinothalamic and spinoreticular tracts. For simplicity, the pathways through the cervical (C) enlargement are not shown. Primary afferents enter the lumbar (L) cord and synapse on tract cells. Second-order projections in the spinothalamic tract (ST) decussate and ascend to end in the medial part of the posterior complex (PO$_m$), the central lateral (CL) intralaminar nucleus, and the ventral posterior lateral (VPL) nucleus (lateral part, l). The spinoreticular tract (SR) is shown decussating also, but in some animals it is a bilateral pathway, and in primates it may be chiefly uncrossed. It terminates in a variety of nuclei of the reticular formation of the brainstem (Med, medulla; P, pons; M, midbrain). The portion of the pathway that ends in the midbrain can also be considered part of the spinotectal projection. The transverse section of the spinal cord shows the location of the spinothalamic tract (STT) and the spinoreticular tract (SR) in the ventral quadrant.

direct projection from the spinal cord to the thalamus in amphibia and in the cat. A number of investigators since Edinger have failed to confirm the presence of a spinothalamic tract in the cat using the Marchi technique or have found just a few fibers (Patrick, 1896; Chang and Ruch, 1947b; Morin et al., 1951). However, it is now known that there is at least a moderate-sized spinothalamic tract in the cat, since terminal degeneration following cordotomy is found in specific diencephalic nuclei when the Glees, Nauta, or Fink–Heimer techniques are used (Getz, 1952; Anderson and Berry, 1959; Mehler, 1966, 1969; Boivie, 1971b; Jones and Burton, 1974). Apparently, the spinothalamic tract is more substantial in the dog than in the cat, since heavy degeneration has been seen with the Marchi technique in dogs following spinal cord lesions (Hagg and Ha, 1970). Other mammalian species that have been shown to have a spinothalamic tract include the marsupial phalanger (Rockel et al., 1972), opossum (Mehler, 1969; Hazlett et al., 1972), rat (Lund and Webster, 1967b; Mehler, 1969), hedgehog (Jane and Schroeder, 1971), pig (Breazile and Kitchell, 1968), sheep (Rao et al., 1969), and primate (Mott, 1895; W. E. L. Clark, 1936; Walker, 1938; Weaver and Walker, 1941; Chang and Ruch, 1947b; Morin et al., 1951; Poirier and Bertrand, 1955; Mehler et al., 1960; Bowsher, 1961; Schroeder and Jane, 1971; Kerr and Lippman, 1974; Kerr, 1975b), including man (Thiele and Horsley, 1901; Collier and Buzzard, 1903; Goldstein, 1910; Foerster and Gagel, 1931; Walker, 1940; Gardner and Cuneo, 1945; Kuru, 1949; Bowsher, 1957; Poirier and Bertrand, 1955; Mehler, 1962, 1969, 1974). Some of these studies, like that of Edinger, failed to take into account damage to the cervicothalamic tract, but in many investigations the lesions used have involved levels below the upper cervical cord.

There is very little evidence about the existence of a direct spinothalamic pathway in nonmammalian vertebrates. No such projection was found in a representative species each of elasmobranch fish, teleost fish, and amphibia by Hayle (1973). However, Burr (1928) claimed to have traced a spinothalamic tract through the brainstem of a teleost (the deep-sea sunfish). Confirmation of such a pathway using experimental techniques is needed before it can be accepted that a true spinothalamic projection occurs in fish. Similarly, Herrick (1939) found a spinothalamic tract in the larvae of the tiger salamander in Golgi-stained preparations. Experimental studies are needed to determine if amphibia do indeed have a spinothalamic tract. As for reptiles, the evidence is divided. Goldby and Robinson (1962) failed to find a spinothalamic projection in one species of lizard, while Ebbesson (1967) could in the tegu lizard. There is a brief report that mentions a spinothalamic tract in a species of bird (Karten, 1963).

Anatomy of the Spinothalamic Tract

The cells of origin of the spinothalamic tract were suggested to be in the dorsal horn, since retrograde chromatolysis is seen in neurons there in monkeys (Fig. 8.2) and man after the contralateral spinothalamic tract is interrupted by cordotomy (Foerster and Gagel, 1931; Kuru, 1949; Morin *et al.*, 1951; Smith, 1976; Kerr, 1975a). Ipsilateral cells also show chromatolysis, but they were regarded as cells of origin of other tracts, since the sensory deficit associated with interruption of the spinothalamic tract is crossed. There were also chromatolytic cells in the contralateral ventral horn, but these were believed to belong to the ventral spinocerebellar or other tracts not ascending to the thalamus. Among the cells considered to project into the spinothalamic tract were neurons in the marginal zone or lamina I (Kuru, 1949; Morin *et al.*, 1951). Kuru (1949) suggested that these were involved in pain and temperature discrimination, while others found in the nucleus proprius region were concerned with touch, since the relative amount of chromatolysis in these two parts of the dorsal horn could be correlated with dissociated sensory losses following partial cordotomies.

Electrophysiological mapping experiments have utilized histologic

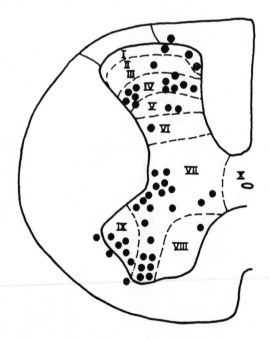

Fig. 8.2. Locations of neurons in the spinal cord gray matter showing retrograde chromatolysis following anterolateral cordotomy at a more rostral level. (From Kerr, 1975a.)

reconstructions of points at which recordings could be made of the activity of cells antidromically activated by stimulation in the contralateral diencephalon. Maps of this kind have been done in the rat, cat, and monkey. In the cervical enlargement of the cat spinal cord, most of the spinothalamic tract cells were found by Dilly et al. (1968) to be in laminae V and VI, although one was in lamina I. The one cell found in the lumbosacral enlargement was in the ventral horn. Trevino et al. (1972) mapped the distribution of spinothalamic tract cells in the lumbosacral enlargement of the cat cord and found most to be in laminae VII and VIII, although some were in laminae V and VI (Fig. 8.3A). The distribution of chromatolytic neurons in the cat lumbosacral spinal cord following spinal cord lesions agrees very well with these findings (Fig. 8.22A) (Molenaar et al., 1974). Trevino and Carstens (1975) succeeded in mapping spinothalamic tract cell distributions in the cat and monkey using the retrograde transport of horseradish peroxidase injected into the diencephalon as a marker. The cells of origin of the spinothalamic tract in the cat had the distribution described by Dilly et al. (1968) in the cervical enlargement and that described by Trevino et al. (1972) in the lumbosacral enlargement (Fig. 8.3B). In addition, many cells in lamina I were also marked. The electrophysiological recordings were evidently biased in favor of the larger neurons found more ventrally than lamina I.

Because of the likelihood of a species difference, Trevino et al. (1973) repeated the mapping study in the monkey lumbosacral spinal cord. Unlike the case of the cat, the greatest concentration of spinothalamic tract neurons in the monkey cord was in the dorsal horn, especially in lamina V (Fig. 8.3C). There were also numerous spinothalamic cells in laminae I, IV, and VI of the dorsal horn, and some in laminae VII and VIII. Albe-Fessard's group (Levante et al., 1973; Albe-Fessard et al., 1974) confirmed the presence of a concentration of spinothalamic tract cells in lamina V of the monkey spinal cord. Although most of the spinothalamic tract cells in the cat and monkey were contralateral to the side of the diencephalon being stimulated, at least a few were found ipsilaterally (Trevino et al., 1972, 1973). The location of spinothalamic tract cells in the monkey has been confirmed in the horseradish peroxidase experiments of Trevino and Carstens (1975). The cells are located chiefly in laminae I, IV and V, but there are some in laminae VI–VIII (Fig. 8.3D). There are more ventral horn spinothalamic tract cells in the lumbosacral than in the cervical enlargement. Most of the cells are contralateral to the site of the thalamic injection, but a few are ipsilateral. These findings were in part confirmed by Albe-Fessard et al. (1975), who found labeled cells in

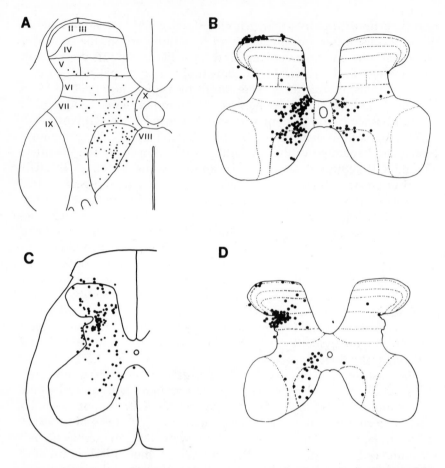

Fig. 8.3. Locations of spinothalamic tract neurons in the lumbosacral enlargement of the cat spinal cord as determined (A) by antidromic activation and (B) by retrograde labeling by horseradish peroxidase. Locations of spinothalamic tract neurons in the monkey lumbosacral spinal cord are shown for antidromic activation experiments in C and for horseradish peroxidase labeling in D. (A from Trevino *et al.*, 1972; B and D from Trevino and Carstens, 1975; C from Trevino *et al.*, 1973.)

lamina I of the contralateral dorsal horn after horseradish peroxidase was injected to the intralaminar nuclei and in laminae I, IV, and V after injections into VPL.

The distribution of spinothalamic tract cells in the rat lumbar cord was mapped electrophysiologically by Giesler *et al.* (1976). Most of the cells were in the base of the dorsal horn, although some were in the marginal zone, intermediate region, and ventral horn. The observation that spinothalamic tract neurons are concentrated in the dorsal horn in the rat has been confirmed by horseradish peroxidase labeling (Giesler *et al.*, 1977). Thus, the distribution of spinothalamic tract cells in the rat more closely resembles the pattern in the primate than in the cat.

The details of how afferent information reaches spinothalamic tract neurons are unknown. Some of the input is undoubtedly by monosynaptic connections of primary afferents with the cells, but part of the input is likely to be polysynaptic (Foreman *et al.*, 1975a). The role of the substantia gelatinosa is at present speculative (Pearson, 1952; Melzack and Wall, 1965; Kerr, 1975a).

The projection path of the axons of spinothalamic tract cells to the contralateral side of the cord is traditionally thought to involve the anterior white commissure. However, Kuru (1949) states that the posteromarginal cells, i.e., lamina I cells, project across the posterior commissure. Ramon y Cajal (1909) illustrated dorsal horn neurons in Golgi material that sent axons across the posterior commissure, but he states that marginal neurons that decussate do so across the anterior commissure. The clinical studies of Foerster and Gagel (1931) led to their suggestion that the crossing must occur within the same segment as that containing the cell body. Gardner and Cuneo (1945) concluded that the decussation is within two segments. However, the axons may remain medially in the ventrolateral white matter for the first several segments of their ascent toward the brain (White *et al.*, 1956). This would help account for the fact that the level of sensory loss following cordotomy in human patients is generally several segments lower than the level of the cordotomy (White and Sweet, 1955). In most cases, the cordotomy does not extend all the way to the midline, so some of the ascending axons from immediately adjacent segments can be expected to remain intact. In addition, pain afferents entering the cord over a particular dorsal root synapse not only at the same segmental level but also over one or two segments rostrally (and caudally). Furthermore, propriospinal connections are then made between neurons of the substantia gelatinosa over several segments; thus, spinothalamic tract cells in several segments may be affected from input originating from a given dermatome (Ranson, 1913b; 1914; Hyndman, 1942; Earle, 1952; LaMotte, 1977). A cordotomy at a particular level will not, therefore, necessarily prevent input from lower levels from reaching spinothalamic tract cells located above the lesion. An additional lesion of Lissauer's fasciculus, not surprisingly, will raise the level of the sensory loss (Hyndman, 1942).

The ascending axons of the spinothalamic tract appear to be myelinated. Lippman and Kerr (1972) examined the region of the ascending degeneration in the ventrolateral quadrant of the monkey spinal cord following multisegmental myelotomies (interrupting spinotha-lamic but, in the monkey, not spinoreticular axons). Degenerating my-elinated axons ranged from less than 2 μm to 7 μm in diameter (not counting the larger axons of the ventral spinocerebellar tract at the pe-riphery of the cord). This spectrum of fiber sizes is somewhat smaller than that predicted from the conduction velocities found for primate spinothalamic tract cells (7–74 m/s, mean 40 m/s) (Willis *et al.*, 1974). Electron microscopy of the region occupied by the spinothalamic tract revealed very few unmyelinated fibers, even in normal control mate-rial (Lippman and Kerr, 1972).

There is at least a rough somatotopic organization of the spinotha-lamic tract in the ventrolateral white matter of the spinal cord (Horrax, 1929; Weaver and Walker, 1941; Foerster and Gagel, 1931). The caudal parts of the body are represented dorsolaterally (Hyndman and Van Epps, 1939; Applebaum *et al.*, 1975) or laterally (Walker, 1940) and the more rostral parts ventromedially or medially in the tract (Fig. 8.4). The spinothalamic tract does not form a compact bundle as was once thought based on the early clinical experience with cordotomies (e.g., Frazier, 1920). Instead, it is presumably widely distributed across the ventrolateral white matter, since adequate pain relief in human pa-tients is produced only by extensive cordotomies (Kahn and Peet, 1948; White *et al.*, 1956). Mapping of the distribution of spinothalamic tract axons in the ventrolateral white matter of the monkey spinal cord (Fig. 8.4) confirms the widespread distribution of the axons, as well as the rough somatotopic organization (Applebaum *et al.*, 1975).

It was suggested by Foerster and Gagel (1931) that there is a com-ponent of the spinothalamic tract mediating touch and pressure lo-cated deep within the ventrolateral white matter. This supported the postulate that there is a separate ventral spinothalamic tract responsi-ble for mediating tactile sensibility. There are undoubtedly spinotha-lamic tract fibers in the ventral funiculus (Kerr, 1975b; Applebaum *et al.*, 1975), but it is not clear that these have a function that is distinct from that of the remainder of the tract. Electrophysiological work suggests that the axons of spinothalamic tract cells activated by tactile stimuli are intermingled with those of cells responding only to high-intensity stimulation, both in the lateral column and probably also in the ventral column (Fig. 8.5) (Applebaum *et al.*, 1975). The only seg-regated axons are those activated by proprioceptive stimuli; they form a band along the ventral margin of the white matter.

The spinothalamic tract ascends through the lower medulla in a position just dorsolateral to the inferior olivary nucleus (Fig. 6.11) and through the remainder of the brainstem dorsolateral to the medial lem-niscus (Walker, 1940, 1942b; Morin *et al.*, 1951; Mehler *et al.*, 1960;

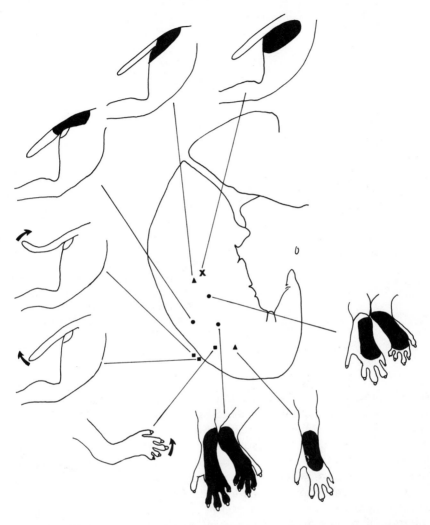

Fig. 8.4. Somatotopic organization of the primate spinothalamic tract at an upper lumbar level. Receptive fields on the skin are indicated by the blackened areas; receptive fields in deep tissues demonstrated by joint movements are indicated by the arrows. (From Applebaum *et al.*, 1975.)

Mehler, 1962; Kerr, 1975b). The somatotopic arrangement is thought to be preserved in the brainstem (Weaver and Walker, 1941; Morin *et al.*, 1951). It is not known what proportion of the axons ascending to the thalamus give off collaterals to the reticular formation, tectum, or to other nuclear groups within the brainstem, but numerous fibers ac-

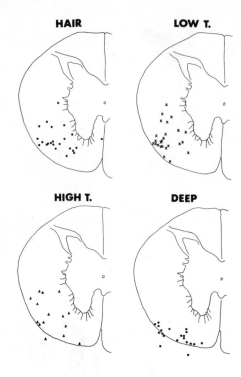

Fig. 8.5. Locations of the axons of spinothalamic tract cells in the monkey spinal cord. Recordings were made at an upper lumbar level. Many of the hair-activated and low-threshold cells responded to a wide dynamic range of inputs. (From Applebaum *et al.*, 1975.)

companying the spinothalamic tract proper do terminate in regions caudal to the diencephalon (Kuru, 1949; Morin *et al.*, 1951; Anderson and Berry, 1959; Mehler *et al.*, 1960; Mehler, 1962; Kerr, 1975b). However, collateralization is presumably uncommon, since commissural myelotomy results in degeneration of only a few terminals within the reticular formation, whereas this procedure produces degeneration of the spinothalamic projection (Kerr and Lippman, 1974).

The areas of termination of the spinothalamic tract within the diencephalon include the ventrobasal complex, the posterior nuclear group and the intralaminar nuclei (Anderson and Berry, 1959; Mehler *et al.*, 1960; Mehler, 1962, 1974; Jones and Burton, 1974). Several investigators (Getz, 1952; Bowsher, 1961; Breazile and Kitchell, 1968) observed terminals in the thalamic reticular nucleus, but this was not confirmed by others (Anderson and Berry, 1959; Mehler *et al.*, 1960; Mehler, 1969; Boivie, 1971b; Jones and Burton, 1974). There is a small component in the monkey which crosses in Gudden's supraoptic commissure (Morin *et al.*, 1951); other fibers cross in the tectal and posterior commissures (Chang and Ruch, 1947b; Mehler *et al.*, 1960; Bowsher, 1961).

Some species differences in termination of the spinothalamic tract have been noted. For instance, the termination of the spinothalamic tract in the ventrobasal complex of the rat is rostral to that of the dorsal column nuclei (Lund and Webster, 1967b). Boivie (1971b) describes the termination of the spinothalamic tract in the cat to involve the medial and rostrolateral parts of the ventral lateral nucleus, rather than the ventral posterior lateral nucleus proper. He indicates that there are terminals in the magnocellular parts of the medial geniculate nucleus, the PO_m part of the posterior nuclear complex, the zona incerta, and several intralaminar nuclei, including centralis medialis, parafascicularis, and centralis lateralis (but not centrum medianum). However, the region he calls parafascicularis is the caudal part of centralis lateralis according to Mehler's terminology. There was no somatotopic organization in the cat thalamic projection. Jones and Burton (1974) obtained similar results in the cat (Fig. 8.6), although they stress that the endings generally assigned to the magnocellular medial geniculate nucleus are on cells that may more properly be considered part of PO_m. Jones and Burton used a combined radioautography and degeneration study to determine if there is any overlap between the areas of termination of the spinothalamic tract and the dorsal column projection in the ventrobasal complex of the thalamus. They conclude that there is not.

The spinothalamic tract of the monkey terminates in a somatotopic fashion (Fig. 8.7) in the ventral posterior lateral nucleus (Chang and Ruch, 1947b; Mehler et al., 1960; however, see Kerr and Lippman, 1974). Mehler et al. (1960) and Mehler (1962, 1974) state that the intralaminar projection in the monkey (Fig. 8.7) and in man (Fig. 8.8) is to the centralis lateralis, rather than to the centrum medianum–parafasciculus complex, as has been suggested by others (Bowsher, 1957, 1961). Bowsher (1961) agrees there is no projection to the centrum medianum in the monkey but feels there is in man. He also believes there is a projection both to the parafascicular and centralis lateralis nuclei in the monkey. Kerr (1975b) indicates that one terminal region of the ventral spinothalamic tract is the paralaminar part of the medialis dorsalis nucleus. The lateral spinothalamic tract, according to Kerr, also has terminals in the medial dorsal nucleus, but by contrast ends in the central lateral nucleus as well (Kerr and Lippmann, 1974; Kerr, 1975b). Mehler (1966, 1969) and Mehler et al. (1960) appear to regard the paralaminar nuclei and centralis lateralis as one entity. There are also endings in the posterior nuclear complex, including the magnocellular part of the medial geniculate body and PO_m, in the monkey as in the cat (Mehler et al., 1960; Kerr, 1975b). The connections to the magnocellular medial geniculate are bilateral (Mehler et

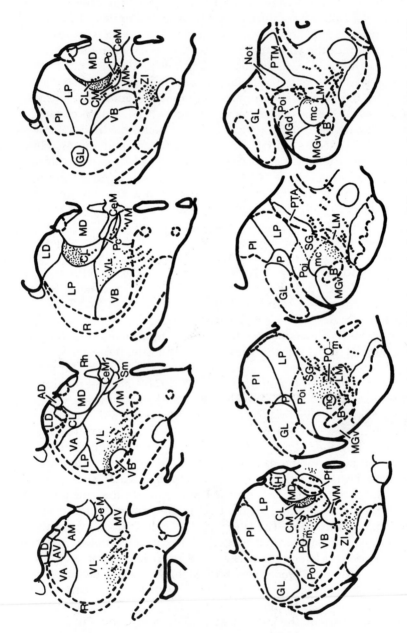

Fig. 8.6. Distribution of degenerating terminals of the spinothalamic tract in the cat following hemisection of the cord at C3. The large dots indicate axons and the small dots terminal areas. Abbreviations: VL = ventral lateral nucleus; CL = central lateral nucleus; ZI = zona incerta; PO_m = medial division of posterior group. (From Jones and Burton, 1974.)

al., 1960). A question must be raised as to the division between the magnocellular medial geniculate and the PO_m, since it has now been shown that the former projects to the auditory cortex (Burton and Jones, 1976). The spinothalamic connections in the monkey are presumably just to PO_m, as in the cat. A few fibers in the monkey end in the posteromedial hypothalamus and possibly the zona incerta (Kerr, 1975b).

An important observation was made by Kerr and Lippman (1974) concerning the spinothalamic and spinoreticular projections in the monkey. The ascending degeneration of these pathways was traced not only following ventrolateral cordotomy (the approach used by previous investigators), but also after median myelotomy over a large number of segments. With the latter approach, the normal pattern of degeneration of spinothalamic fibers was seen (Fig. 8.9), but scarcely any degeneration could be traced into the reticular formation. Thus, in the monkey, the spinoreticular tract is essentially completely uncrossed. Assuming a similar arrangement in man, the crossed sensory deficit produced by cordotomy may be attributed to the interruption of the spinothalamic but not to the spinoreticular tract.

The cortical projections of the posterior thalamic nuclei receiving spinothalamic tract terminals have now been investigated. PO_m has been found to project to the retroinsular cortex (cerebral cortex just posterior to SII) (Burton and Jones, 1976). The intralaminar nuclei project widely over the cerebral cortex (Murray, 1966; Jones and Leavitt, 1974), but it is of interest that the posterior part of centralis lateralis projects to SI (Jones and Leavitt, 1974). The connections of the ventral posterior lateral nucleus to SI and SII have been mentioned previously.

In summary, there are regional and species differences in the distribution of the cells of origin of the spinothalamic tract. The cells in the cervical enlargement of the cat are concentrated in laminae I, V, and VI, while those in the cat lumbar enlargement are in laminae I and V–VIII, but mostly in VII and VIII. In the lumbar cord of the monkey and also the rat, the spinothalamic tract cells are in laminae I and IV–VIII, but mostly in V. Some spinothalamic tract cells project to the ipsilateral diencephalon, but most project contralaterally. The decussation is probably in the same segment as the cell body. The tract has a roughly somatotopic organization, with the caudal body represented dorsolaterally and the rostral body ventromedially. The axons of the spinothalamic tract are myelinated and range in size from small to medium. Although there is a separate ventral component of the tract, at least from cervical levels, it is not evident if there are functionally separate lateral and ventral spinothalamic tracts. The terminations of the

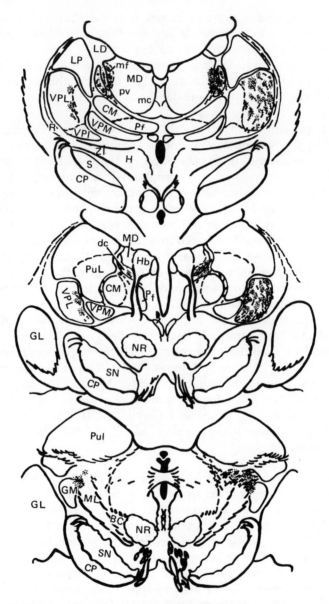

Fig. 8.7. Distribution of terminal degeneration of the spinothalamic tract after cordotomy in the monkey. Abbreviations: VPL = ventral posterior lateral nucleus; CL = central lateral nucleus; MDmf = medial dorsal nucleus, pars multiformis; MDdc = medial dorsal nucleus, pars densocellularis; GM = medial geniculate nucleus. (From Mehler *et al.*, 1960.)

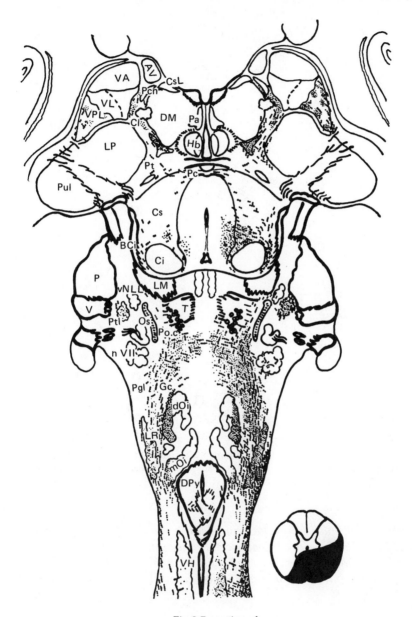

Fig.8.7 continued.

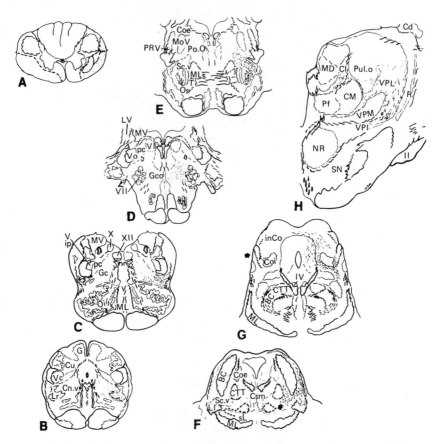

Fig. 8.8. Ascending degeneration in human after cordotomy. The extent of the cordotomy is shown in A. Degenerating fibers are shown by heavy dots and terminal areas by fine stipple. (From Mehler, 1974.)

spinothalamic tract are in the ventrobasal complex (nucleus ventralis posterolateralis in the monkey; boundary between this nucleus and the nucleus ventralis lateralis in the cat), the medial part of the posterior nuclear complex, and the intralaminar nuclei (chiefly centralis lateralis).

Responses of Spinothalamic Tract Neurons to Electrical Stimulation

The activity of axons within the ventrolateral white matter of the spinal cord has been recorded in a number of investigations (Amassian, 1951; Collins and Randt, 1956; Lundberg and Oscarsson, 1962; Oscarsson *et al.*, 1964; Shealy *et al.*, 1966; Manfredi and Castellucci,

1969; Manfredi, 1970; Fields *et al.*, 1970b; Price and Wagman, 1971; Pomeranz, 1973). Although the destination of the axons recorded from was not determined, in several instances the suggestion was made that the fibers belonged to the spinothalamic tract. However, it is likely that the spinoreticular tract was more prominently involved, and so several of these studies will be described later.

Lundberg and Oscarsson (1962) described two pathways in the ventrolateral white matter. One was excited by cutaneous and high-threshold muscle afferents of both hindlimbs, while the other was activated by comparable afferents of just the contralateral hindlimb. The pathways were named the bilateral ventral flexor reflex tract (bVFRT) and the contralateral ventral flexor reflex tract (cVFRT). It was suggested that the bVFRT is a spinoreticulotectal pathway and that the cVFRT could possibly be the spinothalamic tract. A similar crossed pathway was observed in the monkey (Oscarsson *et al.*, 1964), although it was not specifically called the cVFRT.

Price and Wagman (1971) recorded from axons in the dorsolateral column and in the ventrolateral quadrant in monkeys, with the goal of sampling the activity of the spinocervical and spinothalamic tracts. Receptive fields were divided into three size classes—small, interme-

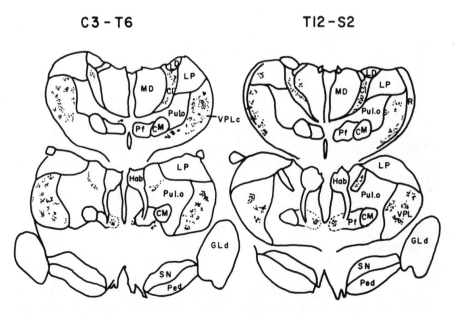

Fig. 8.9. Terminal degeneration in the monkey thalamus following midline myelotomies at the cervical and lumbosacral enlargements. (From Kerr and Lippman, 1974.)

diate, and large. Most of the dorsolateral column units had small receptive fields, and there was often a response both to A and C fiber inputs. Units with small receptive fields had a narrow dynamic range, while those with large receptive fields had a wide dynamic range. Most of the axons in the ventrolateral quadrant had large receptive fields, responded to proprioceptive input and gave a prolonged discharge to A and C fiber stimulation. However, some of the units had small receptive fields. Inhibition was observed for axons in both regions of the cord. Two of the ventrolateral quadrant units had ipsilateral receptive fields.

Pomeranz (1973) found that some axons in the ventrolateral quadrant of the cat spinal cord respond specifically to nociceptive stimulation. Other units were excited by various combinations of tactile, thermal, and noxious stimuli. The units responsive only to noxious stimuli were found to be excited by small myelinated or by unmyelinated afferents, but not by large myelinated afferents, in experiments using electrical stimulation. The receptive fields were large and mostly ipsilateral (40% crossed).

The responses of identified spinothalamic tract cells in the monkey to graded electrical stimulation of peripheral nerves were reported by Foreman et al. (1975a). Hair-activated and low-threshold spinothalamic tract neurons were more readily excited by the largest myelinated afferents than were high-threshold spinothalamic tract cells. However, large afferents could also activate many high-threshold cells. There was a convergence of small myelinated and at least in some cases, of unmyelinated fiber inputs onto spinothalamic tract cells (Fig. 8.10). Monosynaptic connections were demonstrated, at least for some hair-activated and low-threshold cells, but polysynaptic connections were likely for some neurons. Since the major excitatory actions were produced by peripheral nerves contralateral to the axon, it was concluded that the monkey spinothalamic tract forms at least one component of the cVFRT of Lundberg and Oscarsson (1962). The conduction velocities of the afferents that excited the hair-activated and low-threshold spinothalamic tract cells were consistent with those of known sensitive mechanoreceptors of hairy and glabrous skin.

Responses of Spinothalamic Tract Neurons to
Natural Forms of Stimulation

Many of the studies of the response properties of neurons in the dorsal horn of the cat lumbosacral spinal cord done during the 1960s were considered by the investigators (Wall, 1960, 1967; Wall and Cronly-Dillon, 1960) to be relevant to the sensory function of pain

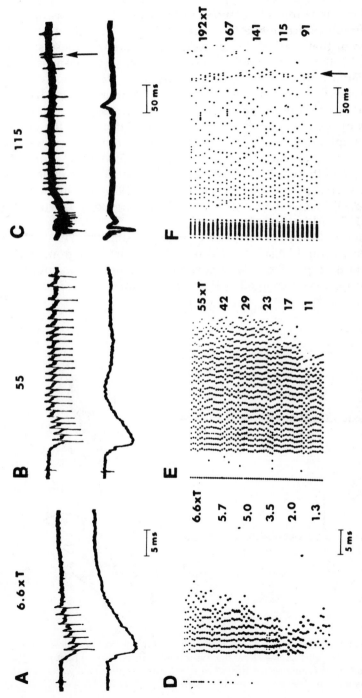

Fig. 8.10. Convergence of myelinated afferents of Aαδ and Aδ size and of unmyelinated afferents upon a primate spinothalamic tract neuron. The stimulus strength was graded in D from near threshold to maximum for the Aαδ fibers; it was graded in E to maximum for the Aδ fibers; in F, C fibers were activated, producing the late discharge indicated by the arrow. (From Foreman et al., 1975a.)

transmission, since the cells responded to noxious as well as to non-noxious stimuli. Since only a few spinothalamic tract cells are in the dorsal horn at that level of the cat cord, it appears that these studies were more likely to provide information about sensory transmission in the spinocervical than in the spinothalamic tract. However, the finding of Christensen and Perl (1970) of a population of neurons in lamina I of the dorsal horn of the cat spinal cord that respond specifically to noxious or thermal stimuli did prove to be pertinent to the operation of the spinothalamic tract. Comparable neurons have now also been found in the monkey (Kumazawa *et al.*, 1975; Willis *et al.*, 1974). At least some of these cells project to the contralateral diencephalon in the cat (Dilly *et al.*, 1968; Trevino and Carstens, 1975) and in the monkey (Fig. 8.11) (Trevino *et al.*, 1973; Willis *et al.*, 1974; Trevino and Carstens, 1975; Albe-Fessard *et al.*, 1975).

The lamina I cells described by Christensen and Perl (1970) in the cat spinal cord could be subdivided into three functional groups. One category of cell responded only to noxious mechanical stimulation, the second group was discharged both by noxious mechanical and nox-

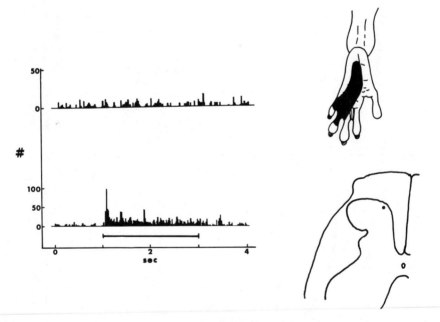

Fig. 8.11. Responses of a spinothalamic tract cell located in lamina I to intense mechanical stimulation. The histograms show the absence of a response to pressure and the brisk response to a very intense mechanical stimulus. The receptive field was on the sole of the foot, as indicated. (From Willis *et al.*, 1974.)

ious thermal stimulation, while the third class of cell was activated by innocuous thermal stimuli, as well as by noxious mechanical and thermal stimuli. The units sensitive to innocuous thermal changes were generally excited by cooling, but some responded to warming. Inhibition was commonly observed from areas of skin adjacent to or perhaps surrounding the excitatory receptive field. Many of these cells were shown by antidromic activation to project contralaterally at least to the upper cervical level by Kumazawa *et al.* (1975) both in the cat and monkey. The units that were found to be antidromically activated responded either to noxious mechanical stimulation (two cat and five monkey units) or to innocuous thermal stimulation (cooling: one cat and four monkey units; warming: one monkey unit). The third class of unit described by Christensen and Perl (1970), cells responsive to noxious mechanical and thermal stimulation, were not represented in the sample of Kumazawa *et al.* (1975). However, it is possible that the sample size was too small. Such neurons were found by Willis *et al.* (1974) to be antidromically activated from the contralateral diencephalon in the monkey. A few such units were recently described by Kumazawa and Perl (1978).

The response properties of spinothalamic tract cells in the cat in regions other than lamina I have been described in a few studies. Dilly *et al.* (1968) state that most of their cells in the cervical cord responded to a wide range of cutaneous stimuli, from light brush to heavy pinch. Some of the ventral cells responded to joint bending. The lamina I cell had a small field and responded to weak mechanical stimuli but not to pressure. The cell in the ventral horn of the lumbar region was activated to touch and pressure in a large bilateral receptive field. Trevino *et al.* (1972) obtained responses to tap, pressure, and pinch in a limited number of cells. In a sample of ten spinothalamic tract cells in the thoracic spinal cord of the cat, Hancock *et al.* (1975) observed responses to cutaneous stimulation that fell into three categories: low-threshold mechanical stimulation, noxious mechanical stimulation, and a combination of the two. All of the cells studied received a convergent input from small myelinated fibers of the splanchnic nerve. Finally, McCreery and Bloedel (1975, 1976) found that cat spinothalamic tract cells could respond to weak mechanical stimuli, to strong mechanical stimuli, or to both, much like primate spinothalamic tract cells (see below).

Antidromically activated spinothalamic tract cells were found in the dorsal horn of the monkey by Albe-Fessard's group (Levante *et al.*, 1973; Albe-Fessard *et al.*, 1974). These neurons were said to respond like the lamina V cells of the cat dorsal horn. They had restricted tactile receptive fields, but they could also be excited by pinch or pricking in a larger area. The cells were discharged both by large and small myel-inated fibers when electrical stimuli were applied to the receptive field.

Willis *et al.* (1974) examined the responses of spinothalamic tract cells in the monkey lumbosacral cord to natural stimulation of the hind limb. The cells were identified by antidromic activation from the con-tralateral diencephalon. They divided the cells into four classes—hair-activated, low-threshold, high-threshold, and deep—according to the weakest form of mechanical stimulation required to activate them (Fig. 8.12). However, the hair-activated and low-threshold cells could often also be excited by intense mechanical or thermal stimulation (that is, many were wide-dynamic-range neurons) (Fig. 8.13). These cells were located in laminae IV–VI. The high-threshold cells were generally ex-cited by intense mechanical and thermal stimulation, and they were located in laminae I and IV–VI. The cells with deep receptive fields were often activated by joint movement or by probing exposed mus-cle; they were located in laminae IV–VIII. There was a somatotopic relationship between the locations of the spinothalamic tract cells in laminae I and IV that was like that described previously for cells of the spinocervical tract (Bryan *et al.*, 1973, 1974). Cells in the lateral part of the dorsal horn had receptive fields on the dorsal surface of the limb, while cells in the medial dorsal horn had receptive fields on the ventral surface of the limb. Inhibition of some of the cells could be demon-strated from inhibitory receptive fields in areas of the skin adjacent to the excitatory fields or in a complementary position on the contrala-teral hind limb. Similar observations were made by Wagman and Price (1969) for unidentified dorsal horn neurons in the monkey.

Price and Mayer (1974) obtained very similar results in a study of the receptive field properties of lumbosacral dorsal horn neurons in the monkey that could be antidromically activated by stimulation in the ventrolateral quadrant on the contralateral side at an upper cervical level. The neurons were presumably spinothalamic tract cells. The animals were unanesthetized, but pain was prevented by bilateral carotid artery ligations. The cells were divided into five classes accord-ing to their response characteristics: (I) touch, (II) touch–pressure, (III) touch–pressure–pinch, (IV) pressure–pinch, and (V) pinch. No class I or II cells responded to noxious heat; class III and IV cells could re-spond to warming and noxious heat, just noxious heat, or neither. Some class V cells were activated by noxious heat, but not all. No cells were found that were excited by heat but not by mechanical stimuli. The receptive field sizes of class I, II, and V cells were small; medium-sized fields were found for class III and IV cells; and large fields all belonged to class III cells. The locations of the cells proved to be as

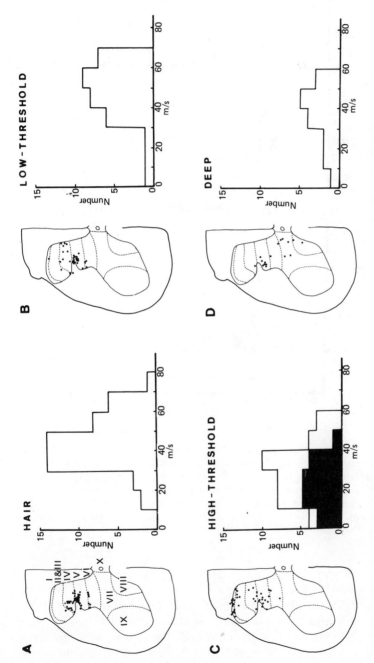

Fig. 8.12. The drawings in A–D show the locations of the spinothalamic tract cells classified according to the weakest mechanical stimuli that excited them. Many of the hair-movement and low-threshold cells had a wide dynamic range of responsiveness. The histograms show the conduction velocities of cells of the same classes. The blackened area in C represents the conduction velocities of lamina I cells. (From Willis *et al*, 1974.)

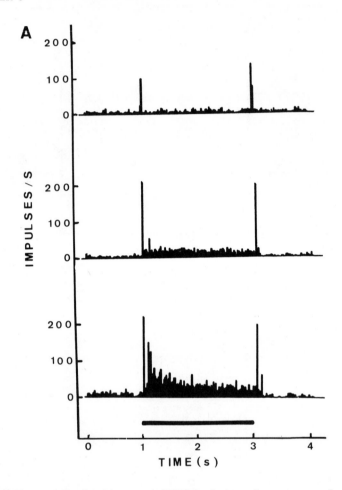

Fig. 8.13. The poststimulus histograms (PSTs) in A show the responses of a primate spinothalamic tract neuron to several intensities of mechanical stimulation (period of stimulation indicated by the bar under the lower histogram). (From Willis *et al.*, 1974.)   The PST in B shows the excitation of another spinothalamic neuron by noxious heat. The discharges triggered the pulses shown below, and the lowermost trace is the temperature monitor. The thermal change was from an adapting temperature of 35°C to 50°C and back. (From Kenshalo, Leonard, and Willis, unpublished.)

follows: class V were in lamina I; class I, II, and some III cells with small receptive fields were in lamina IV; class III and IV cells were in laminae V and VI, but those cells with medium-sized receptive fields were in lamina V and those with large fields in lamina VI.

The receptive fields of monkey spinothalamic tract neurons were analyzed by Applebaum *et al.* (1975). The largest receptive fields were

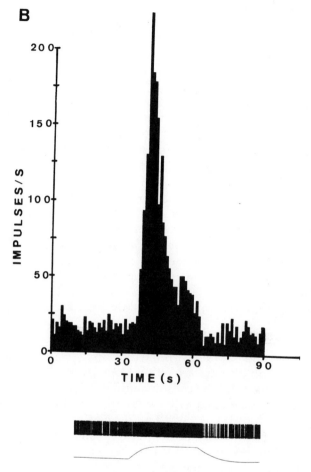

Fig. 8.13 continued.

those of hair-activated units (mean 44.6 cm², median 26.2 cm²), while the smallest belonged to high-threshold cells (mean 17.8 cm², median 9.3 cm²). Low-threshold cells had intermediate-sized receptive fields (mean 38 cm², median 19.7 cm²). The receptive field size was correlated with the positions of the fields on the hind limb and with the location of the neurons within the dorsal horn. The smallest fields were located distally on the limb. Furthermore, the receptive fields were progressively larger for neurons in laminae I, IV, and V.

Willis *et al.* (1975) examined the effects of mechanical stimulation upon spinothalamic tract neurons. The responses were divided into static and dynamic ones. Noxious mechanical or thermal stimuli were found to produce a marked excitation and typically a bursting pattern of discharge in most spinothalamic tract neurons. Graded indentation of the skin generally produced a graded maintained response. It was suggested that the slowly adapting response signaled either pressure or displacement of the skin. The responses continued to increment with increases in pressure well into the noxious range. The dynamic responses of hair-activated and low-threshold spinothalamic tract neurons were also studied. The hair-activated cells tended to signal stimulus acceleration (or a higher derivative of position), while the low-threshold units tended to signal stimulus velocity.

Price and Mayer (1975) recorded from neurons of the monkey dorsal horn that were antidromically activated from the contralateral ventrolateral white matter of C1. It can be presumed that these cells belonged to the spinothalamic tract. The receptive field properties were as described by the same authors in a previous publication (Price and Mayer, 1974). Almost all of the lamina I cells were activated by noxious mechanical stimulation, while most of the lamina IV cells were best activated by tactile stimuli. The cells that were discharged by noxious mechanical stimuli had the following responses to heating of the skin: some were fired by noxious heat, others by warming and noxious heating, and still others were not sensitive to heating. The lamina IV cells either failed to respond to heat or were discharged by warming. The absolutely and relatively refractory periods were determined using repetitive antidromic activation. Lamina I cells had longer refractory periods than did the cells in laminae IV–VI. Lamina I cells also had axons with slower conduction velocities and higher thresholds to electrical stimulation (Fig. 9.18). These properties were compared with the properties of axons within the ventrolateral quadrant of humans that produced pain responses (see Chapter 5 and Chapter 9) (Mayer *et al.*, 1975). It was concluded that spinothalamic tract neurons with wide dynamic responses were sufficient to cause pain. Participation of lamina I cells in pain transmission was not excluded, however. One criticism of this study is that the conduction velocities and refractory periods of human lamina I cells are unknown.

The effect of stimulation of the dorsal column upon spinothalamic tract cells in the monkey was examined by Foreman *et al.* (1976a). A single dorsal column volley depressed the activity of all types of spinothalamic tract cells for some 150 ms (Fig. 8.14). However, there was an initial excitation of hair-activated and low-threshold spinothalamic neurons, as might be expected from the fact that the kinds of large myelinated fibers that terminate on these cells also project up the dorsal column. A similar depression could be produced by stimulation of large afferents in a peripheral nerve (see also Willis *et al.*, 1974). The depression was thought to be mediated by collaterals of the dorsal col-

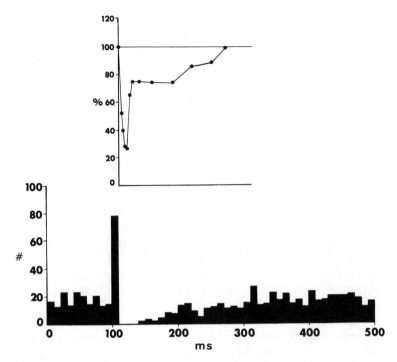

Fig. 8.14. Inhibition of the responses of the spinothalamic tract neurons to electrical (graph) stimulation of peripheral nerves or to noxious mechanical stimulation of the skin (histogram) by dorsal column volleys. (From Foreman *et al.*, 1976a.)

umn that were invaded by the descending volley, since the effect was abolished by a lesion of the dorsal column between the stimulation and the recording sites. However, the possibility that the effects were due to axons descending in the dorsal column from the dorsal column nuclei (Burton and Loewy, 1977) was not ruled out. The mechanism of the depression probably involved collision of the dorsal column volley with incoming activity in large afferents, at least in the cases of hair-activated and low-threshold spinothalmic tract cells, and pre- and postsynaptic inhibition. An action at the level of interneurons could not be excluded. The excitation of hair-activated and low-threshold neurons argues against their involvement in signaling pain, since dorsal column stimulation in humans does not evoke pain (Nashold *et al.*, 1972). However, it is possible that the volley ascending in the dorsal columns or in other sensory pathways may interfere with responses evoked by the wide-dynamic-range spinothalamic tract cells. The depression of spinothalamic tract discharges may help account for the effectiveness of dorsal column stimulation in relieving pain, although an additional action at higher levels of the nervous system is likely.

Many spinothalamic tract cells respond to electrical stimulation of peripheral cutaneous nerves or of the skin with a double burst discharge (Albe-Fessard *et al.*, 1974; Foreman *et al.*, 1975a). The earlier of the two burst discharges can be attributed to $A\alpha\beta$ afferents and the latter to $A\delta$ afferents (Albe-Fessard *et al.*, 1974; Beall *et al.*, 1977), as shown by experiments using graded stimulus strengths, measurements of conduction delays, and also anodal block of the large myelinated fibers.

In addition to receiving input from a variety of types of cutaneous afferents (Willis *et al.*, 1974, 1975) and of visceral afferents (Hancock *et al.*, 1975), it has recently been shown that spinothalamic tract cells also receive a convergent input from muscle afferents (Foreman *et al.*, 1977). The muscle afferents were excited by algesic chemicals (K^+, bradykinin, serotonin) injected into the arterial circulation of the triceps surae muscles (Fig. 8.15). It appears that the muscle input is to wide-dynamic-range spinothalamic trace cells, since none of the lamina I cells examined was activated by chemical stimuli. It is suggested that spinothalamic tract cells that can be excited both by cutaneous and by muscle nociceptors might signal poorly localized pain, while more specific spinothalamic tract cells, like those of lamina I, might be concerned with discretely localized pain.

In summary, the response properties of spinothalamic tract neurons are currently under investigation. The cells need to be identified by antidromic activation, since they must be distinguished from interneurons and the cells of origin of other tracts. Spinothalamic tract cells have been studied in the cat and the monkey, but considerably more information is known about those in the monkey. Some spinothalamic tract cells respond only to noxious or near noxious stimuli; many of these are located in lamina I, although high-threshold cells are also found deeper in the dorsal horn. Other spinothalamic tract cells can be activated by tactile forms of stimulation and often also by noxious stimuli. In addition, there is a class of spinothalamic tract cells that is fired by joint movements or pressure applied to muscle. There is a somatotopic relationship between receptive field position and the location of spinothalamic tract cells, at least in laminae I and IV. The receptive fields of spinothalamic tract cells tend to be intermediate to large in size, but the smallest fields are those of high-threshold spinothalamic tract cells. The receptive fields are larger for cells in deeper laminae. Although all of the cells in laminae IV–VI appear to have receptive fields to mechanical stimuli, some are also activated by noxious heat. The thresholds and refractory periods of the spinothalamic tract cells of laminae IV–VI are like those

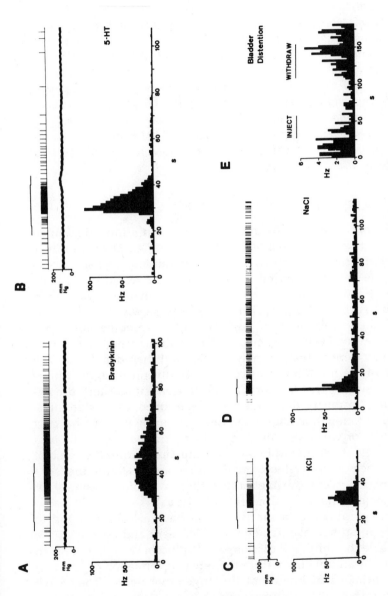

Fig. 8.15. (A–C) The responses of a spinothalamic tract neuron to the injection of algesic chemicals (bradykinin, 5-HT (serotonin), and KCl) into the arterial circulation of the triceps surae muscles. (D) The response to the injection of hypertonic NaCl into the muscle. (E) The inhibition produced by bladder distention. For A–D, the records include window discriminator pulses representing cell discharges and histograms indicating firing rate. The systemic arterial blood pressure is also shown in A–C. (From Foreman *et al.*, 1977.)

of the axons in the human ventrolateral quadrant that produce pain, and so the cells with response properties of wide dynamic range may be sufficient to produce pain, although the high-threshold cells may also contribute. However, dorsal column stimulation both excites and inhibits these cells while just inhibiting the high-threshold cells. Since dorsal column stimulation is not painful, a role for the hair-activated and low-threshold cells with wide dynamic range in pain transmission requires further explanation. However, the fact that many spinothalamic tract cells respond to input over Aδ afferents and receive a convergent input from a variety of cutaneous receptors, including nociceptors, and from muscle nociceptors suggests a role for wide-dynamic-range cells in nociception. Perhaps such cells are involved in poorly localized pain, whereas more specific cells, like those of lamina I, signal discretely localized pain.

Descending Control of Spinothalamic Neurons

One of several studies of the effects of brain stimulation upon spinothalamic tract cells is that of Coulter *et al.* (1974). The sensorimotor region of the cerebral cortex was stimulated in monkey, and it was found that the rapidly adapting component of the responses of hair-activated and low-threshold spinothalamic tract neurons was often inhibited by such stimulation (Fig. 8.16). The slowly adapting discharges of these cells and of high-threshold spinothalamic tract neurons were unaffected. Some of the hair-activated and low-threshold cells were initially weakly excited and then depressed. The time course of the inhibition was consistent with presynaptic inhibition. The possibility that the cortical effects were similar to those expected during "corollary discharge" was mentioned, as was an alternative interpretation that the action resulted in switching the cells from detectors of weak stimuli to detectors of intense stimuli. In a follow-up study, it was found by microstimulation within the cerebral cortex that each of several cytoarchitectural areas within the sensorimotor region were capable of exerting corticofugal control of spinothalamic tract neurons (Coulter *et al.*, 1976a).

Pathways originating in the brainstem have also been found to alter activity in spinothalamic neurons. McCreery and Bloedel (1975, 1976) were able to inhibit the discharges of spinothalamic tract cells in the cat either by stimulating within the reticular formation or by stimulating the infraorbital branch of the trigeminal nerve. They were inclined to attribute the inhibitory effects to reticulospinal pathways. Interestingly, they found an effect opposite to that described by Coulter *et al.* (1974) following cortical stimulation. Volleys in the infraorbital nerve resulted in a selective inhibition of the slowly adapting re-

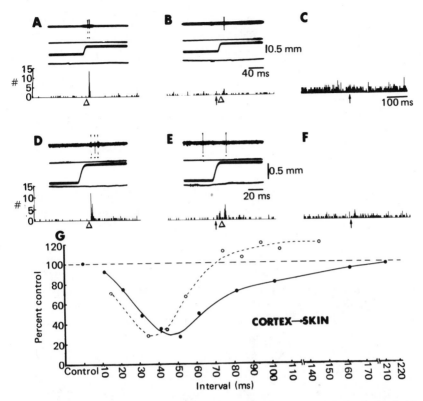

Fig. 8.16. Inhibition of the rapidly adapting responses of primate spinothalamic tract neurons by stimulation of the sensorimotor cortex. The inhibition is demonstrated using test responses to step indentations of the skin in A–B and D–E for two different cells. The time course of inhibition is shown in G. The cell in D–F was weakly excited by the corticofugal volley prior to the inhibition. There was no apparent effect of the cortical volleys upon the responses of the cells to noxious stimuli, D and F. (From Coulter et al., 1974.)

sponses of spinothalamic neurons to pressure, with sparing of the rapidly adapting component of the response at the time of contact with the skin by the mechanical stimulator (Fig. 8.17).

A great deal of recent work has been concerned with one or more systems of neurons in the region of the periaqueductal gray and the brainstem raphe, which when stimulated produce behavioral signs of analgesia or when destroyed result in increased responsiveness to noxious stimuli (Reynolds, 1969; Mayer et al., 1971; Balagura and Ralph, 1973; Liebeskind et al., 1973; Oliveras et al., 1974a,b, 1975; Mayer and Liebeskind, 1974; Melzack and Melinkoff, 1974; Proudfit and Anderson, 1975; Giesler and Liebeskind, 1976; Mayer and Price,

1976; however, cf. Melzack *et al.*, 1958; Kelly and Glusman, 1968). There is evidence that at least part of the analgesia is mediated by serotonergic neurons (Fig. 8.18), although other nonserotonergic neurons are likely to be involved as well (Akil and Mayer, 1972; Guilbaud *et al.*, 1973a; Akil and Liebeskind, 1975; Hayes *et al.*, 1977; see also Messing and Lytle, 1977). Furthermore, the serotonin system appears to play a major role in the production of analgesia by opiates (see Chapter 9).

At least a part of the analgesic effects of brainstem stimulation is likely to be mediated by descending, rather than ascending, pathways (Mayer and Price, 1976). A major relay in the descending system seems to be in the nucleus raphe magnus, since stimulation of this nucleus produces analgesia (Oliveras *et al.*, 1975; Proudfit and Anderson, 1975) and its destruction (but not of the adjacent nucleus reticular gigantocellularis) reduces the analgesia due to morphine injections (Proudfit and Anderson, 1975). An anatomic link exists between the periaqueductal gray and adjacent dorsal raphe nucleus (both candidates for producing analgesia) and the nucleus raphe magnus (Ruda, 1975; Taber-Pierce *et al.*, 1976). The nucleus raphe magnus projects to the spinal cord through the dorsolateral fasciculi and terminates in the

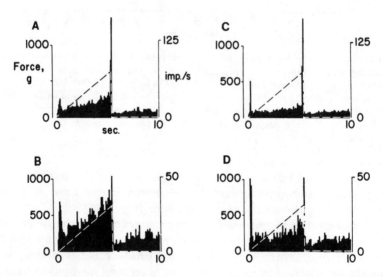

Fig. 8.17. Inhibition of the responses of cat spinothalamic tract neurons to intense ramp stimuli by electrical stimulation of the infraorbital nerve. A and B are control responses, while the inhibition is shown in C and D. Note that the effect is on the slowly adapting response, rather than upon the initial rapidly adapting response. (From McCreery and Bloedel, 1976.)

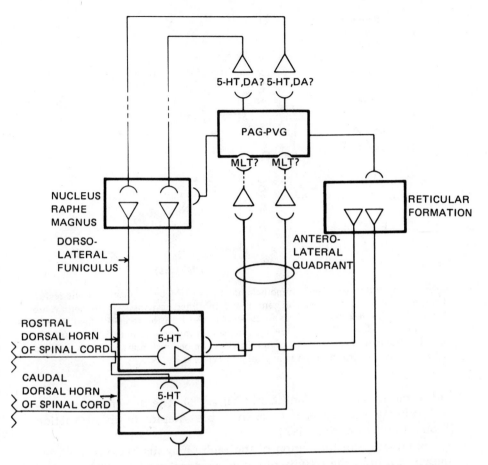

Fig. 8.18. Scheme of the hypothetical intrinsic analgesia system. Abbreviations: MT = morphine-like transmitter; PAG-PVG = periaquaductal and periventricular gray; 5-HT = serotonin; DA = dopamine. (From Mayer and Price, 1976.)

dorsal horn (Brodal *et al.*, 1960a; Kuypers and Maisky, 1975; Basbaum *et al.*, 1976, 1977; Martin *et al.*, 1977, 1978; however, cf. Bobillier *et al.*, 1976). Since the serotonin-containing axons of the spinal cord (Carlsson *et al.*, 1964) originate from neuronal cell bodies in the raphe nuclei (Dahlström and Fuxe, 1965; Pin *et al.*, 1968; Hubbard and DiCarlo, 1974; Felten *et al.*, 1974), it seems reasonable to suppose that the serotonin-mediated component of the analgesia system involves a raphe–spinal projection. The effects of serotonin released iontophoretically at the cord level include inhibition of the discharges of many interneurons, including cells in lamina I (Engberg and Ryall, 1966; Weight

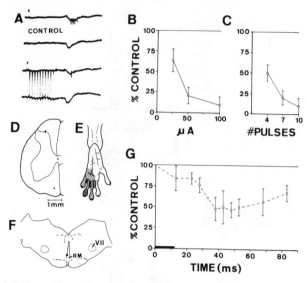

Fig. 8.19. Inhibition of lamina I spinothalamic tract neuron by stimulation in the region of the nucleus raphe magnus. The control and inhibited responses of the neuron are shown in A; the test response was to an electric shock in the receptive field, E. The location of the cell is in D and of the stimulus site in the brainstem in F. The effects of graded stimulus strengths and of variations in the number of stimuli are shown in B and C. The time course of inhibition is in G. (From Willis *et al.*, 1977.)

and Salmoirhagi, 1966; Randić and Yu, 1976). The descending seroto-nin pathway also appears to exert a presynaptic inhibitory action (Proudfit and Anderson, 1974).

Stimulation in the region of the raphe magnus nucleus has been shown to inhibit the activity of spinal cord interneurons that respond to noxious stimuli (Fields *et al.*, 1977a; Guilbaud *et al.*, 1977b), as does stimulation in the periaqueductal gray (Liebeskind *et al.*, 1973; Oliveras *et al.*, 1974a). In addition, it has been found (Fig. 8.19) that stimulation in the area of the nucleus raphe magnus results in an inhibition of the activity of primate spinothalamic tract neurons (Beall *et al.*, 1976; Willis *et al.*, 1977). The pathway for inhibition descends in the dorsolateral fasciculus. In the case of primate spinothalamic tract cells, the stimulation inhibits not only the responses to noxious stimuli but also spontaneous activity and the responses to tactile stimuli (Fig. 8.20). It was suggested that the same pathway might be the one responsible for the tonic inhibition of the flexion reflex pathways in the spinal cord (Job, 1953; R. M. Eccles and Lundberg, 1959b; Kuno and Perl, 1960; Holmqvist and Lundberg, 1959, 1961; Carpenter *et al.*, 1963a; Wall, 1967; Engberg *et al.*, 1968a,b,c,d; Chambers *et al.*, 1970; Handwerker *et al.*, 1975; Cervero *et al.*, 1976).

To determine whether or not spinothalamic neurons in the primate might be susceptible to a postsynaptic action of serotonin, Jordan *et al.* (1978) applied serotonin iontophoretically to such neurons. Most high-threshold and wide-dynamic-range spinothalamic neurons were depressed. Since the excitatory action of glutamate was antagonized by serotonin (Fig. 8.21), it was concluded that at least part of the action of serotonin was postsynaptic.

In summary, the spinothalamic tract is subject to descending control from the brain. Stimulation of the sensorimotor cortex selectively inhibits rapidly adapting responses to tactile stimuli without affecting the slowly adapting responses to noxious stimuli. Brainstem pathways originating in the reticular formation have the converse effect. A powerful inhibition results from stimulation in the region of the nucleus raphe magnus. The pathway descends in the dorsolateral fasciculus and may utilize serotonin as an inhibitory transmitter.

THE SPINORETICULAR TRACT

Projections ascend from the spinal cord through the ventrolateral white matter to the brainstem reticular formation. These projections are collectively called the spinoreticular tract. However, at least two major components of the spinoreticular tract should be distin-

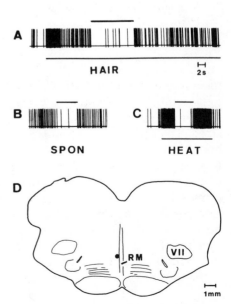

Fig. 8.20. Inhibition of the discharges of a spinothalamic tract neuron by stimulation in the region of the raphe magnus nucleus. The activity in A was enhanced by hair movement prior to the conditioning stimuli. The discharges in B were spontaneous, while those in C were enhanced by a noxious stimulus. (From Willis *et al.*, 1977.)

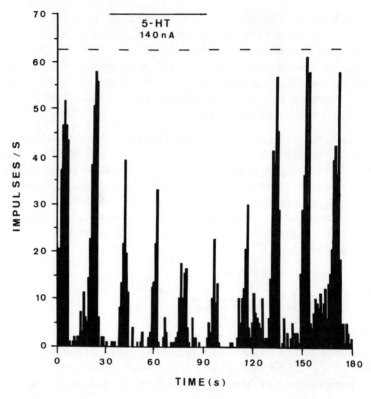

Fig. 8.21. Depression of the responses of a spinothalamic tract cell to glutamate pulses by the iontophoretic application of 5-hydroxytryptamine (serotonin). (From Jordan *et al.*, 1978).

guished—a projection to the lateral reticular nucleus and one to the medial reticular formation. The first of these forms part of the spinoreticulocerebellar pathway (see Oscarsson, 1973) and presumably has no role in sensation; for this reason, this pathway will not be emphasized. The other pathway ends in part on neurons of the reticular formation that project either back down into the spinal cord in the reticulospinal tracts or rostrally to higher levels, including the midbrain and diencephalon. A spinoreticulothalamocortical pathway is often proposed as a possible sensory pathway, especially with reference to pain mechanisms. In addition to connections with reticular neurons, fibers ascending from the spinal cord also synapse with neurons in a number of other nuclei of the rhombencephalon. Of these, brief mention will be made of the effects of such connections on neurons of the raphe nuclei.

Phylogeny of the Spinoreticular Tract

Spinoreticular projections are prominent in all mammalian species examined, including the opossum (Mehler, 1969; Hazlett *et al.*, 1972), rat (Lund and Webster, 1967b; Mehler, 1969), cat (Morin *et al.*, 1951; F. H. Johnson, 1954; Rossi and Brodal, 1957; Anderson and Berry, 1959; Bowsher and Westman, 1970), pig (Breazile and Kitchell, 1968), sheep (Rao *et al.*, 1969), hedgehog (Jane and Schroeder, 1971), tree shrew (Schroeder and Jane, 1971), monkey (Morin *et al.*, 1951; Mehler *et al.*, 1960; Kerr, 1975b; Kerr and Lippman, 1974), and man (Bowsher, 1957; Mehler, 1974).

Mehler (1966), emphasized the similarity in the projections of spinoreticular fibers in the various mammalian species. The most significant change in the more "advanced" species is the greater number of fibers that ascend past the pons to end in midbrain and diencephalic structures.

Spinoreticular fibers are also prominent in other vertebrates than mammals. They have been described in fish, amphibia, reptiles, and birds (Goldby and Robinson, 1962; Karten, 1963; Ebbesson, 1967, 1969; Hayle, 1973).

Anatomy of the Spinoreticular Tract

Molenaar *et al.* (1974) investigated the distribution of neurons projecting into the ventral and lateral funiculi in the cat, using the technique of retrograde chromatolysis (Fig. 8.22). Lesions of the cord at an upper lumbar level produced the following pattern of chromatolysis. Ipsilaterally, chromatolytic cells were located chiefly in lamina IV at the level of the lumbosacral enlargement (below segments containing large numbers of altered propriospinal neurons). These cells of lamina IV presumably contribute to the spinocervical tract. Contralaterally, cells undergoing chromatolysis were concentrated in laminae VII and VIII, although there were also some in the dorsal horn. This distribution resembles that of the cells of origin of the spinothalamic tract described earlier; presumably these and the spinoreticular neurons originate from neurons in the same region.

The locations of spinal neurons that could be activated antidromically following stimulation in the reticular formation were mapped by several groups (Levante and Albe-Fessard, 1972; Fields *et al.*, 1975, 1977b). In most of these studies, the cells were concentrated in laminae VII and VIII or VI–VIII, although some were also found in the motor nucleus. In one study (Fields *et al.*, 1977b), some spinoreticular neurons were also found in the superficial layers of the dorsal

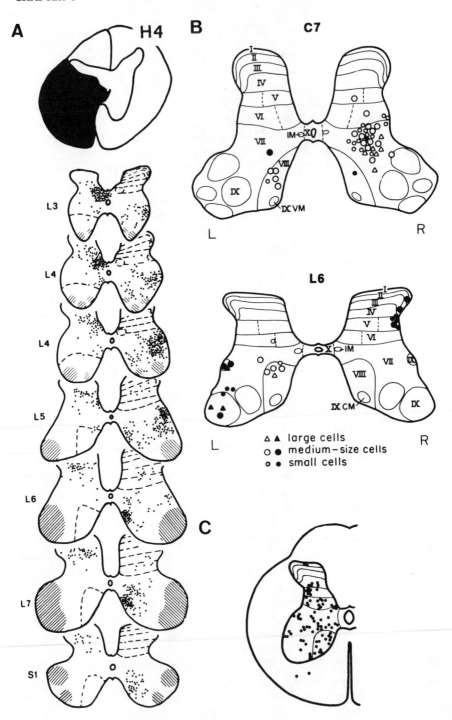

A   H4

B   C7

L3

L4

L4

L5

L6

L7

S1

L6

△ ▲ large cells
○ ● medium-size cells
○ ● small cells

L   R

C

horn (Fig. 8.22C). Although the cells studied by Levante and Albe-Fessard (1972) projected contralaterally, Fields and his associates found contra- and ipsilaterally projecting cells to be about equally abundant (Fields *et al.*, 1975, 1977b).

Recently, Corvaja *et al.* (1977) have demonstrated the locations of the cells of the spinal cord that project to the lateral reticular nucleus, using small injections of horseradish peroxidase into the latter (Fig. 8.22B). Although the cells of origin of the spinoreticular neurons projecting to the medial reticular formation were not investigated, it is possible that they have a similar distribution. The cells in the cervical enlargement that were retrogradely labeled by horseradish perioxidase injected into the lateral reticular nucleus were usually ipsilateral and either in the lateral part of laminae V and VI or in the central part of lamina VII. Contralateral cells were in laminae VII and VIII. In the lumbar enlargement, labeled cells were usually contralateral to the injection and in laminae VII–IX. However, a few ipsilateral cells were found in laminae I–V, especially after an injection into the lateral part of the lateral reticular nucleus. The cells in the contralateral ventral horn were often as large as motoneurons.

Spinoreticular axons ascend in the ventral part of the lateral funiculus and in the ventral funiculus (Bohm, 1953; Rossi and Brodal, 1957; Anderson and Berry, 1959; Mehler *et al.*, 1960; Kerr, 1975b). They are intermingled with spinocerebellar, spinotectal, and spinothalamic fibers (Bohm, 1953; Anderson and Berry, 1959). As the spinoreticular fibers enter the medulla, they form a prominent bundle lateral in the brainstem (Fig. 8.23). Fibers leave this bundle, coursing medially into the reticular formation. Terminals are found in the following reticular nuclei* after interruption of the ventral quadrant of the spinal cord: nucleus medullae oblongatae centralis, the lateral reticular nucleus, nucleus reticular gigantocellularis, nucleus reticularis pontis

---

* For terminology applied to the various nuclei of the reticular formation, see Meessen and Olszewski, 1949; Olszewski and Baxter, 1954; Olszewski, 1954; Brodal, 1957; Rossi and Zanchetti, 1957; and Taber, 1961.

←──────────────────────────────────

Fig. 8.22. Locations of neurons that may contribute to the spinoreticular pathway. (A) Distribution of neurons that are labeled by horseradish peroxidase injected into the lateral and ventral funiculi of the spinal cord; the cells would include propriospinal as well as tract cells of various kinds. (From Molenaar *et al.*, 1974). (B) Distribution of spinoreticular neurons that were labeled after injections of horseradish peroxidase into the lateral reticular nucleus. (From Corvaja *et al.*, 1977.) (C) Locations of spinoreticular neurons identified by antidromic activation from the nucleus gigantocellularis. (From Fields *et al.*, 1977b.)

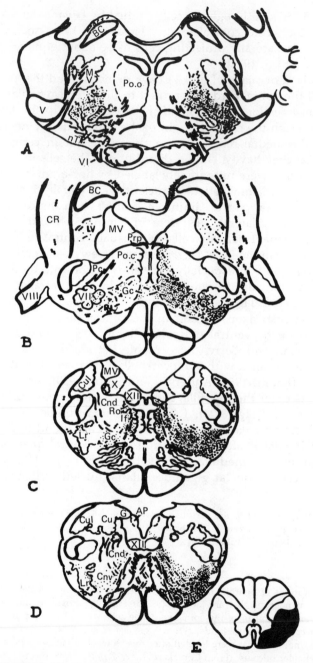

Fig. 8.23. Terminal degeneration of the reticular formation of the medulla and pons following cordotomy at a high level. (From Mehler *et al.*, 1960.)

caudalis and oralis, nucleus paragigantocellularis dorsalis and lateralis, nucleus subcoeruleus (Anderson and Berry, 1959; Mehler *et al.*, 1960; Westman and Bowsher, 1971; Bowsher and Westman, 1970; Jane and Schroeder, 1971; Schroeder and Jane, 1971; Kerr, 1975b).

There are also spinal projections to the raphe nuclei (Fig. 8.24), including the nucleus raphe pallidus and magnus (Mehler *et al.*, 1960; Bowsher, 1957; Brodal *et al.*, 1960b; Breazile and Kitchell, 1968).

Although there is evidence of a bilateral spinal cord projection to the reticular formation of the cat (Fields *et al.*, 1975, 1977b; Corvaja *et al.*, 1977), the arrangement appears to be different in primates. Kerr and Lippman (1974) compared the ascending degeneration resulting from cordotomies with that produced by multisegmental median com-

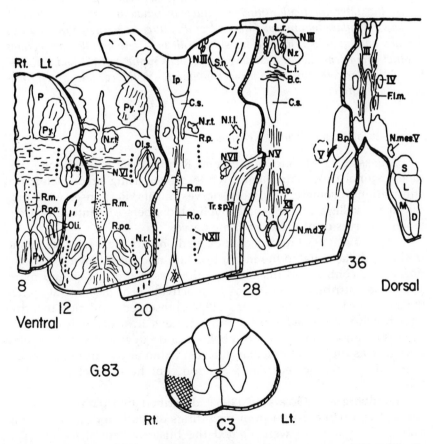

Fig. 8.24. Terminal degeneration in the nuclei raphe magnus and pallidus following anterolateral cordotomy. (From Brodal *et al.*, 1960b.)

missurotomies in the monkey. Whereas spinothalamic degeneration was similar following either procedure, there was very little spinoreticular degeneration after commissurotomy in contrast to cordotomy. It was concluded that the spinoreticular pathway is largely uncrossed in the primate.

Spinoreticular axons terminate both on cell bodies and on dendrites of reticular neurons (Bowsher and Westman, 1970; Westman and Bowsher, 1971).

In summary, the cells of origin of the spinoreticular tract are concentrated in laminae VII and VIII in the cat spinal cord, although there are also spinoreticular cells in the dorsal horn. The axons ascend to the brainstem in the ventral quadrant of the cord and terminate on somata and dendrites of cells in a number of nuclei, including the nucleus medullae oblongata centralis, the lateral reticular nucleus, nucleus reticularis gigantocellularis, nucleus reticularis pontis caudalis and oralis, nucleus paragigantocellularis dorsalis and lateralis, and nucleus subcoeruleus. There are also projections to other brainstem nuclei, including the nucleus raphe magnus and pallidus. Spinoreticular cells appear to project bilaterally in the cat but largely ipsilaterally in the monkey.

Responses of Spinoreticular Neurons

Amassian (1951) and Collins and Randt (1956) evoked potentials in the spinal cord ventrolateral white matter using graded electrical stimulation of somatic or visceral nerves in cats. Responses were produced by volleys in the small myelinated fibers of contralateral cutaneous nerves or of the splanchnic nerve.

Berry *et al.* (1950) recorded an evoked potential in a restricted zone in the medulla lateral to the inferior olivary nucleus following stimulation of the contra- and ipsilateral saphenous nerve in cats and monkeys. They attributed the response to activation of the ventral spinothalamic tract. However, Bohm (1953) presented evidence that the response was recorded from a relay nucleus in a pathway en route from the spinal cord to the cerebellum and suggested that the relay nucleus was the lateral reticular nucleus. Bohm also noticed slower activity in the nearby reticular formation, but he did not investigate this.

Lundberg and Oscarsson (1962) described two pathways in the ventrolateral white matter from recordings of discharges in ascending axons. The pathways were named the bilateral ventral flexor reflex tract (bVFRT) and the contralateral ventral flexor reflex tract (cVFRT), according to the pattern of their input from the "flexion reflex afferents." It was suggested that the bVFRT is the initial part of a spin-oreticulotectal pathway. However, the axons of the bVFRT seem to terminate in the region of the lateral reticular nucleus, and the bVFRT has now been identified as a spinoreticulocerebellar path (Oscarsson, 1973).

Shealy et al. (1966) found that electrical stimulation of small myelinated and unmyelinated afferents in peripheral nerves evoked potentials bilaterally in the ventrolateral white matter in the vicinity of the ventral horn in cats and monkeys. Although it was not shown what pathway(s) were involved, the authors were inclined to think that the fibers were propriospinal.

Manfredi and Castellucci (1969) showed that a C fiber volley (A fibers blocked by anodal polarization) in a peripheral nerve evoked a late potential in the ventrolateral white matter of the contralateral spinal cord. The wave was conducted up the cord at a velocity of about 14–30 m/s, indicating that the ascending axons were myelinated. Manfredi (1970) recorded activity from ventrolateral quadrant axons that could be evoked by Aβ or Aδ input; he thought the axons might terminate in the reticular formation, tectum, or thalamus.

Fields et al. (1970b) recorded from axons in the ventrolateral white matter in the cat spinal cord. Some of the axons were directly activated by stimulation at the junction between the cord and the medulla and also synaptically; these were judged to be the axons of ascending tracts. The somatic receptive fields of the axons were classified as restricted or as convergent. The ascending axons included examples of each class. Many of the restricted field axons were activated from the ipsilateral hindlimb, but some were excited from the contralateral hindlimb or from various regions on the trunk. Some of these cells also had visceral input. Inhibitory receptive fields were also commonly found, but in only a few cases were these of the surround type. The convergent class of axon generally had bilaterally symmetrical receptive fields. Most units also received an input from one or more viscera. The identity of the tract(s) to which the axons belonged was not determined, but the authors suggested that they were probably spinoreticular.

Fields et al. (1975) recorded from spinal neurons that were activated antidromically following stimulation in the region of the nucleus reticularis gigantocellularis. Most of the cells examined were in laminae VI–VIII, either contra- or ipsilateral to the stimulating electrode, although a few were in the motor nucleus. Receptive fields were usually ipsilateral and excitatory, although contralateral and inhibitory receptive fields were seen. Many of the receptive fields were bilateral. Often, deep structures had to be activated to excite spinoreticular

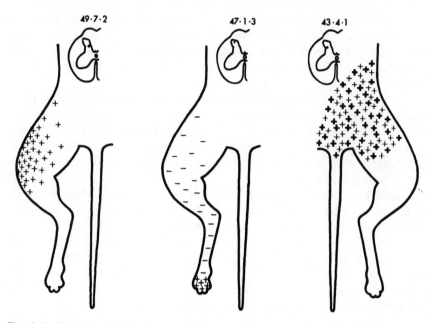

Fig. 8.25. Receptive fields of spinorecticular neurons (identified by antidromic activation). Excitation indicated by + and inhibition by −. Bold symbols indicate that noxious levels of intensity were required. (From Fields *et al.*, 1977b.)

neurons, although some cells responded to such weak tactile stimuli as hair movement. Cells of the latter type had a wide dynamic range, since they responded additionally to noxious stimuli, such as pinch. Some spinoreticular neurons responded just to noxious stimuli.

A similar but more extensive study has been reported recently by Fields *et al.* (1977b). To resolve the question of possible antidromic activation of axons ascending past the stimulating electrode in the reticular formation, electrodes were placed not only at several levels of the reticular formation but also across the midbrain. A given neuron could then be tested for activation just from the reticular formation, just from the midbrain, or both. There was a possibility of stimulus spread in the case of cells of the latter type, although alternatively, some neurons may project both to the reticular formation and to higher levels. Cells antidromically activated from the reticular formation were located in a wider area of the spinal gray matter than in the previous study. Some spinoreticular neurons were found in the most superficial layers of the dorsal horn, as well as in laminae VI–IX. Ipsilaterally and contralaterally projecting neurons were seen in about equal numbers. The conduction velocities of the axons ranged from 2 to 93 m/s (mean 45 m/s). Receptive fields were categorized as (1) superficial, restricted; (2) deep, restricted; and (3) complex, extensive. Spinoreticular cells with excitatory receptive fields on part of an extremity and activated best by hair movement or light touch were in the first category (Fig. 8.25). These cells were located chiefly in laminae IV and V. Cells activated by deep receptors and also often by strong stimuli applied to skin were categorized as having deep, restricted receptive fields. These cells could be in laminae IV–IX but usually were in the ventral horn. The other spinoreticular neurons had large or multiple receptive fields. Cells with complex, extensive receptive fields were located deep within the gray matter. At least some neurons in each category responded maximally to noxious stimuli (Fig. 8.26). Some of these neurons projected to the level of the midbrain in addition to being activated antidromically from the reticular formation.

In summary, spinoreticular neurons often receive a highly convergent input. Cells of the bilateral ventral flexor reflex tract (bVFRT) presumably correspond to spinoreticular neurons with bilateral receptive fields; other spinoreticular neurons, however, can have relatively restricted fields on part of an extremity. It is likely that many spinoreticular neurons receive inputs from cutaneous and subcutaneous receptors and also from visceral receptors. Some spinoreticular neurons are best excited by tactile stimuli, but others have a wide dynamic range of responsiveness or are excited only by noxious stimuli.

Descending Control of Spinoreticular Neurons

Using recordings of multiunit discharges in a dissected half of the spinal cord following stimulation of contralateral peripheral nerves, Holmqvist *et al.* (1960a) demonstrated that activity in the bVFRT was subject to a tonic descending inhibition, since the discharge increased when the dorsal half of the cord was sectioned in the decerebrate preparation. The activity could also be released by cold block of the

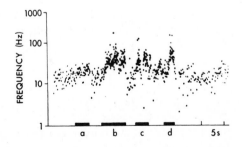

Fig. 8.26. Responses of a spinoreticular neuron to noxious stimuli. The skin was pricked in a, a toe pad squeezed in b and c, and the webbing between two toes was pinched in d. (From Fields *et al.*, 1977b.)

cord or following a lesion at the level of the obex. Ascending activity could be inhibited by stimulation of a dissected dorsolateral fasciculus. The same inhibitory pathway appears to be involved in the tonic descending inhibition of other ascending tracts and of the flexion reflex pathways at the spinal cord level. It is probably also responsible for the phasic depression of the activity of bVFRT axons that occurs during bursts of eye movements during desynchronized sleep (Pompeiano et al., 1967).

Descending excitation of the bVFRT was also demonstrated by Holmqvist et al. (1960b). The descending pathway traveled in the ventral quadrant and ended monosynaptically on contralateral cells of origin of the bVFRT. The descending pathway originated in the brainstem near the lateral vestibular nucleus. Grillner et al. (1968) found evidence that at least part of the pathway was the lateral vestibulospinal tract; however, propriospinal and reticulospinal tracts also contributed.

The axons of spinoreticular neurons were impaled in the cervical spinal cord in a study by Coulter et al. (1976b). Many of the axons could be activated antidromically following stimulation in the ipsilateral lateral reticular nucleus and thus can be presumed to belong to the spinoreticulocerebellar pathway. The remaining axons presumably terminated in the medial reticular formation; these responded to peripheral inputs like axons of the bVFRT. The activity of axons of both categories was affected by tilt; this suggested a convergent input to spinoreticular neurons from the macula of the labyrinth. Presumably, the macular input was transmitted to the spinoreticular neurons by way of the lateral vestibular nucleus and the lateral vestibulospinal tract.

The bVFRT has also been shown to be excited after stimulation of the sensorimotor cortex (Magni and Oscarsson, 1961; Lundberg et al., 1963). Inhibition by corticofugal volleys was not noted.

In summary, spinoreticular neurons are subject to a tonic descending inhibitory control similar to that which affects the spinocervical and spinothalamic tracts. The cells of the spinoreticular tract are excited by volleys descending from the lateral vestibular nucleus in the lateral vestibulospinal tract and perhaps also from the reticular formation. Stimulation of the sensorimotor cortex produces an excitation; inhibition by corticofugal volleys has not been described.

Responses of Reticular Formation Neurons to Somatic Stimuli

Much of the activity recorded from reticular neurons in response to stimulation of receptive fields on the body surface or of peripheral nerves can be attributed to activity ascending in the spinoreticular tract. However, it is likely that part of the responses seen in animals with an intact neuraxis is influenced by other pathways and by input from the cerebellum, cerebral cortex, and other centers. Thus, it cannot be assumed that the responses recorded in the reticular formation represent a faithful transmission of activity ascending directly from the spinal cord, even after taking into account the possibility of convergence of spinoreticular axons from different levels of the cord upon a given reticular neuron.

The investigations that will be reviewed are those that emphasize inputs to the reticular formation from somatosensory stimulation. There are few studies that have employed stimulation of visceral receptors. Emphasis will also be given to investigations in which recordings were made in regions known to be rich in neurons having long ascending or descending axons, since these are the most likely to play a role in sensory processing. Such areas include the nucleus reticularis gigantocellularis and nucleus reticularis pontis caudalis and oralis, as well as the nucleus reticularis ventralis and nucleus reticularis lateralis (Brodal and Rossi, 1955; Torvik and Brodal, 1957; Nauta and Kuypers, 1958; Scheibel and Scheibel, 1958; Valverde, 1961; Magni and Willis, 1963; Wolstencroft, 1964; Nyberg-Hansen, 1965; Petras, 1967; Peterson et al., 1974; Kuypers and Maisky, 1975). Note that some reticulocerebellar projections also originate in the nucleus reticular gigantocellularis, according to Avanzino et al. (1966).

Early studies employing single-unit recordings from reticular neurons consisted essentially of surveys of reticular activity, since the levels of recording encompassed much of the extent of the reticular formation, and no attempt was made to distinguish the neurons according to their projection path. It was found that many reticular neurons could be excited or inhibited by peripheral nerve stimulation or by activation of receptive fields on the body. Convergence of excitation from as wide an area as all four limbs could be seen (Amassian and DeVito, 1954), although the degree of convergence varied from unit to unit, and some kinds of input were more likely to participate in convergence than others (Scheibel et al., 1955). No evidence of a somatotopic organization was detected in these or later investigations. Volleys descending from the sensorimotor cortex often excited reticular neurons monosynaptically and inhibited the responses of reticular neurons to peripheral inputs (Amassian and DeVito, 1954).

Palestini et al. (1957) tried to detect differences in the responses of neurons located in different parts of the reticular formation. Convergent inputs were more prominent for cells in the medial reticular formation, whereas single inputs (especially trigeminal) were more common for neurons of the lateral reticular formation. No differences were found in recordings from regions that were rich in reticular neurons projecting either to the spinal cord or rostrally.

Pompeiano and Swett (1963a) simplified the neural circuitry available for altering the discharges of reticular neurons by recording from decerebrate, cerebellectomized cats. Graded volleys in peripheral cutaneous and muscle nerves were used to characterize the kinds of input reaching reticular neurons (presumably by way of the spinoreticular tract). Of the reticular units affected by cutaneous nerve volleys, most were excited, although some were inhibited. Responses were about the same following stimulation of nerves on either side of the body. One group of units could be excited by low stimulus intensities, while another required higher strengths of stimulation (sufficient to activate Aδ fibers). The low-threshold units were most commonly found in the medulla and caudal pons (in the region of the medial lemniscus, nucleus reticularis gigantocellularis, and nucleus reticularis paramedianus), while the high-threshold units were more often found in the pons and midbrain (nucleus reticularis pontis caudalis and oralis, periaqueductal gray, midbrain reticular formation). Fewer units responded to muscle afferent volleys than to cutaneous volleys, and those that did also responded to cutaneous volleys. Generally, the muscle nerve volleys had to include group II fibers to be effective, although for forelimb nerves high-threshold group I fibers were sometimes able to excite reticular neurons. In experiments on decerebrate cats having intact cerebella (Pompeiano and Swett, 1963b), high-threshold group I muscle afferents were more commonly effective, even for hindlimb muscle nerves; cutaneous nerve thresholds were also lower, and the response patterns were more complex than when the cerebellum was absent. These differences were presumed to be due to activity reaching the reticular formation by way of cerebellar circuitry. The apparent absence of effects on reticular neurons by group Ia muscle afferents, even when the cerebellum was intact, was confirmed in experiments utilizing sinusoidal stretch of muscle to activate primary endings selectively (Barnes and Pompeiano, 1971; Pompeiano and Barnes, 1971). However, group Ib and possibly group II afferents from secondary endings could affect the discharges of some reticular neurons.

Intracellular recordings from reticular neurons revealed the presence of resting and action potentials, excitatory and inhibitory postsynaptic potentials (Limanskii, 1961, 1962; Magni and Willis, 1963, 1964a,b; Segundo et al., 1967a; Ito et al., 1970; Udo and Mano, 1970). Convergent inputs from a variety of sources (including volleys in cutaneous, muscular, and visceral afferents; also vestibular, tectal, and cortical volleys) were demonstrated by recordings of synaptic activity

(Limanskii, 1963, 1966; Magni and Willis, 1964a,b; Udo and Mano, 1970; Peterson and Felpel, 1971; Peterson et al., 1974).

The identification of reticular neurons according to their rostral or caudal projections was initiated by Magni and Willis (1963) and Wolstencroft (1964). Although many of the records of Magni and Willis (1963) were likely to have been from axons (Ito et al., 1970), the fact that synaptic potentials could be recorded from most of the units indicated that the cell bodies were nearby. Stimulation of cutaneous and muscle nerves of the forelimb resulted in excitatory postsynaptic potentials (EPSPs) or combinations of EPSPs and inhibitory postsynaptic potentials (IPSPs) in many reticulospinal neurons (Magni and Willis, 1964b). Most of the reticulospinal neurons studied by Wolstencroft (1964) could be excited by such stimuli as pinch or pressure over much of the body surface. Some cells had inhibitory as well as excitatory receptive fields. A wide convergence of input was also demonstrated when peripheral nerves were stimulated electrically. Thermal stimuli had no effect. Hair movement or other tactile stimuli seldom produced a discharge; the best stimuli were noxious ones, such as pinching the skin with serrated forceps. There was also evidence of an input from muscle receptors.

Segundo et al. (1967b) examined the responsiveness of reticular neurons scattered in many nuclei of the pons and medulla to somatic stimuli. Most of the neurons responded to stimulation of the face or body. The best stimuli were touch or tap. The sizes of the receptive fields varied from widespread (more than half the surface of the skin) to highly restricted (a few square centimeters). Inhibitory receptive fields were also seen. Bilateral receptive fields predominated. Unilateral fields were usually ipsilateral. Highly restricted receptive fields were usually on the face.

Burton (1968) also examined the responses of reticular neurons of the medulla of the cat to somatic stimuli. His sample of cells was in the lateral tegmental field of Berman (1968). Most of the cells responded to trigeminal inputs, either bilateral or ipsilateral. Noxious mechanical or thermal stimuli were required to activate most of the cells. Comparable responses have been reported for units in the ventral reticular nucleus of the rat (Benjamin, 1970).

Bowsher et al. (1968) recorded evoked potentials and unit activity in the nucleus gigantocellularis produced by stimulation of the skin. A lesion of the dorsal column did not affect the evoked potential, whereas bilateral sectioning of the ventral quadrants of the cord eliminated it. The units were activated by brusque but not necessarily noxious mechanical stimuli, but not by touch or joint movement. Since stimulation in the nucleus gigantocellularis produced an evoked potential in the center median nucleus and cooling this part of the reticular formation reduced the center median potential evoked from peripheral stimulation, it was suggested that the nucleus gigantocellularis might be a relay for information ascending to the center median from the spinal cord. In contrast to these results, it was found that many units in the reticular formation of the caudal medulla could be activated by hair movement, although the most effective stimulus was tapping (Bowsher, 1970).

The possibility that neurons of the medullary reticular formation might respond primarily to noxious levels of stimulation was pursued by Casey (1969), using decerebrate, cerebellectomized cats. He recorded unitary activity from the nucleus reticularis gigantocellularis, as well as evoked potentials. Confirming Bowsher *et al.* (1968), Casey found that dorsal column lesions and also lesions of the dorsolateral fasciculi failed to alter potentials evoked in the nucleus reticularis gigantocellularis (NGC) by stimulation of cutaneous nerves, while lesions of the ventral quadrant reduced or abolished the evoked potentials. Dorsal column stimulation did not evoke a potential in the NGC. Of the units that responded to peripheral stimuli, a minority was activated by innocuous stimuli, including joint movement. The majority of units was excited just by noxious stimulation or both by innocuous and noxious stimulation. The receptive fields were large, varying from the surface of one limb to the whole body. Electrical stimulation of cutaneous nerves showed that most units fired maximally only when all the Aδ fibers were stimulated, although some units could be discharged by large afferents (see also Goldman *et al.*, 1972; LeBlanc and Gatipon, 1974). The excitation by Aδ afferents remained after the larger afferents were blocked by anodal current.

Recordings from the nucleus reticularis gigantocellularis were also made by Casey (1971a) in awake, freely moving cats trained to escape noxious stimuli. Many units discharged only in response to noxious stimuli or in association with escape, although some units could be excited by innocuous stimuli. Stimulation in the same area elicited escape or avoidance behavior (Casey, 1971b).

The responses of neurons in the NGC to intraarterial injections of the algesic chemical bradykinin were investigated by Guilbaud *et al.* (1973b). Most cells (82%) were affected. The usual response was an excitation. More than half of the affected cells were also activated by noxious mechanical stimulation of the skin, although the others could be activated just by innocuous stimuli. Electrocortical arousal was either absent or followed the onset of the changes in neural activity. The authors suggest three possible roles for the cells of the NGC that respond to noxious stimuli: (1) they may evoke arousal; (2) they may elicit reflex responses, perhaps through reticulospinal projections; or (3) they may participate in sensory processing. Of course, combinations of these roles would also be possible.

The role of the reticular formation in synchronizing and desynchronizing the electroencephalogram and in altering motor activity is reviewed by Pompeiano (1973).

In summary, neurons of the reticular formation typically receive a convergent input from ascending pathways conveying information from wide areas of the body. Convergence is greater for neurons of the medial than of the lateral reticular formation. The fibers of cutaneous nerves that are responsible for activating reticular neurons include Aαβ axons for some neurons but Aδ fibers for others. The muscle afferents that are most effective in activating reticular neurons belong to groups II and III, although high-threshold group I afferents can excite some cells. These are not group Ia fibers. Antidromic activation of reticular neurons can be used to identify the cells by their projection path. Reticulospinal neurons can best be activated by strong somatic stimuli, such as pinch or pressure, over much of the body surface. Other, unidentified reticular neurons respond to weaker stimuli and may have more restricted receptive fields, especially on the face. Neurons in the lateral tegmental field appear to respond best to noxious stimuli in the trigeminal distribution. On the other hand, the nucleus reticularis gigantocellularis contains numerous cells that respond best to noxious stimulation of the body or to volleys in Aδ fibers. Such neurons discharge in awake, freely moving cats in response to noxious stimuli or in association with escape behavior. Stimulation in the nucleus reticularis gigantocellularis is aversive. Intraarterial injections of the algesic chemical bradykinin activates neurons of the nucleus reticularis gigantocellularis. Such cells may (1) help trigger arousal, (2) assist in reflex responses, or (3) contribute to the sensory experience of pain.

RESPONSES OF NEURONS IN THE RHOMBENCEPHALIC RAPHE NUCLEI

Only a few studies describe the responses of neurons in the raphe magnus and pallidus nuclei (Moolenaar *et al.*, 1976; Menzies, 1976; Anderson *et al.*, 1977; West and Wolstencroft, 1977). Many of the cells can be antidromically activated following stimulation of the spinal cord. Conduction velocities have been reported to range from 1 to 67 m/s (West and Wolstencroft, 1977); cells having the slowest conduction are concentrated in the nucleus raphe pallidus and the ventral part of the raphe magnus, while the faster-conducting neurons are in raphe magnus.

Most raphe neurons have somatic receptive fields, often to innocuous stimuli, especially deep pressure or tapping, although some require noxious stimuli before they respond (Moolenaar *et al.*, 1976; Anderson *et al.*, 1977). There is generally a spontaneous discharge. Receptive fields are large, often involving all four limbs. The cells responding to noxious stimuli appear to be concentrated in the rostral part of the nucleus raphe magnus (Moolenaar *et al.*, 1976).

THE SPINOTECTAL TRACT

Loosely speaking, the spinotectal tract consists of the spinal projections to the midbrain. However, several different components should be distinguished. There is a "spinotectal" tract proper, which ends in the deep layers of the superior colliculus. Somatosensory afferents also terminate in nuclear groups adjacent to the inferior colliculus or between the superior and inferior colliculi in areas known as the external nucleus of the inferior colliculus and the intercollicular nucleus. A notable projection is to the periaqueductal gray, an area implicated in pain mechanisms. Finally, some authors describe a direct spinal projection to the midbrain reticular formation.

Phylogeny

Spinotectal fibers are found in the same vertebrate forms mentioned previously as having spinoreticular projections (see description and references; refer also to Antonetty and Webster, 1975; Robards *et al.*, 1976).

Anatomy of the Spinotectal Tract

The locations of the cells of origin of the spinotectal tract have not been studied extensively. For the cat, it may be presumed that they are in the same area of the cord gray matter as the cells of origin of the spinoreticular and spinothalamic tracts (see Figs. 8.3 and 8.22). In the monkey, there are large numbers of spinotectal cells in lamina I, and others are found in laminae IV–VII (Fig. 8.27) (Trevino, 1976).

The spinotectal tract ascends in the ventral part of the lateral funiculus and in the ventral funiculus, along with the spinoreticular, spinothalamic, and ventral spinocerebellar tracts (Anderson and Berry, 1959; Mehler *et al.*, 1960). The fibers ascend with the spinothalamic tract into the midbrain, turning medially to cross the dorsolateral border of the brachium conjunctivum. Terminal fields have been de-

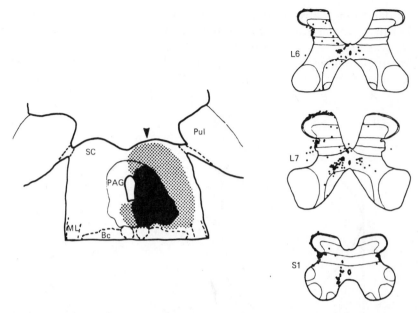

Fig. 8.27. Horseradish peroxidase was injected into the midbrain of a monkey in the area shown at the left. Cells that were labeled in the enlargements are shown at the right on composite plots at each segmental level. (From Trevino, 1976.)

scribed in the following midbrain structures: external nucleus of the inferior colliculus, the intercollicular nucleus (lateral area between the inferior and superior colliculi), the periaqueductal gray (especially rostrally), deep layers of the superior colliculus, the cuneiform nucleus, the nucleus of Darkschewitz, the red nucleus, and the midbrain reticular formation (Morin et al., 1951; Anderson and Berry, 1959; Mehler et al., 1960; Lund and Webster, 1967b; Breazile and Kitchell, 1968; Rao et al., 1969; Schroeder and Jane, 1971; Jane and Schroeder, 1971; Hazlett et al., 1972; Antonetty and Webster, 1975; Kerr, 1975b; Robards et al., 1976).

Particular attention was given to the spinal projections to the superior colliculus in the rat (Fig. 8.28) by Antonetty and Webster (1975). The axons leave the area of the medial lemniscus and spinothalamic tract at the level of the caudal superior colliculus and enter the latter through its ventral aspect. Terminals were abundant in the caudal half of the stratum album intermedium bilaterally after a unilateral cord lesion. Degeneration extended across the entire mediolateral extent of the layer. Terminal degeneration was also seen in the stratum album profundum and stratum griseum profundum. There was a rostrocaudal topography—spinotectal fibers from different cord levels ended in bands across the caudal half of the superior colliculus. Evidence was given for a pattern of projection of fibers ascending in two different pathways, one ipsilateral and the other contralateral, with different areas of termination (as shown in Fig. 8.28).

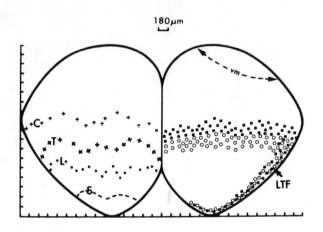

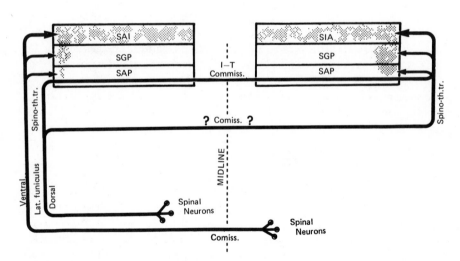

Fig. 8.28. Diagram above shows the extent of degeneration of the spinotectal tract from the cervical (C), thoracic (T), lumbar (L), and sacral (S), cord on the left side and the extent of distribution of the tract from the upper five cervical segments on the right side. LTF = lateral terminal field. The scheme below shows the proposed organization of two components of the spinotectal pathway with reference to terminations in different layers of the superior colliculus. (From Antonetty and Webster, 1975.)

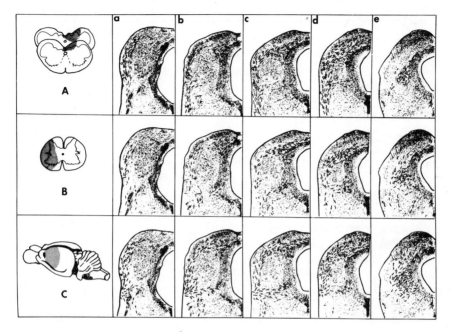

Fig. 8.29. Terminal degeneration in the intercollicular nucleus following lesions of (A) the dorsal column nuclei, (B) the spinal cord, or (C) the sensorimotor cortex in the opossum. (From Robards *et al.*, 1976.)

The projection to the intercollicular region was described in the opossum by Robards *et al.* (1976). Following cordotomy, terminal degeneration was found in the external nucleus of the inferior colliculus and in the intercollicular nucleus. There was also degeneration in the periaqueductal gray, the deep layers of the superior colliculus, and in the cuneiform nucleus. Decussating fibers ended in the contralateral external and intercollicular nuclei. Much of the same region received terminals from the dorsal column nuclei and from the sensorimotor cortex (Fig. 8.29).

Responses of Midbrain Neurons to Somatic Stimuli

No recordings have as yet been made from spinotectal neurons, and so the properties of these cells must be inferred from the response characteristics of neurons in the midbrain. However, since midbrain units can be influenced by a variety of pathways in addition to the direct spinotectal tract, such inferences must be made with caution.

Evoked potentials were recorded by Morin (1953) from the midbrain tegmentum of cats following stimulation of cutaneous, muscle, or joint nerves. The potentials were largest in a lateral area just dorsal to the medial lemniscus. Since the potentials remained after the dorsal columns were sectioned, it was concluded that the potentials were due to activity in the spinotectal or spinothalamic tract. A separate potential was seen in recordings from the area of the central tegmental tract. Morin felt that this might reflect activity relayed to the midbrain through the reticular formation.

Collins and O'Leary (1954) also recorded an evoked potential in the medial part of the midbrain tegmentum. The potential reached its maximum size only when the peripheral nerve volley included the Aδ fibers. The ascending activity traveled in the ventrolateral quadrant of the cord on the side opposite the stimulated nerve. A later study of Collins and Randt (1960) showed that C fibers could also contribute to the activity recorded in this area.

Evoked potentials have been observed in recordings from the superior colliculus following electrical stimulation of the skin. The fastest component of the activity is conveyed in fibers of the ventrolateral funiculi (Jassik-Gerschenfeld, 1966). Stimulation in the bulbar reticular formation evoked similar potentials in the superior colliculus, suggesting the possibility that some of the ascending activity is relayed in the reticular formation.

Responses of single units to somatic stimuli were recorded in the midbrain tegmentum of the goat by Cooper et al. (1953). They also found occasional responses in recordings from the deep layers of the superior colliculus. Mancia et al. (1957) found that many units in the midbrain reticular formation and periaqueductal gray could be affected by stimulation of all four limbs. Pomeiano and Swett (1963a) observed that a high proportion of the units they studied in the periaqueductal gray and midbrain reticular formation were activated by cutaneous Aδ fibers but not by larger afferents. Cells in the tectum received a convergent input from cutaneous myelinated afferents of all sizes.

Bell et al. (1964) mapped the receptive fields of neurons in the midbrain reticular formation. Somatic stimuli produced responses in well over half the cells. Tapping or hair movement excited most of the cells, although a few required strong pressure. The receptive fields of half the units activated by somatic stimuli were widespread (half to all of the body surface). However, 20% of the units had "highly restricted" receptive fields (a few square centimeters). When a receptive field was unilateral, it was almost always contralateral to the unit. Many neurons showed responses to several different sensory modalities.

A number of investigators have reported responses of units in the superior colliculus, usually in its deeper layers, to somatic stimuli (Horn and Hill, 1966; Straschill and Hoffmann, 1969; Stein and Arigbede, 1972; B. Gordon, 1973; Abrahams and Rose, 1975a,b). In the experiments of Straschill and Hoffman (1969) and of Stein and Arigbede (1972), the receptive fields were most often contralateral; their sizes ranged from a paw to several limbs. Some units were activated by hair movement, but many required tapping, squeezing, or electrical stimulation of the skin. In B. Gordon's (1973) experiments, done on cats, the receptive fields were also contralateral, but they were restricted in size, and hair movement was the best stimulus for most cells. Strong stimuli seldom increased the discharges.

While most other workers emphasized the effects of cutaneous stimuli on units in the superior colliculus, Abrahams and Rose (1975a,b) were impressed by the strength of the input from muscle afferents, both of the neck and of the limbs. The effective afferents were generally of group II and III size, although group I afferents were sometimes effective. Many of the collicular neurons receiving an input from muscle afferents are cells of origin of the tectospinal tract (Abrahams and Rose, 1975b). The spinal pathway conveying muscle input proved to be largely in the dorsolateral fasciculus contralateral to the unit.

Descending Control

Nothing is known about possible descending control of the spinotectal tract.

In summary, the locations of the cells of origin of the spinotectal tract are unknown but can be presumed to be similar to those of the spinothalamic and spinoreticular tracts. The spinotectal tract ascends in the ventral quadrant to the midbrain, where different components of the pathway end in the following nuclei: external nucleus of the inferior colliculus, intercollicular nucleus, deep layers of the superior colliculus, cuneiform nucleus, nucleus of Darkschewitz, periaqueductal gray, red nucleus, and midbrain reticular formation. No responses have been recorded from spinotectal neurons. Activity in the midbrain tegmentum can be evoked in response to stimulation of cutaneous, muscle, or joint nerves. The maximum potentials are produced by Aδ and C fibers. Single units in the midbrain reticular formation are often best activated by Aδ fibers. Many cells, however, can be excited by weak mechanical stimuli. Most units have very large receptive fields, although some have restricted ones located on the contralateral body. Neurons in the deep layers of the superior colliculus are often activated by stimulation of large cutaneous afferent or by weak mechanical stimulation *of the skin. The receptive fields can be large, but they are often small and contralateral. Muscle afferents of the limbs and neck are also effective in activating tectal neurons. The best excitation is produced by group II and III afferents, but sometimes group I fibers can activate cells. Many of the responsive units in the tectum give rise to tectospinal fibers.*

CONCLUSIONS

1. The spinothalamic tract is present in a variety of mammalian species, and it is particularly prominent in monkeys and in man. It is likely that there is a spinothalamic projection in some reptiles and in birds.

2. The cells of origin of the spinothalamic tract are both in the dorsal horn, as traditionally believed, and in the ventral horn. In the cat lumbosacral enlargement, the ventral horn component is more prominent than the dorsal horn one, but in the monkey and rat, the majority of the cells are in the dorsal horn. The laminar distribution includes laminae I and IV–VIII.

3. Although most spinothalamic tract cells project to the contralateral diencephalon, a few project ipsilaterally.

4. It is not yet certain whether the decussation of spinothalamic tract axons is in the posterior or anterior commissure of the cord nor is it known at what level relative to the cell body.

5. The spinothalamic tract appears to consist of small to intermediate-sized myelinated fibers; there do not seem to be any unmyelinated fibers, at least in the monkey.

6. The spinothalamic tract has at least a roughly somatotopic organization, with the caudal levels of the body represented dorsolaterally and the rostral parts ventromedially. The axons are not in a compact bundle, but spread widely over the ventral quadrant.

7. The traditional view that pain and temperature fibers are in a lateral spinothalamic tract and tactile fibers in a ventral spinothalamic tract does not appear to hold for the hindlimb portion of the monkey spinothalamic tract. The only distinctly segregated axons are those belonging to cells responding to proprioceptive stimuli, and these axons are in a band along the ventral margin of the cord.

8. The spinothalamic tract ends in the diencephalon. In the rat and the cat, the terminals in the ventrobasal complex are rostral to those of the dorsal column nuclei; in fact, in the cat they are in the ventral lateral nucleus. In addition, there are endings in the PO_m and in intralaminar nuclei (centralis lateralis, centralis medialis, and parafascicularis), as well as the zona incerta. However, in the monkey the

spinothalamic tract ends in the VPL nucleus in the same zone as the dorsal column nuclear projections. The intralaminar projection is to the centralis lateralis nucleus, although possible terminals in other intralaminar nuclei have been claimed, and there are endings in the PO_m and in the zona incerta and posteromedial hypothalamus.

9. Some spinothalamic tract neurons, including many of those located in lamina I, respond specifically to intense mechanical or mechanical and thermal stimuli. Most spinothalamic tract cells are of the wide dynamic range variety and can be activated both by innocuous and noxious stimuli. Some spinothalamic tract cells are responsive just to innocuous mechanical stimuli or to proprioceptive stimuli.

10. A convergence of input from $A\alpha\beta$, $A\delta$, and C fibers can be demonstrated for at least some spinothalamic tract cells. However, the proportion of such cells has not been determined.

11. The receptive fields of spinothalamic tract neurons are on the average larger for neurons in lamina IV than for cells in lamina I, and they are larger for cells in lamina V than for those in IV.

12. Many spinothalamic tract cells are activated in a slowly adapting fashion by mechanical stimuli. The responses grow as the intensity is graded from innocuous to noxious pressure.

13. Spinothalamic tract cells with rapidly adapting responses appear to signal stimulus acceleration or velocity.

14. Volleys descending in the dorsal columns generally inhibit spinothalamic tract neurons. In the case of wide-dynamic-response cells, the inhibition is preceded by an excitation.

15. Electrical stimulation of peripheral cutaneous nerves or of the skin can result in a double-burst discharge in spinothalamic tract cells. The initial burst is due to $A\alpha\beta$ and the later burst to $A\delta$ fibers.

16. Many spinothalamic tract cells can be excited by visceral afferents or by high-threshold muscle afferents, as well as by cutaneous afferents. The muscle input can be demonstrated by the injection of algesic chemicals into the arterial circulation of skeletal muscles.

17. The rapidly adapting responses of spinothalamic tract cells to innocuous mechanical stimulation of the skin can often be inhibited following stimulation of the sensorimotor cortex. However, the same stimuli fail to affect the slowly adapting responses to noxious mechanical or thermal stimuli.

18. Spinothalamic tract cells can be inhibited by stimulation in the reticular formation.

19. Another descending pathway that inhibits spinothalamic tract cells can be demonstrated by stimulation in the region of the raphe magnus nucleus. The pathway appears to descend in the dorsolateral fasciculus. It may be a raphe–spinal tract, and it may be serotonergic.

However, other nonserotonergic descending axons could play a role as well. This pathway is a candidate path to account for stimulus-produced analgesia.

20. There is a prominent spinoreticular pathway in all vertebrate classes.

21. The spinoreticular pathway includes a component that is part of a pathway from the spinal cord to the cerebellum and another component that terminates in the medial part of the reticular formation.

22. The cells of origin of the spinoreticular pathway in the cat are located both ipsilaterally and contralaterally to the region of termination of the axons, and the cells are found both in the dorsal horn and in the ventral horn.

23. The spinoreticular tract ascends in the ventral quadrant and ends in a number of nuclei of the reticular formation, including the lateral reticular nucleus (a cerebellar relay nucleus), the nucleus gigantocellularis, the nuclei reticularis pontis caudalis and oralis, and others. There are also spinal projections to the bulbar raphe nuclei.

24. In the primate, there is evidence that the spinoreticular projection is largely uncrossed.

25. Many spinoreticular neurons have bilateral receptive fields. However, others have restricted fields.

26. Some spinoreticular neurons are excited by innocuous mechanical stimuli. Others are of the wide dynamic range variety. Still others are excited just by intense stimuli. Some receive an input from visceral receptors.

27. Spinoreticular neurons are under the control of the tonic descending inhibitory pathway that alters transmission in the spinal cord flexion reflex pathways. There is also a descending excitatory pathway that originates in part in the lateral vestibular nucleus and in part in the reticular formation.

28. Neurons in the reticular formation have been found that respond to somatic stimuli. Many of these cells are in areas that give rise to long descending or ascending projections.

29. Reticular neurons may have large or restricted receptive fields. They may respond to $A\alpha\beta$ fibers or primarily to $A\delta$ fibers when cutaneous nerves are stimulated. Effective muscle afferents include group II and group III fibers; in some circumstances, high-threshold group I fibers (but not group Ia muscle spindle afferents) help excite reticular neurons. This may require an intact cerebellum.

30. Reticulospinal neurons in the nucleus gigantocellularis are generally best excited by intense mechanical stimuli, although some unidentified neurons in the same nucleus respond to innocuous cutaneous stimuli or even to joint movement.

31. Neurons in the nucleus gigantocellularis have been shown to discharge in response to noxious stimulation or during escape behavior in awake, freely moving cats. Stimulation in the same area produces escape or avoidance behavior.

32. Intraarterial injections of the algesic chemical bradykinin produce an excitation of many neurons in the nucleus gigantocellularis.

33. The nucleus gigantocellularis appears to play a role in pain mechanisms. Particular functions may include one or more of the following: (1) production of arousal, (2) reflex responses, (3) sensory processing.

34. Neurons in the raphe magnus and pallidus have been studied. Some are activated by innocuous stimuli, while others require intense stimulation.

35. The spinotectal tract consists of several components, including projections to the superior colliculus, the external nucleus of the inferior colliculus and intercollicular nucleus, the periaqueductal gray, and the midbrain reticular formation.

36. The cells of origin of the spinotectal tract appear to be located in laminae I and IV–VII in the monkey.

37. The projection to the superior colliculus in the rat has been mapped; the projection is very precise.

38. The spinotectal projection to the intercollicular region ends in the same area as do connections from the dorsal column nuclei and the sensorimotor cortex, suggesting that this is an important somatosensory integrative center.

39. No recordings have been made from identified spinotectal neurons.

40. Neurons of the midbrain reticular formation and periaqueductal gray seem to be excited best by Aδ fibers. However, many of the units respond to innocuous stimuli. The receptive fields are often very large, but sometimes they are restricted and contralateral.

41. Neurons in the deep layers of the superior colliculus often have small, contralateral receptive fields and respond to innocuous mechanical stimuli. There is also an important input from muscle afferents, especially groups II and III. This is true for cells of origin of the tectospinal tract.

9 The Sensory Channels

As discussed in Chapter 1, the mechanism for transmission of information concerning a specific form of sensation can be referred to as a sensory channel. The sensory channel includes the receptors, any spinal cord processing circuits, and the sensory pathways transmitting the information to the thalamus and cerebral cortex, as well as the parts of the brain that then process the data to produce perception. This chapter will consider what is known or can be deduced about the initial parts of the sensory channels for several of the kinds of somatic sensation. Emphasis will be placed on information derived from human subjects and from primates.

TOUCH–PRESSURE

The first sensory channel to be considered is that responsible for the sensations of touch and of pressure. These are often thought to reflect a continuum of stimulus intensity, and so they are sometimes referred to as touch–pressure. The sensation meant here is one that has a low threshold and that is maintained as long as the stimulus is applied (up to 1–2 min) (Horch *et al.*, 1975). The tactile experiences associated with mechanical transients will be discussed under the heading of flutter–vibration.

Receptors

The sensory receptors thought to be involved in signaling information about the duration of low intensity, maintained mechanical contact, and about the degree by which skin is indented include the type I and type II slowly adapting sensitive mechanoreceptors

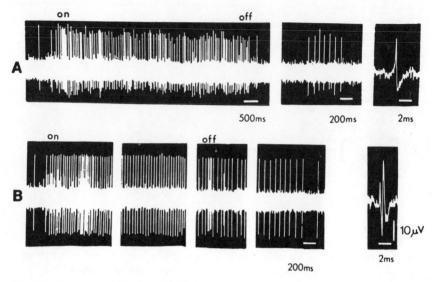

Fig. 9.1. Responses of (A) type I and (B) type II units in human skin. (From Hagbarth *et al.*, 1970.)

(Chapter 2). The type I receptors are associated with Merkel cells, sometimes in a recognizable tactile dome (Tapper, 1965; Burgess *et al.*, 1968; K. R. Smith, 1968; Iggo and Muir, 1969). Domelike structures are not seen in glabrous skin, and they are difficult to recognize in the skin of primates (K. R. Smith, 1970). However, type I endings are found in the skin of monkeys and of man (Fig. 9.1) (Werner and Mountcastle, 1965; Perl, 1968; Harrington and Merzenich, 1970; Knibestöl and Vallbo, 1970; Knibestöl, 1975; Johansson, 1976). Type I endings are very sensitive to stimuli applied directly to the ending, but they are relatively insensitive to stimuli applied to immediately adjacent areas of skin (Fig. 9.2). Type II endings are associated with Ruffini endings and are found in hairy and glabrous skin and in cats, monkeys, and man (Fig. 9.1) (Chambers *et al.*, 1972; Burgess *et al.*, 1968; Knibestöl and Vallbo, 1970; Harrington and Merzenich, 1970; Knibestöl, 1975; Johansson, 1976). They respond to small displacements of the skin, both over the receptor and adjacent to it, and are sensitive to skin stretch (Fig. 9.2). Both type I and type II endings have a degree of velocity responsiveness that might assist the nervous system in stimulus localization (Békésy, 1967).

Werner and Mountcastle (1965) found that slowly adapting mechano-receptors in the hairy skin of the cat or monkey responded to skin indentations of less than 15 μm (their data undoubtedly included the responses of both type I and type II endings). The stimulus–response relationships proved to be fitted best by a power function of the form

$$Response = K \ (stimulus \ intensity)^n$$

The exponent n had a mean value of 0.52 for ten selected fibers (Fig. 9.3). A calculation based on information theory suggested that the information transmitted by such fibers would allow the discrimination of only about six or seven steps of stimulus intensity, an estimate that is consistent with values obtained in human psychophysical experiments (Fig. 9-3B) (Miller, 1956; Jones, 1960; Mountcastle *et al.*, 1966; Harrington and Merzenich, 1970). Werner and Mountcastle concluded that the overall neural transfer between the level of the first-order tactile neurons and the level of perception must be linear to give such good agreement between the stimulus–response properties of the receptors and sensory experience.

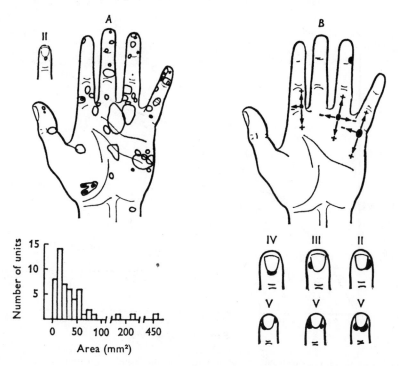

Fig. 9.2. Receptive fields of slowly adapting mechanoreceptors in human skin. The receptive fields in A are for type I receptors, and the histogram shows the distribution of receptive field sizes for them. The receptive fields in B are for type II endings. The arrows indicate responses to stretching (+ = excitation, − = reduced firing). (From Knibestöl, 1975.)

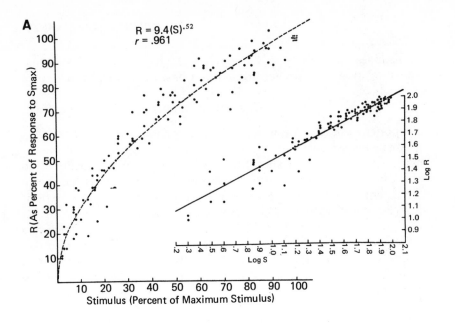

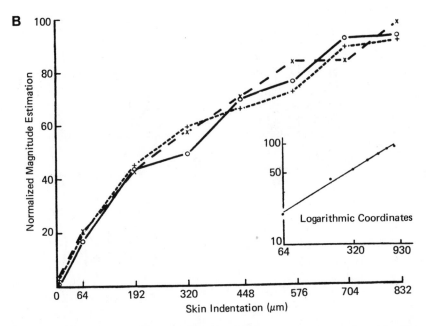

Fig. 9.3. (A) Input–output curves for slowly adapting receptors in monkey skin. (From Werner and Mountcastle, 1965.) (B) Relationship between estimates of stimulus intensity and the amount of skin indentation in human subjects. Three different rates of skin indentation are shown to give similar results. The pooled results are plotted on logarithmic coordinates in the inset (slope 0.59). (From Harrington and Merzenich, 1970.)

Harrington and Merzenich (1970) also found that a power function provided a good fit for the stimulus–response relationships of both type I and type II receptors in hairy skin (the ranges of n were 0.35–0.77 and 0.39–0.75 for type I and type II fibers, respectively). However, slowly adapting receptors in the glabrous skin are fitted best by linear functions (see Mountcastle et al., 1966; Werner and Mountcastle, 1968). Harrington and Merzenich observed that the sensation of pressure was lost when the skin was anesthetized, suggesting that subcutaneous receptors were not involved in the sensation being studied. Rapidly adapting receptors could not account for the maintained sensation of pressure, and in their experience type I receptors when activated in human subjects did not produce any sensation (see also Järvilehto et al., 1976). They concluded that type II slowly adapting receptors are responsible for pressure sensation (the sensation referred to here as touch–pressure), and they agreed that the central nervous system must operate linearly on the data provided by these receptors.

Kruger and Kenton (1973) criticized some of the propositions put forward by Mountcastle and his associates. Kruger and Kenton obtained linear relationships for most of the slowly adapting receptors in their sample from hairy skin. They contested the notion that the central nervous system necessarily operates upon the data from the slowly adapting cutaneous mechanoreceptors in a linear way. And they calculated that a type I fiber is capable of signaling 17 or 18 levels of stimulus intensity (Fig. 9.4). It appears that it may be premature to stress the closeness of correspondence between the activity of the type I and II endings and the results of psychophysical experiments. However, it can be said that the information transmitted by the receptors is more than sufficient to account for the human sensation.

For human type I and type II receptors, a log tanh function (Naka and Rushton, 1966) provided a better fit for the overall stimulus–response relationship than did a power function (Knibestöl, 1975), although a power function often provided the best fit for the static response. The responses were far from linear, despite being from receptors in glabrous skin (cf. Mountcastle et al., 1966). Furthermore, different functions can be obtained in the same subject for the stimulus–response relationships in psychophysical tests and in the activity recorded from slowly adapting mechanoreceptors (Fig. 9.5) (Knibestöl and Vallbo, 1976). This suggests that at least in some individuals the central nervous system processing of sensory data is not an overall linear transform.

Type I endings should not be ruled out as contributors to the sensation of touch–pressure. Tapper (1970) found that cats can be trained to respond to activation of individual type I endings. Type I receptors

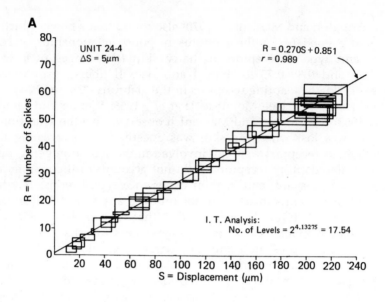

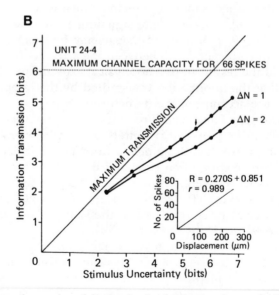

Fig. 9.4. A shows the number of discrete levels of activation that can be identified in the discharge of a type I receptor, using a graphical solution. The information theory analysis in B indicated that seventeen to eighteen discrete levels can be recognized. (From Kruger and Kenton, 1973.)

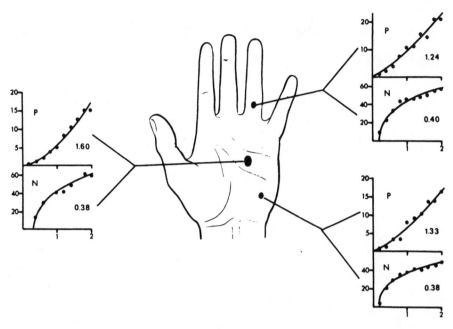

Fig. 9.5. Psychophysical (P) and neural (N) function in the same subject from stimulation at several different positions on the hand. The neural activity was recorded from three different type I slowly adapting mechanoreceptors. (From Knibestöl and Vallbo, 1976.)

appear to represent the bulk of the slowly adapting receptor population in the human hand (Knibestöl, 1975). Finally, there is no reason to assume that tactile stimuli (apart from small laboratory stimulators) would activate just single type I endings; a stimulus involving contact with a few square centimeters of skin would probably stimulate a number of type I receptors nearly simultaneously (Burgess *et al.*, 1974), allowing the possibility of spatial summation in the central pathway.

Spinal Pathways

Some information is available about spinal cord processing of input from type I receptors. These fibers appear to project directly into the deeper layers of the dorsal horn, rather than follow the recurrent course used by hair-follicle afferents, which are responsible for the candelabra endings (Fig. 9.6) (A. G. Brown, 1977). Interneuronal responses to type I input have been investigated in Tapper's laboratory. Some interneurons can be discharged by the excitatory input from a single type I afferent (Tapper and Mann, 1968). In fact, a single type I

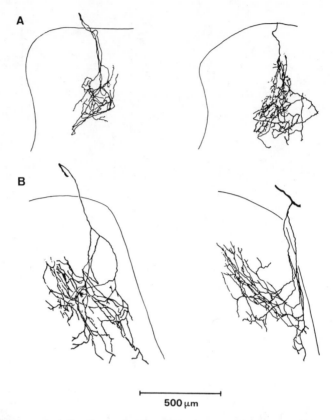

500 μm

Fig. 9.6. The terminal distribution of two collaterals of a type I afferent are shown in A and of a type II afferent in B. (From A. G. Brown, 1977.)

fiber can produce either excitation, inhibition, or combinations of these in dorsal horn interneurons (P. B. Brown *et al.*, 1973). Although some interneurons are affected just by type I fibers, many receive a convergent input also from hair-follicle afferents (Tapper *et al.*, 1973).

Transmission of touch–pressure information seems to involve several different parts of the cord white matter (Fig. 9.7). The dorsal column alone appears to be sufficient for transmission of tactile information (Myers *et al.*, 1974; Frommer *et al.*, 1977; however, cf. Wall, 1970), but type I activity from the hindlimb depends upon the dorsolateral fasciculus (Tapper, 1970; Mann *et al.*, 1972). The profound tactile deficits that result from sectioning the dorsal column plus the dorsolateral fasciculus in cats suggest that the critical pathways for touch–pressure in this animal ascend in the dorsal half of the cord. It is not clear if some touch–pressure information can also use the ventral quadrant pathways in the cat, since most studies of the effects of lesions did not distinguish between touch–pressure (a slowly adapting sensation) and flutter–vibration (a rapidly adapting sensation). It is probable that touch–pressure information does reach the brain by way of the ventral half of the cord in primates and in man. For instance, the patient of Noordenbos and Wall (1976) could sense touch and pressure bilaterally despite a transection of all of the cord except one anterolateral quadrant.

Several sensory pathways are activated by type I and type II endings. A. G. Brown (1968) found axons within the fasciculus gracilis with the properties of type I receptors, as well as others having the properties of type II endings. Petit and Burgess (1968), on the other hand, found only type II primary afferents in the dorsal columns, not type I afferents. Type I receptors have been reported to activate cells of the second-order dorsal column pathway (Angaut-Petit, 1975b), and Angaut-Petit suggests that Brown recorded the responses of these second-order fibers. On the other hand, there appears to be a direct projection of type I primary afferents from the forelimb up the fasciculus cuneatus (Pubols and Pubols, 1973; Bromberg and Whitehorn, 1974). In any case, information from both type I and type II fibers reaches the dorsal column nuclei. Furthermore, responses have been recorded from neurons in the dorsal column nuclei that are consistent with the activation of type I and II receptors (Kruger *et al.*, 1961; Perl *et al.*, 1962; Gordon and Jukes, 1964a; A. G. Brown *et al.*, 1974).

Brown and Franz (1969) did not find any evidence that type I or II receptors activate neurons of the spinocervical tract. However, Mann

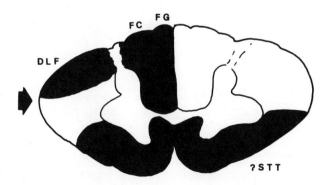

Fig. 9.7. The blackened areas show the locations of the pathways that appear to transmit touch–pressure. The arrow at the left indicates the side of the input. The pathways include the fasciculus cuneatus and gracilis (FC, FG), the dorsolateral fasciculus (DLF) and possibly the spinothalamic tract (STT).

et al. (1971) recorded from axons in the L6–S1 region that were antidromically activated from the dorsolateral column, but not from the restiform body, and that were discharged by type I receptors. They were not certain that these axons belong to the spinocervical tract, but they do give evidence for an alternative route to the dorsal column for such information. It is conceivable that the axons project to the dorsal column nuclei (cf. Gordon and Grant, 1972; Rustioni, 1973, 1974; Dart and Gordon, 1973). Lesions interrupting the dorsal column did not alter the cortical evoked potential produced by activation of a single type I receptor, whereas a discrete lesion of the dorsolateral fasciculus eliminated the evoked potential (Mann *et al.*, 1972). This suggests that the pathway in the dorsolateral column is more important for the transmission of type I activity than is the dorsal column route.

Spinothalamic tract cells in the monkey were often found to respond with a maintained discharge to pressure stimuli (Willis *et al.*, 1974), but the thresholds for such responses were high enough to cause doubt that type I or II receptors were involved. However, the possibility that the stimuli stretched the skin enough to activate type II receptors in adjacent areas was not ruled out.

In summary, it seems likely that the sensation of touch–pressure depends upon input to the central nervous system from type I and type II slowly adapting cutaneous mechanoreceptors. There is a synapse in the pathway from type I afferents of the hindlimb, allowing sensory processing to occur within the spinal cord. The ascending pathways are in the dorsal columns and the dorsolateral fasciculus in the cat and probably also in the ventral quadrants in monkeys and in man. The tracts include the fasciculus gracilis (second-order fibers carrying type I information, primary afferents from type II receptors), the fasciculus cuneatus (primary afferents from both type I and type II receptors), an unidentified pathway (the spinocervical tract?) of the dorsolateral fasciculus (second-order fibers carrying type I information), and in monkeys possibly the spinothalamic tract (second-order axons carrying type II information?).

FLUTTER–VIBRATION

When an oscillating stimulus is applied to human skin, two different sensations are felt, depending upon the frequency of the oscillation. In the range of 5–40 Hz, the sensation is described as "flutter," whereas oscillations at frequencies over 60 Hz produce a sensation of "vibration." The two sensations together can be called "flutter–vibration" (Talbot *et al.*, 1968).

Receptors

It is clear from human psychophysical studies that two different receptor populations are responsible for the sensations of flutter and of vibration. The sense of flutter is localized accurately to an area of skin, and the threshold is elevated by an order of magnitude when the skin is anesthetized. Vibration is poorly localized to deep tissues and remains intact after the skin is anesthetized (Talbot *et al.*, 1968). Therefore, the receptors that are responsible for flutter are to be found within the skin, while those responsible for vibration are in tissue deep to the skin. Furthermore, the thresholds are sufficiently low to make it evident that sensitive mechanoreceptors must be involved.

The most obvious types of receptors that are candidates for the sense of flutter are the rapidly adapting sensitive mechanoreceptors—Meissner's corpuscles in glabrous skin (Figs. 9.8 and 9.9) and hair-follicle and field receptors in hairy skin. However, C mechanoreceptors and the slowly adapting mechanoreceptors should also be considered, since these all have discharge patterns with a velocity-sensitive component (see Chapter 2). The obvious candidate receptor for vibration is the Pacinian corpuscle (Fig. 9.8), but muscle and joint receptors should also be considered.

Talbot *et al.* (1968) compared the curve relating threshold for flutter–vibration sensation to stimulus frequency in the glabrous skin of the human hand to the tuning curves of "quickly adapting" and Pacinian corpuscle afferents of the monkey hand (Fig. 9.10). Tuning curves consisted of plots of thresholds for one-to-one entrainment of a receptor at different frequencies of sinusoidal stimulation. The quickly adapting (Meissner) receptors had best frequencies of about 30 Hz (20–40 Hz), whereas the Pacinian corpuscles had best frequencies of about 250 Hz. The tuning curves for the quickly adapting receptors overlay the low-frequency end of the curve based on human psychophysical data (Fig. 9.10A), whereas the tuning curve for the Pacinian corpuscles overlay the high-frequency end (Fig. 9.10B). This finding suggests that flutter in glabrous skin results from the input to the central nervous system from Meissner's corpuscles and vibration from Pacinian corpuscles. There is also a sensation of "roughness" at amplitudes of vibration below those that produce one-for-one entrainment of the receptors but that do produce a phase-locking of responses to the stimuli. Frequency or "pitch" discrimination is poor in human skin, presumably because individual members of the receptor populations have similar tuning curves. The significant signal is location, rather than frequency. One major question that was left unanswered by Talbot *et al.* (1968) was how stimulus intensity is coded in the

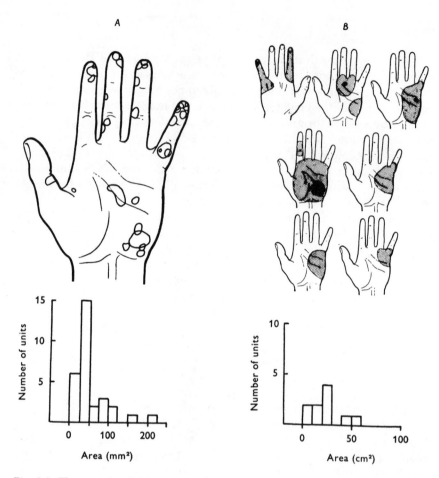

Fig. 9.8. The receptive fields in A are for rapidly adapting receptors (Meissner's corpuscles) in the glabrous skin of the human hand, while those in B are for Pacinian corpuscles. Note the change in scale for the abscissas in the graphs. (From Knibestöl, 1973.)

flutter–vibration system. Intensity of sensation was found to vary linearly with the amplitude of the stimulus in the human psychophysical experiments, yet the discharges of individual receptors increased along a discontinuous curve. One possibility that was suggested is that the number of receptors that participate in the response grows in proportion to stimulus intensity.

Merzenich and Harrington (1969) extended the findings of Talbot *et al.* to the hairy skin. Thresholds for vibration applied to the distal ventral forearm were higher than on glabrous skin, and the minimum threshold was at 200 Hz, which is a lower best frequency than that for glabrous skin. Exploration of the hairy skin revealed low-threshold spots over hair follicles; furthermore, oscillatory stimuli at 100 Hz applied to touch corpuscles did not produce a sensation of vibration. The responses of both rapidly and slowly adapting afferents of the hairy skin were investigated. G2 hair-follicle afferents could be excited by

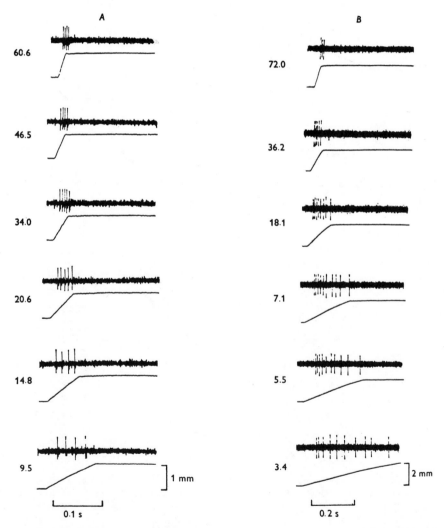

Fig. 9.9. Discharges of two different rapidly adapting receptors in the glabrous skin of the human hand in response to graded ramp displacements (velocities given in mm/s). Note the constant number of spikes for the unit in A and the increased number for lower velocity stimuli in B. (From Knibestöl, 1973.)

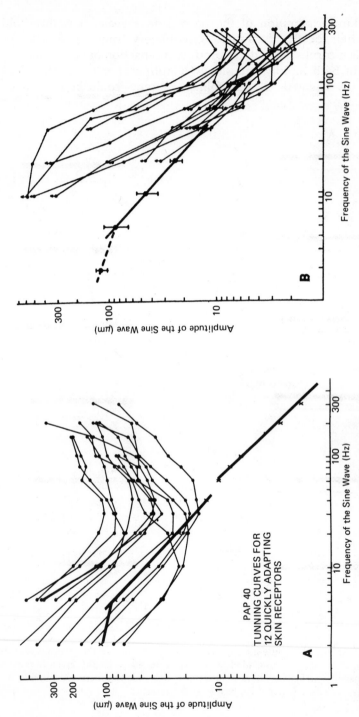

Fig. 9.10. Tuning curves for afferent fibers of the monkey glabrous skin superimposed on a human frequency-intensity function (heavy line) derived from a psychophysical study in which sinusoidal stimuli were applied to the fingertip. The tuning curves in A were from rapidly adapting receptors (Meissner's corpuscles) and overlie the low-frequency end of the human function. The tuning curves in B were from Pacinian corpuscles and overlie the high-frequency end of the human function. (From Talbot *et al.*, 1968.)

the vibratory stimuli, whereas G1 receptors could not. D hair-follicle afferents were quite sensitive to vibratory stimuli over a wide range of frequencies. Pacinian corpuscles behaved like those under glabrous skin. Tuning curves showed the following best frequencies: G2 hair-follicle receptors, 10–40 Hz; Pacinian corpuscles, 100–400 Hz; D hair-follicle afferents, 5–100 Hz. Evidently, G2 hair-follicle receptors account for flutter and Pacinian corpuscles for vibration in hairy skin. The D hair follicle receptors have a much lower threshold than is appropriate for flutter sensation, and so they presumably do not contribute to this sensation. Similarly, it was found that the discharges of slowly adapting receptors are modulated sinusoidally by the stimuli used at thresholds much below those that evoke the sensation of flutter, and so these receptors, too, can be discounted as candidates to explain this sensation. Furthermore, slowly adapting receptors in humans do not follow high-frequency stimuli that elicit a sensation of vibration (Järvilehto et al., 1976).

The question of how the receptors for flutter–vibration code for stimulus intensity was addressed by K. O. Johnson (1974). The study was limited to the population of rapidly adapting receptors in the glabrous skin. The responses of single units were defined, both with 40-Hz stimuli of variable amplitude applied to the point of maximal sensitivity and with the same stimuli at varying distances from this point. Based on a mathematical analysis, it was possible to predict the behavior of the population of receptors to stimuli of varying amplitude (Fig. 9.11). Several ways in which the stimulus intensity could be coded by the receptor population were considered: (1) total number of active fibers, (2) total activity of the receptor population, and (3) total activity of the receptors under or near the stimulus probe. All of these measures were linearly related to stimulus intensity and provided a good fit to the psychophysical data. A further outcome of this study was the finding that the size and position of the stimulus is well represented by the activity of the receptor population (Fig. 9.11).

The assumption underlying the experiments of the Mountcastle group outlined above was that the receptor apparatus is very similar in the human and in the monkey and that recordings of afferent discharges in the monkey can be related in a direct way to the outcome of human psychophysical tests. Further work by the Mountcastle group has shown in animal psychophysical experiments that such an assumption is valid, since detection thresholds, amplitude, and frequency discrimination are very similar in humans and in monkeys (Mountcastle et al., 1972; LaMotte and Mountcastle, 1975).

One apparent disagreement with the results of the Mountcastle group is the finding of Knibestöl (1973) that the stimulus–response

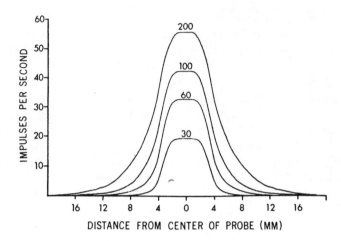

Fig. 9.11. Average firing rate at various distances from the center of the stimulus probe for different stimuli (displacements given in microns). The curves indicate the form of the expected spatial recruitment at sites away from the probe. (From K. O. Johnson, 1974.)

relationship of human rapidly adapting receptors (and some Pacinian corpuscles) is a log tanh function (Naka and Rushton, 1966). The Mountcastle group found a discontinuous relationship between the amplitude of indentation and the number of spikes generated per cycle of their sinusoidal stimulus (Talbot *et al.*, 1968; Merzenich and Harrington, 1969; K. O. Johnson, 1974). The reason for the discrepancy is that Knibestöl used ramp stimuli and found that the discharge frequency reflected stimulus velocity. However, for a given skin displacement, the total number of spikes evoked by each stimulus could remain constant or even decrease as stimulus intensity increased (Fig. 9.9). The central nervous system would have to decode the information contained in the discharge rate of the first few spikes in order to determine stimulus velocity. The experiments of K. O. Johnson (1974) support an alternative hypothesis that stimulus intensity is coded by the population of receptors, rather than by individual receptors.

Other receptors that should be considered in relation to their possible role in flutter–vibration are field receptors, C mechanoreceptors, and muscle and joint receptors. Field receptors have apparently not been studied with respect to their responses to sinusoidal stimuli. C mechanoreceptors respond best to slowly moving stimuli, and so they are unlikely candidates (Bessou *et al.*, 1971); they may instead be involved in tickle (Zotterman, 1939). However, there are so far no reports of these receptors in humans (Van Hees and Gybels, 1972;

Torebjörk, 1974). Muscle receptors are also unlikely to be involved. Muscle spindle primary afferents are very sensitive to small-amplitude stretches of the muscle containing them (Bianconi and van der Meulen, 1963; M. C. Brown *et al.*, 1967). However, it is doubtful that small-amplitude vibrations of the skin would activate them under normal circumstances. The controversy surrounding the question of the sensory contribution of muscle spindle afferents will be reviewed in the section on position sense. The only joint receptors that are likely to play a role in flutter–vibration are the paciniform corpuscles. These undoubtedly contribute to the sensation of vibration in the same fashion as do subcutaneous Pacinian corpuscles.

Spinal Pathways

The pathways carrying information from Pacinian corpuscles and from rapidly adapting receptors and hair-follicle afferents will be discussed in that order. It is not known with certainty if input from Pacinian corpuscles activates interneurons in the dorsal horn, and it is not evident that any second-order ascending tracts originating from cell bodies in the spinal cord convey information from Pacinian corpuscles to the brain.

The notion that vibratory sensibility in the human depends upon the dorsal columns is rooted in tradition, although this idea has been challenged (Calne and Pallis, 1966). The fact that vibratory sensation remains intact after surgical interruption of the dorsal column (Cook and Browder, 1965) must be regarded with reservation until autopsy data confirms the completeness of the interruption. The buzzing sensation reported by patients during repetitive stimulation of the dorsal columns (Shealy *et al.*, 1970; Nashold *et al.*, 1972) is not interpretable, since impulses in axons of the dorsal columns activate not only neurons in the dorsal column nuclei but also the cells of origin of several parallel ascending tracts (Taub and Bishop, 1965; Foreman *et al.*, 1976a). Vibratory sensation apparently cannot be conveyed by a single anterolateral quadrant (Noordenbos and Wall, 1976).

Behavioral experiments in animals have done little to shed light on the pathways involved in vibratory sensation. Dorsal column lesions produced little alteration in vibratory sensibility (Schwartzman and Bogdonoff, 1968, 1969). However, the lesions may not have been complete, and it is known that at least 90% of the dorsal columns must be sectioned before behavioral changes are seen (Dobry and Casey, 1972a). Evoked potential studies have been more helpful. Pacinian corpuscles evoke substantial potentials in the sensory cortex, and these depend upon the dorsal column pathway (McIntyre, 1962; Norrsell and

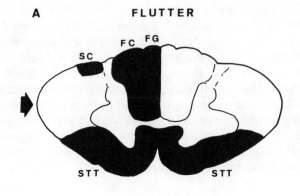

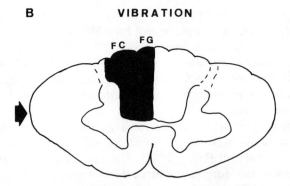

Fig. 9.12. Pathways for flutter and for vibration. The pathways for flutter are in A and include the fasciculus cuneatus and gracilis (FC, FG), the spinocervical tract (SC) and the spinothalamic tract (STT). The pathways for vibration in B are the dorsal column pathways, FC and FG. The arrows indicate the side of the input.

Wolpow, 1966; McIntyre *et al.*, 1967; Silfvenius, 1970). The presence of Pacinian corpuscle afferents in the dorsal columns is well documented (A. G. Brown, 1968; Petit and Burgess, 1968; Uddenberg, 1968a; Pubols and Pubols, 1973; however, cf. Horch *et al.*, 1976). Furthermore, cells have been found in the dorsal column nuclei that respond as if they received an input from Pacinian corpuscles (Amassian and DeVito, 1957; Perl *et al.*, 1962; Gordon and Jukes, 1964a; Bystrzycka *et al.*, 1977). The best available evidence, therefore, indicates the vibratory sensibility depends upon the dorsal column pathway (Fig. 9.12B).

The pathways convening information from the rapidly adapting receptors of glabrous skin and from hair-follicle afferents are more complex than those involved in mediating the information from Pacinian corpuscles. Not only the dorsal columns, but also other ascending

pathways must be considered, since stimulation of the rapidly adapting receptors or of hair-follicle afferents evokes activity in many
neurons of the dorsal horn (e.g., Kolmodin and Skogland, 1960; Wall,
1960; Wagman and Price, 1969; Tapper et al., 1973), including neurons
contributing to a number of ascending tracts (see below).

Clinical observations indicate that "touch" is mediated not only
by the dorsal columns but also by pathways in other parts of the cord
white matter, including the anterolateral quadrant (Head and Thompson, 1906; Foerster and Gagel, 1931; White et al., 1950). In fact,
"touch" was intact in a patient who had only a single anterolateral
quadrant intact (Noordenbos and Wall, 1976). One problem with such
evidence is that it is generally not clear what is meant by "touch" in
clinical evaluations. It would be useful to test specifically for the sensations of flutter and vibration in patients.

Animal behavioral studies indicate that "touch" depends both
upon the dorsal column and the dorsolateral fasciculus (Levitt and
Schwartzman, 1966; Norrsell, 1966b; Kitai and Weinberg, 1968; Dobry
and Casey, 1972a; Vierck, 1973, 1974; Azulay and Schwartz, 1975;
Frommer et al., 1977). Evoked potential studies support this evidence
(Morin, 1955; Mark and Steiner, 1958; Norrsell and Voorhoeve, 1962;
Norrsell, 1966a; Norrsell and Wolpow, 1966; however, cf. Whitehorn et
al., 1969; and Ennever and Towe, 1974). For primates, evoked potential experiments suggest the possibility that tactile information may
also reach the cerebral cortex by way of the ventral quadrant (Gardner
and Morin, 1953, 1957; Eidelberg and Woodbury, 1972; Andersson et
al., 1972). Studies employing single-unit recordings in the thalamus or
cortex are consistent with the evoked potential work (e.g., Whitlock
and Perl, 1959, 1961; Perl and Whitlock, 1961; Andersson, 1962; Levitt
and Levitt, 1968; Millar, 1973b; Dreyer et al., 1974; Andersson et al.,
1975).

The types of axons present in the dorsal columns include the ascending collaterals of hair-follicle afferents and of rapidly adapting
receptors of glabrous skin (A. G. Brown, 1968; Petit and Burgess, 1968;
Uddenberg, 1968a; Pubols and Pubols, 1973; Bromberg and Whitehorn, 1974). Furthermore, units that respond as if they receive inputs
from these receptors have been described in the dorsal column nuclei
(Kruger et al., 1961; Yamamoto and Miyajima, 1961; Perl et al., 1962;
Gordon and Jukes, 1964a; A. G. Brown et al., 1974). In addition to the
dorsal column pathway, hair follicle, and glabrous skin, rapidly adapting afferents excite neurons in the spinocervical and spinothalamic
tracts (Taub, 1964; A. G. Brown and Franz, 1969; Bryan et al., 1973;
1974; Willis et al., 1974, 1975). Furthermore, some spinoreticular
neurons are activated by hair movement or by light touch (Fields et

al., 1977b). Therefore, the sensation of flutter probably depends on a number of pathways ascending in all spinal funiculi (Fig. 9.12A).

In summary, the sensation of flutter–vibration depends upon several sets of receptors. Flutter in the glabrous skin is produced by activation of the rapidly adapting glabrous skin receptors (Meissner's corpuscles), while that in hairy skin is due to hair-follicle afferents (type G2). Vibration is mediated by Pacinian corpuscles. The coding for stimulus intensity is attributable to a progressive increase in the activity of the population of rapidly adapting receptors, rather than upon information conveyed by individual members of the population. The spinal cord pathway most likely to convey vibratory sensibility is the dorsal column pathway. Flutter is probably the result of information transmitted not only in the dorsal columns but also in the spinocervical tract, the spinothalamic tract, and perhaps other pathways as well.

PAIN

Pain will be treated here as a specific sensation (Perl, 1971; Kerr, 1975a; Zimmermann, 1976; Price and Dubner, 1977), albeit a complex one (Melzack and Wall, 1965; Melzack, 1973). Several types of pain can be recognized. Lewis (1942) described two basic kinds of pain—superficial and deep. Superficial pain results from intense stimulation of the skin and can be well localized. Deep (or aching) pain arises from skeletal muscles, tendons, periosteum, and joints and is poorly localized. Visceral pain shares many of the attributes of deep pain, including a tendency to be referred to superficial structures and to induce powerful autonomic responses. Many authors further subdivide superficial pain into bright (pricking) pain and burning pain. Synonyms are first and second pain, since a noxious stimulus will evoke the two kinds of superficial pain in temporal succession (early evidence is reviewed by Lewis, 1942). It has been proposed that first and second pain are produced by activation of Aδ and C fibers and that the temporal lag between the pains is due in part to different peripheral conduction velocities (Lewis, 1942; Price *et al.*, 1977).

In addition to the sensory experience called pain, strong stimuli produce other behavioral events. Besides autonomic responses (Schmidt and Weller, 1970), there are somatic motor responses, such as the flexion reflex (Sherrington, 1906). In addition, there are strong motivational–affective responses, resulting in arousal and aversive behavior (Magoun, 1963; Melzack and Casey, 1968). These more global consequences of painful stimuli will not be discussed in detail here, but they are very important aspects of the full reaction to painful stimulation, in many respects more important (e.g., in human disease states) than the sensation proper.

Stimuli that evoke the pain reaction are said to be noxious (Sherrington, 1906), meaning that they threaten damage or actually produce damage. This is an important consideration in experiments designed to investigate the neural basis for pain mechanisms. Animal subjects cannot report pain, nor can neurons. It is reasonable to expect that neural responses will occur in the pain channel when strong but not overtly damaging stimuli are applied, since such responses can serve as a warning to the individual that harm is imminent. However, maximum activity in the pain system is likely to result only when frank damage is produced. Observations consistent with these suppositions have been made in studies of peripheral nociceptors (Burgess and Perl, 1967).

Another major consideration in experiments on nociceptive neurons is that some neurons may play a role in one aspect or another of the total pain reaction, but not all such neurons need contribute to all aspects of the reaction. Thus, it is possible to separate the sensory mechanism from the motivational–affective system and these from the reflex and arousal systems. For example, patients who have had a frontal lobotomy feel pain but are not concerned by it (White and Sweet, 1969), and the flexion reflex is vigorous below the level of a spinal cord transection (Sherrington, 1906).

Receptors

Nociceptors, whether in the skin, muscle, or viscera, all seem to terminate in free endings. There is no obvious structural distinction between the endings of various kinds of nociceptors, yet several have quite distinctive response properties. The cutaneous mechanical nociceptors respond just to intense mechanical stimuli, and polymodal nociceptors can be activated by noxious mechanical, thermal, or chemical stimuli (Fjällbrant and Iggo, 1961; Iggo, 1962; Burgess and Perl, 1967; Perl, 1968; Bessou and Perl, 1969; Beck et al., 1974; Beck and Handwerker, 1974; Croze et al., 1976; Georgopoulos, 1976). All of the nociceptors are supplied by small-sized afferent fibers, including both Aδ and C fibers (Zottermann, 1939; Burgess and Perl, 1973). It should be noted, however, that the largest nociceptive afferents have conduction velocities as fast as 40–50 m/s (Burgess and Perl, 1967; Georgopoulos, 1976).

Recordings from human cutaneous or mixed nerves have shown the presence of several of the types of nociceptors that have been iden-

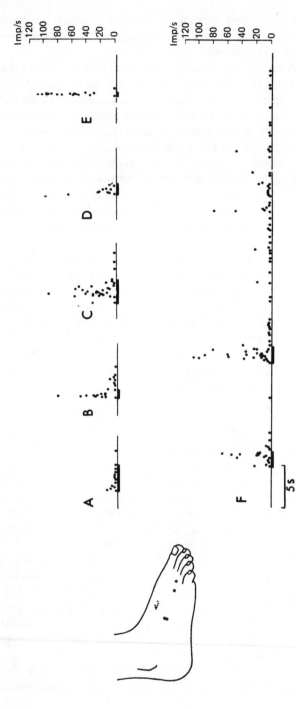

Fig. 9.13. The drawing shows the receptive fields of several C polymodal nociceptors in the human foot. The circles indicate the locations of four receptive fields in a schematic way, while the dots show seven foci of sensitivity for a single receptor that had the largest receptive field of the units studied. The responses in the graph were from a single unit and resulted from the following stimuli: (A) pointed stimulus probe, 2 g, (B) firm stroke, (C) squeezing skin with forceps, (D) needle prick, (E) touching skin with glowing match, (F) puncturing skin with hypodermic needle at left and then injection of 0.02 ml of 5% KCl. The heavy bars under the records indicate times when the subject reported a sensation, generally pain. (From Torebjörk, 1974.)

tified in animal experiments, including Aδ mechanoreceptors, Aδ heat nociceptors, and C polymodal nociceptors (Fig. 9.13) (Van Hees and Gybels, 1972; Torebjörk, 1974; Torebjörk and Hallin, 1974). It appears that single impulses or even a few impulses in a nociceptive afferent are insufficient to evoke a sensation of pain (Van Hees and Gybels, 1972; Torebjörk and Hallin, 1973). However, activation of a population of Aδ or C fibers in the human produces considerable pain, especially if the activity of Aαβ fibers is blocked (Fig. 9.14) (Heinbecker et al., 1933, 1934; D. Clark et al., 1935; Pattle and Weddell, 1948; Collins et al., 1960; Torebjörk and Hallin, 1973; Hallin and Torebjörk, 1976). Conversely, pain is abolished when Aδ and C fiber activity is blocked, e.g., by local anesthetic (Fig. 9.15).

Nociceptors are also found in muscle nerves. They were named pressure–pain endings by Paintal (1960). They are generally supplied by group III and group IV afferents, but sometimes the afferent is of group II or even group I size. Unmyelinated afferents form a large proportion of the axons in muscle nerves (Stacey, 1969). Muscle pressure–pain endings can be activated by mechanical stimulation, by injection of algesic chemicals into the arterial circulation of the muscle, by ischemia, and even by thermal stimulation (Paintal, 1960; Bessou and Laporte, 1961; Iggo, 1961; Lim et al., 1962; Guzman et al., 1962; Hník et al., 1969; Mense and Schmidt, 1974; Franz and Mense, 1975; Fock and Mense, 1976; Hiss and Mense, 1976; Hertel et al., 1976; Mense, 1977; Kumazawa and Mizumura, 1977b).

Visceral nociceptors seem to respond best to mechanical stimuli, although chemical agents may also be effective (Gernandt and Zotterman, 1946, Guzman et al., 1962; Lim et al., 1962; A. M. Brown, 1967; Uchida and Murao, 1974; Kumazawa and Mizumura, 1977a). Some C fibers have been found that innervate the mucous membrane of the rectal canal and that behave like polymodal nociceptors in the skin (Clifton et al., 1976). The pain that results from excessive distention or contraction of hollow viscera may be due to activity in the "in series" tension receptors (Leek, 1972).

Graded stimulation of polymodal nociceptors reveals a linear relationship between stimulus strength (noxious heat) and response in the cat (Beck et al., 1974), but a power function with an exponent greater than 1 in the monkey (Fig. 9.16) (Croze et al., 1976). Psychophysical tests in human subjects have yielded comparable power functions with exponents of 1 or more (Melzack et al., 1963; Adair et al., 1968; Stevens, 1970). It seems probable that such an accelerating response helps account for the overwhelming nature of pain reactions.

Repeated applications of a noxious stimulus may sensitize the receptors (Fig. 9.16) (Bessou and Perl, 1969; Beck et al., 1974; Croze et

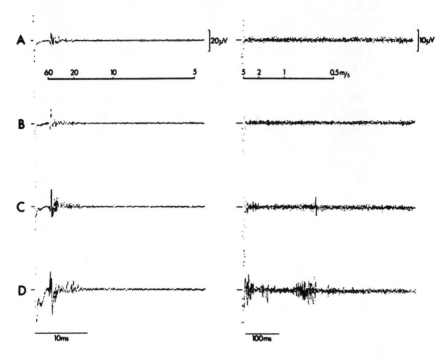

Fig. 9.14. Signal averaged records of activity in the radial nerve of a human subject evoked by electrical stimulation of the dorsum of the hand (conduction distance 15 cm). The records in the left column were a higher sweep speed than those in the right column (scales beneath records in A show conduction velocities). In A, the stimulus activated just A fibers, but the subject noticed no sensation. In B, more A fibers were activated, and the subject reported a barely perceptible sensation. In C, as Aδ and C fibers began to appear in the volley, the subject had a prickling sensation. In D, the addition of A and C fibers cause pain. (From Hallin and Torebjörk, 1976.)

al., 1976; Fitzgerald and Lynn, 1977) or suppress their responses (Price *et al.*, 1977). The sensitization phenomenon is undoubtedly important in terms of the hyperalgesia of the skin in areas of damage due to repeated noxious stimulation (Hardy *et al.*, 1951). It is likely that sensitization plays a significant role in the pathology of inflammation.

It has been proposed that nociceptors are activated by a chemical substance released in the vicinity of free nerve endings when tissue is damaged (Lim, 1970). The damage could be produced by any insult, and the released agent might be K^+, a polypeptide like bradykinin, or a monoamine like serotonin. A special arrangement of the receptor might prevent particular forms of noxious stimulation from having an effect; this would permit some specialization of nociceptors. Several observations tend to argue against the theory that nociceptors are basically chemoreceptors. For example, the responses of group III and IV muscle afferents to serotonin show tachyphylaxis, while the effects of bradykinin may or may not; however, there is no cross-tachyphylaxis between serotonin and bradykinin (Beck and Handwerker, 1974; Mense and Schmidt, 1974; Hiss and Mense, 1976). Therefore, the mechanism of action of these algesic chemicals is at least in part different. Second, in a population of nociceptors, some respond to one set of algesic chemicals, while others respond to a different set (Fock and Mense, 1976). Finally, slowing adapting cutaneous mechanoreceptors are activated in addition to nociceptors (Fjällbrant and Iggo, 1961; Beck and Handwerker, 1974). This suggests a nonspecific effect of the chemicals. However, it is reasonable to suppose that the release of algesic agents in an area of damage might contribute to the sensitization process (Fig. 9.17) (Beck and Handwerker, 1974; Zimmermann, 1976).

Spinal Pathways

The afferents from nociceptors end in the dorsal part of the dorsal horn. Many Aδ fibers terminate in lamina I, but some branches end in

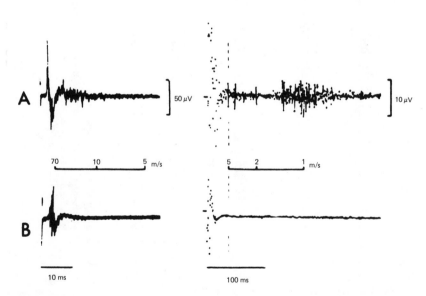

Fig. 9.15. Signaled averaged records of activity recorded from the human radial nerve in response to electrical stimulation of the dorsum of the hand. In A, the volley is seen to include Aδ and C fibers (note the two different sweeps speeds and the bars indicating conduction velocity). The stimulus was painful. In B, the Aδ and C fiber activity was abolished by local anesthetic, but some Aαβ activity remains. The subject no longer feels pain, but he still feels touch. (From Hallin and Torebjörk, 1976.)

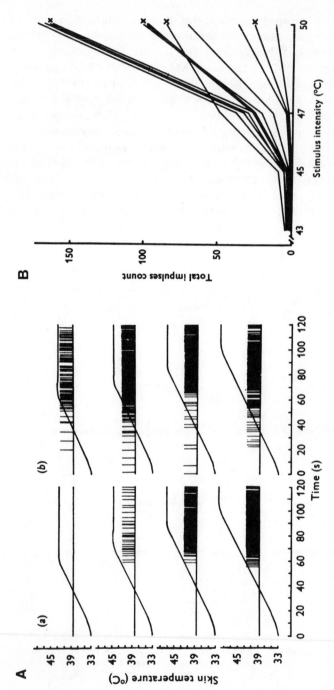

Fig. 9.16. The responses in A were recorded from a polymodal nociceptor. In the first column (a), a series of heat stimuli were applied to the receptive field (successively to 43, 45, 47, and 50°C) from an adapting temperature of 33°C). The series was repeated in the second column. Note that the unit was sensitized, since the threshold was lower and discharged at a higher rate for a given temperature. The graph in B shows the relationship between the total number of discharges during the dynamic responses of ten polymodal nociceptors as a function of stimulus intensity. The curve of the mean response for all the fibers is shown by the heavy line. This can be fitted with a power function: $R = 10^{-45}T^{27}$. (From Croze et al., 1976.)

lamina V as well (Light and Perl, 1977). C fibers appear to end in laminae II and III (Réthelyi, 1977). There are spinothalamic tract neurons in lamina I, but the small cells of laminae II and III do not appear to project for long distances (Trevino et al., 1973; Trevino and Carstens, 1975). The details of how these small cells interact with tract cells are still unclear, although it has been suggested that they are inhibitory interneurons (Kerr, 1975a).

Experiments employing natural forms of stimulation have shown that there are interneurons in lamina I that respond specifically to noxious mechanical and sometimes also to noxious thermal stimuli (Christensen and Perl, 1970; Kumazawa et al., 1975; Cervero et al., 1976). In addition, there are similar interneurons in deeper layers of the dorsal horn (Kolmodin and Skoglund, 1960; Gregor and Zimmermann, 1972; Heavner and DeJong, 1973; Price and Browe, 1973; Menétrey et al., 1977). These nociceptive specific, narrow-dynamic-range cells are quite likely to be involved in the reaction to painful stimulation (Price and Dubner, 1977).

In addition to nociceptive specific cells, there are many wide-dynamic-range interneurons in the dorsal horn; these respond to both innocuous and noxious stimuli (Kolmodin and Skoglund, 1960; Wall, 1960, 1967; Fetz, 1968; Wagman and Price, 1969; Besson et al., 1972; Gregor and Zimmermann, 1972; Price and Browe, 1973; Heavner and DeJong, 1973; Handwerker et al., 1975; Fields et al., 1977a; Menétrey et al., 1977). It has been proposed that wide-dynamic-range cells contribute importantly to pain sensation (Price and Dubner, 1977). For example, there is evidence that such neurons may account for the pain resulting from electrical stimulation of the anterolateral quadrant in human patients undergoing cordotomy (Fig. 9.18) (Mayer et al., 1975). Wide-dynamic-range neurons, like many peripheral nociceptors, are activated maximally by noxious stimuli, although they have thresholds in the nonnoxious range. The activity of wide-dynamic-range neurons shows many parallels with second-pain sensation (Price, 1972; Price et al., 1977). For instance they show windup (Mendell, 1966; Wagman and Price, 1969), which could account for the increment in second-pain sensation produced by repetitive stimulation of C fibers. Stimulation of the axons of presumed wide-dynamic-range neurons in the human results in sensations of burning, aching, cramping, but sometimes sharp pain (Mayer et al., 1975). Finally, many spinothalamic tract cells are of this type (Willis et al., 1974).

One reservation about the involvement of wide-dynamic-range cells in pain transmission is that these cells are activated at rates of at least 50 per second by repetitive stimulation of the dorsal columns (Foreman et al., 1976b), and yet dorsal column stimulation in humans

unmyelinated fiber
unit 372-7

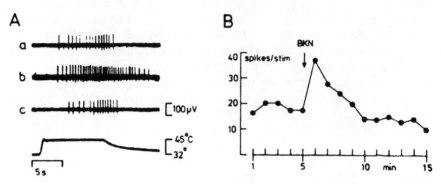

Fig. 9.17. The discharges of a C polymodal nociceptor are shown in A (a) before, (b) 1 min after, and (c) 6 min after an intraarterial injection of bradykinin (10 μg). The stimulus is a heat pulse to 45°C. The graph in B shows the increase in discharge as a result of the bradykinin injection. (From Zimmermann, 1976.)

is not painful (Shealy *et al.*, 1970; Nashold *et al.*, 1972). Possibly the ascending information conveyed by the wide-dynamic-range tract cells is ineffective in activating the pain system in the brain because of interactions with the activity of the dorsal column–medial lemniscus system or other ascending pathways (Dong and Wagman, 1976).

Clinical studies indicate that the chief pathway carrying nociceptive information to the human brain is crossed and ascends in the anterolateral quadrant (Fig. 9.19) (e.g., Foerster and Gagel, 1931; Hyndman and Van Epps, 1939; Kuru, 1949; White and Sweet, 1955, 1969). There are presumably also alternative pathways, since cordotomies may produce only temporary pain relief, even though the surgical lesion interrupts all of an anterolateral quadrant (White and Sweet, 1969). In other species, such as the cat, there appear to be important pathways for nociception in other parts of the spinal cord, including the dorsolateral fasciculus (Kennard, 1954).

The usual presumption in the case of the human is that pain is the result of information transmitted by the spinothalamic tract. However, this term is frequently meant to include not only direct projections from the spinal cord to the thalamus, but also indirect projections via the reticular formation. There is a possibility that the spinotectal tract is also involved in pain mechanisms. The alternative pain pathways in the cat appear to include the spinocervical tract and the second-order dorsal column pathway (Fig. 9.19).

Experiments on animals, such as the monkey, that have a neural organization like that of man, provide evidence concerning the tracts likely to be involved in pain mechanisms. To date, a number of studies have been done on the spinothalamic tract in monkey, but little is known about the primate spinoreticular or spinotectal tracts. The spinothalamic tract in the monkey includes neurons with narrow dynamic response ranges either to innocuous or to noxious stimuli. The noci-

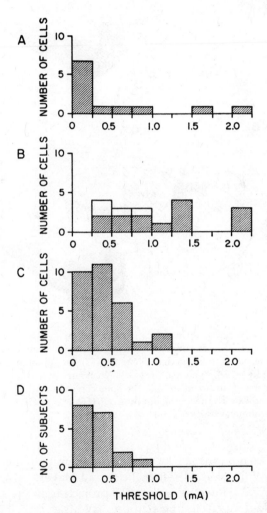

Fig. 9.18. Electrical thresholds for antidromic activation of (A) nonnociceptive cells in laminae IV–VI of the monkey spinal cord, (B) nociceptive-specific cells (those in lamina I are shown by shading), (C) and wide-dynamic-range cells. The thresholds for inducing pain in human patients by stimulation in the anterolateral quadrant are shown for comparison in D. (From Price and Mayer, 1975.)

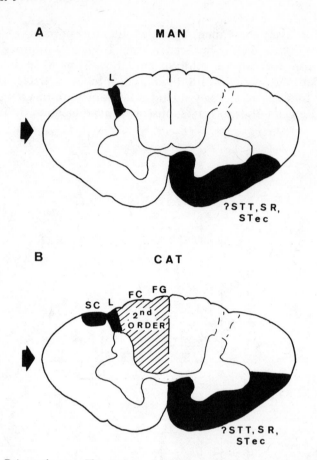

Fig. 9.19. Pain pathways. The major pain pathways in man as shown in A are in Lissauer's tract (L) on the side stimulated (arrow) and in the ventral quadrant contralaterally, possibly including the spinothalamic tract (STT), the spinoreticular tract (SR), and the spinotectal tract (STec). Other pathways, which assume more significance in animals like the cat, are shown in B and include the spinocervical tract (SC) and second-order dorsal column pathway in the fasciculus cuneatus (FC) and fasciculus gracilis (FG) ipsilaterally to the stimulus.

ceptive-specific neurons are located both in lamina I and in the region of lamina V (Willis *et al.*, 1974; cf. Price and Mayer, 1974, 1975; Kumazawa *et al.*, 1975). However, most cells projecting in the spinothalamic tract are wide-dynamic-range neurons (Willis *et al.*, 1974; Albe-Fessard *et al.*, 1974).

It is relatively easy to evoke substantial responses in spinothalamic tract neurons by procedures that produce pain in man. For example, in addition to responses to noxious cutaneous stimuli, spinothalamic tract cells show vigorous responses to the injection of algesic chemicals into the arterial circulation (Fig. 8.15) (Levante *et al.*, 1975; Foreman *et al.*, 1977).

The likelihood that spinothalamic tract neurons participate in pain sensation in primates is supported by the fact that the axons of these cells terminate in several thalamic nuclei, including the ventral posterior lateral and the medial part of the posterior, known to project to sensory receiving areas of the cerebral cortex (Mehler *et al.*, 1960; Burton and Jones, 1976). However, the spinothalamic tract may also contribute to arousal, since another thalamic termination zone is in the intralaminar complex, specifically the nucleus centralis lateralis. Although this nucleus does project to the sensory cortex, it also projects diffusely to many other cortical areas (Murray, 1966; Jones and Leavitt, 1974).

Little is known about the response properties of the spinoreticular tract in the monkey. Kerr and Lippman (1974) feel that most of the spinoreticular projection is uncrossed in primates. If this is the case, the spinoreticular tract would not be a good candidate to mediate pain sensation, since cordotomies show that the human pain transmission system is crossed at the spinal cord level. However, Kerr and Lippman did find a few crossed spinoreticular terminals, and so it is conceivable that the spinoreticular tract contributes to pain sensation. Neurons have been found in the nucleus gigantocellularis, which receives an input from the spinoreticular tract, that respond specifically to noxious stimuli, at least in the cat (Wolstencroft, 1964; Casey, 1969, 1971a). Many of these cells are reticulospinal tract cells (Wolstencroft, 1964), but ascending projections from the same neurons cannot be ruled out (cf. Scheibel and Scheibel, 1958). Little is known about reticulothalamic projections in the monkey, but comparable projections in the cat appear to end in the intralaminar nuclei (Nauta and Kuypers, 1958). This suggests that the spinoreticulothalamic system may function more as an arousal mechanism than as a sensory pathway. The reticulospinal projection may be involved in the reflex and autonomic adjustments of the pain reaction.

Even less is known about the spinotectal tract in the monkey. Spinotectal fibers have been traced into the periaqueductal gray and to the intercollicular nucleus and the external nucleus of the inferior colliculus (e.g., Mehler *et al.*, 1960; Schroeder and Jane, 1971; Kerr, 1975b). Stimulation in the periaqueductal gray is known to produce analgesia, depending upon the exact location of the electrodes (Reynolds, 1969; Mayer and Liebeskind, 1974) and so an involvement of this structure in pain mechanisms is highly likely.

The spinocervical tract exists in the monkey and probably also in the human (Ha and Morin, 1964; Truex *et al.*, 1965; Mizuno *et al.*, 1967; Kircher and Ha, 1968; Ha, 1971; Bryan *et al.*, 1974). However, the dorsolateral fasciculus is not adequate to convey nociceptive information in the human. On the other hand, the spinocervical tract may well be utilized for nociception by cats and other mammalian species (Kennard, 1954; Cervero *et al.*, 1977a). A similar possibility exists for the second-order dorsal column pathway in the cat (Uddenberg, 1968b; Angaut-Petit, 1975a,b) and for propriospinal pathways in the rat (Basbaum, 1973). Conceivably, these or other pathways account for the restoration of pain transmission in some patients following an initially successful cordotomy (White and Sweet, 1969).

A clinically important aspect of pain phenomena is the tendency for patients to refer visceral or deep pain to superficial structures (Lewis, 1942). A number of theories have been proposed to account for pain referral (Head, 1893; MacKenzie, 1893; Ruch, 1947; Sinclair *et al.*, 1948). The evidence that is available at present suggests that the convergence–projection theory of Ruch is most likely to prove correct. This theory assumes that somatic and visceral afferents converge on a common pool of neurons in the spinal cord. These neurons transmit information to the brain concerning noxious stimuli. Normally, visceral pain occurs only rarely, whereas somatic pain is common. Information transmitted by the neurons in question is associated through learning with somatic stimuli, and so when visceral pain does occur, the information is misinterpreted. There is now ample evidence for convergent activation of spinal cord neurons, including spinothalamic tract cells, by somatic and visceral afferents (Pomeranz *et al.*, 1968; Selzer and Spencer, 1969; Fields *et al.*, 1970a,b, 1975; Hancock *et al.*, 1970, 1973, 1975; Foreman *et al.*, 1975b, 1977; Guilbaud *et al.*, 1977a). In addition to pain referral, viscerosomatic convergence can help explain the superficial tenderness that may develop secondary to visceral disease (Zimmermann, 1976).

Inhibitory interactions at the spinal cord level are undoubtedly of importance in pain reactions. It is well known that strong stimulation of the skin (sometimes called "counterirritation") helps alleviate pain. Phenomena of this kind were explained by the gate theory of pain (Melzack and Wall, 1965) (see Chapter 4), and the gate theory led to the reintroduction (Kane and Taub, 1975) (Fig. 9.20) of electrical stimulation of peripheral nerves or of the skin for the treatment of pain (Wall and Sweet, 1967; Sweet and Wepsic, 1968; Long and Hagfors, 1975; Long, 1973; Loeser *et al.*, 1975; Sternbach *et al.*, 1976). An efficient means of stimulating large numbers of cutaneous afferents is by stimulating the ascending collaterals of these fibers in the dorsal columns; thus, dorsal column stimulation was given a clinical trial and found to

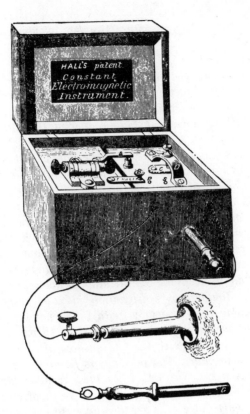

Fig. 9.20. Commercial magnetoelectric machine used for electroanesthesia in the mid-1800s. (From Kane and Taub, 1975.)

be useful in selected patients (Shealy *et al.*, 1967, 1970; Nashold and Friedman, 1972; Nielson *et al.*, 1975; however, see Fox, 1974).

It is still not clear exactly how pain relief is achieved by stimulation of large afferent fibers. The details of the gate theory are in question; for example, it appears that Aδ nociceptive afferents are not subjected to primary afferent depolarization following stimulation of Aαβ fibers, although they are if other Aδ fibers are activated (Whitehorn and Burgess, 1973). Nothing is known about presynaptic inhibition of C fibers. There is evidence that large afferent fibers do produce inhibition of spinal cord interneurons, including spinothalamic tract cells; this is shown most clearly by the results of stimulation of the dorsal colums (Fig. 8-2) (Hillman and Wall, 1969; Beck *et al.*, 1974; Foreman *et al.*, 1976a). However, it was not ruled out that fibers descending from the dorsal column nuclei could have been involved (Burton and

Loewy, 1977). Other sites of interaction at the level of the brain are also likely.

In summary, there are several types of pain, including superficial bright and burning pain, deep pain, and visceral pain. Besides the sensation of pain, the pain reaction includes somatic and autonomic reflexes and mo-tivational-affective responses, including aversive behavior and arousal. Painful stimuli are noxious, i.e., they threaten damage. Neurons involved in the pain reaction may contribute to one or more aspects of the total reac-tion. The receptors involved in signaling painful stimuli are the nociceptors. There are several kinds of cutaneous nociceptors that are activated by one or more kinds of noxious stimuli—mechanical, thermal, or chemical. Other nociceptors are found in muscle and in viscera. These can also be activated by particular forms or sets of noxious mechanical or chemical stimuli. The psychophysical response to a painful stimulus is a power function with an exponent of 1 or more; a similar curve relates stimulus strength to the responses of certain nociceptors. Sensitization of nociceptors may occur fol-lowing repeated stimulation; sensitization may be responsible for hy-peralgesia, including that associated with inflammation. There are argu-ments against the theory that all nociceptors are chemoreceptors, but it is likely that algesic substances released in an area of damage may result in sensitization of nociceptors. The nociceptors terminate in the dorsal horn and activate cells there. The details of the neural circuits are unclear. Nociceptive specific cells are highly likely to be involved in pain mecha-nisms. Wide-dynamic-range cells are also likely to play a similar role, and some authors argue that these cells are sufficient to produce the sensation of pain, especially second pain. The main pathway(s) for pain transmission in the human cross at the segmental level and ascend in the anterolateral quadrant. In other animals, such as the cat, there is an important pain pathway in the dorsolateral fasciculus. The spinothalamic tract is a good candidate to be the chief pain pathway in man, since it is crossed and as-cends in the anterolateral quadrant and ends in several thalamic nuclei that project to the somatosensory regions of the cerebral cortex. Spinothalamic neurons include nociceptive specific and wide-dynamic-range types. The projections to the intralaminar nuclei suggest that the spinothalamic tract may also evoke arousal. The spinoreticular and spinotectal tracts may also be involved in the pain reaction. It is not clear what contribution these tracts make to sensory experience, but other potential roles include arousal, aversive behavior, and somatic and autonomic reflex adjustments. The spin-ocervical tract and the second-order dorsal column pathway are unlikely to be very important in human pain transmission under normal circumstances, but they may play a role in the return of pain after an initially successful cordotomy. These pathways may be involved in pain mechanisms in ani-

mals like the cat. Pain referral seems to be accounted for by viscerosomatic convergence upon spinal neurons, including the cells of origin of the spinothalamic tract. Inhibitory effects of large afferent fibers have proved useful in the clinical treatment of pain. The mechanism of this inhibition is unknown, although at the spinal cord level there is inhibition of interneurons and of spinothalamic tract cells following dorsal column stimulation. However, there may also be inhibitory interactions in the brain.

TEMPERATURE

There are two distinct thermal sensations—cold and warm (Hensel, 1973a, 1974). These sensations can be evoked by focal stimulation of cold and warm spots (Fig. 1.1) (Blix, 1884; Donaldson, 1885; Frey, 1906; Dallenbach, 1927), as well as by changing the temperature of broad areas of the skin. When the skin is kept at 32–34°C, no thermal sensation is noted (Hensel, 1973a). However, when the temperature is altered in either direction from this indifferent level, a sense of warming or of cooling results. The threshold for thermal sensation depends upon a number of factors, including the rate of temperature change, the amount of change, the surface area affected, and the original or "adapting" temperature. At the extremes of the temperature range (above 45°C and below 13°C), the subject feels either heat pain or cold pain. Thermal pain is evoked by a different set of receptors than those responsible for thermal sensation.

In addition to thermal sensation, changes in surface temperature result in thermoregulatory responses in homothermic animals (Hensel, 1973b; Dykes, 1975). Despite their importance, such thermoregulatory responses will not be considered here. The activity of reptilian infrared detectors will also not be discussed (see Hartline, 1974).

Receptors

Thermal sensation depends upon two kinds of specific thermoreceptor, the cold receptor and the warm receptor. Cold receptors are innervated either by Aδ or by C fibers, while warm receptors are supplied by C fibers (Table 2.1) (Hensel, 1973a, 1974). Myelinated cold fibers are common in primate skin and also in the trigeminal distribution in the cat and dog. Thermoreceptors are completely insensitive to mechanical stimuli or respond feebly to strong mechanical stimuli (Hensel *et al.*, 1960; Perl, 1968; Hensel and Kenshalo, 1969; Iggo, 1969; Darian-Smith *et al.*, 1973). The receptive fields of most thermoreceptors are small spots about 1 mm in diameter, and generally a given

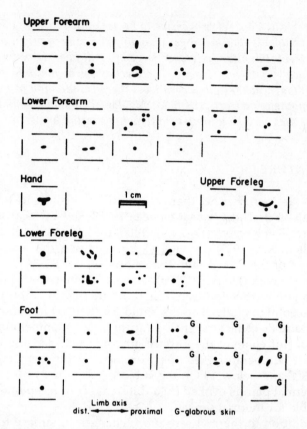

Fig. 9.21. Receptive fields of cold receptors in monkey. (From Kenshalo and Duclaux, 1977.)

thermoreceptor supplies just one spot (Perl, 1968; Hensel and Ken-shalo, 1969; Iggo, 1969; Hensel and Iggo, 1971). However, in primates a thermoreceptive afferent may innervate two to five spots, and the largest dimension of a spot may be as great as 5 mm (Fig. 9.21) (Du-claux and Kenshalo, 1973; Darian-Smith *et al.*, 1973; Dubner *et al.*, 1975; Kenshalo and Duclaux, 1977; Long, 1977; Duclaux and Kenshalo, 1978). The spotlike receptive fields of the specific thermoreceptors appear to correlate well with the cold and warm spots of human psychophysical experiments.

Anatomic findings indicate that the receptors responsible for cold spots have a distinctive morphology (Hensel *et al.*, 1974). Terminals that can be identified as cold receptors are in the basal layer of the epidermis (Fig. 2.10), an observation that is consistent with the prediction that cold receptors are located about 0.1–0.2 mm from the surface of the skin, based upon human psychophysical studies (Bazett and McGlone, 1930; Bazett *et al.*, 1930) and upon stimulation of thermoreceptors in the cat's tongue by known thermal gradients (Hensel *et al.*, 1951). Warm receptors are located deeper in the skin of the human (0.3–0.6 mm), but as yet no specific morphological entity has been described which corresponds to a warm receptor.

The afferent fibers of both cold and warm fibers have a background discharge at neutral skin temperatures. When the temperature is lowered, the discharges of cold receptors increase in frequency, while those of warm receptors decrease (Fig. 9.22). Conversely, when the temperature is elevated, cold receptors show a slowed discharge and warm receptors fire more vigorously (Hensel and Zotterman, 1951a,b,c; Hensel and Boman, 1960; Hensel *et al.*, 1960; Iriuchijima and Zotterman, 1960; Hensel and Kenshalo, 1969; Hensel and Iggo, 1971; Darian-Smith *et al.*, 1973; Konietzny and Hensel, 1975; Kenshalo and Duclaux, 1977; Duclaux and Kenshalo, 1978).

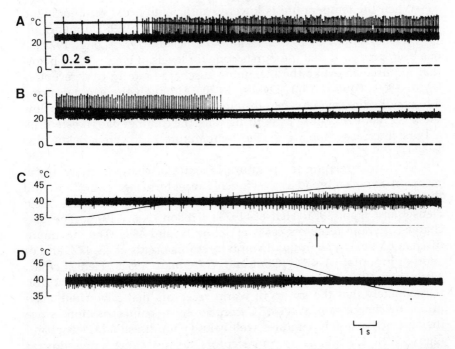

Fig. 9.22. (A and B) Response of a cold receptor in human skin during cooling from 34 to 26°C and then rewarming. (From Hensel and Boman, 1960.)   (C and D) Activity of a warm receptor from human skin during warming from 35 to 45°C and recooling. The arrow in C is the time at which the subject reported a warm sensation. (From Konietzny and Hensel, 1975.)

The curve relating the static discharge rate to temperature is not monotonic for either type of receptor (see Fig. 2.12). The curve for cold receptor static discharges is a very broad one, with discharges in some cold receptors at temperatures as low as 5°C and as high as 43°C; however, most cold receptors cease discharging at 10° and at 40°C. The maximum discharge rate occurs for a given receptor at a temperature somewhere between 18° and 34°C (Dodt and Zotterman, 1952a; Hensel et al., 1960; Iggo, 1969; Poulos and Lende, 1970a; Hensel, 1973a, 1974). Some cold fibers also discharge when the skin temperature exceeds 45°C, with a maximum frequency at 50°C. This response is called the "paradoxical response" of cold receptors (Dodt and Zotterman, 1952b; Kenshalo and Duclaux, 1977), and it may account for the "paradoxical cold" sensation which is reported when the skin is heated above 45°C (Hensel, 1973a). The tendency for a given cold receptor to show a paradoxical response appears to be related to the core body temperature, an effect apparently mediated by changes in vasomotor tone (Long, 1977).

When the temperature is lowered sufficiently, cold receptors tend to discharge in bursts (Fig. 2.10) (Dodt, 1952; Iggo, 1969; Dubner et al., 1975; Hellon et al., 1975; Kenshalo and Duclaux, 1977; Long, 1977). It has been proposed that the bursts code for levels of temperature below that required to evoke the maximum discharge rate in cold receptors (Iggo, 1969; Poulos, 1971; Dykes, 1975). Although the average firing rate may be the same for two different temperatures above and below the level that evokes the peak firing rate, the number of spikes within a burst increases linearly as the temperature is lowered below this level (Fig. 9.23).

The curve relating temperature to static discharge rate for warm receptors is not so broad as that for cold receptors (Fig. 2.12) (Dodt and Zotterman, 1952a; Hensel et al., 1960; Hensel and Kenshalo, 1969; Hensel and Iggo, 1971; Hensel, 1973a; Hellon et al., 1975). The discharges of warm receptors cease at about 30° and 48°C. The maximum discharge rate of one group of warm receptors occurs at 45–47°C and of another group at 41–43°C (Dodt and Zotterman, 1952a; Hensel et al., 1960; Iggo, 1969; Hensel and Iggo, 1971; Duclaux and Kenshalo, 1978). It is unlikely that the group of warm receptors that have their maximum discharge rate at 45–47°C contribute to pain sensation, since they are active at temperatures well below pain threshold (Hensel and Iggo, 1971). Cutaneous warm receptors do not show a paradoxical response to extreme cooling (Hensel et al., 1960; Hensel, 1973a).

Complete adaptation of thermal sensation can occur at temperatures between about 28° and 38°C over an area of 1 cm² or 30° to 36°C for 15 cm²; this range is called "physiological zero" (Kenshalo and

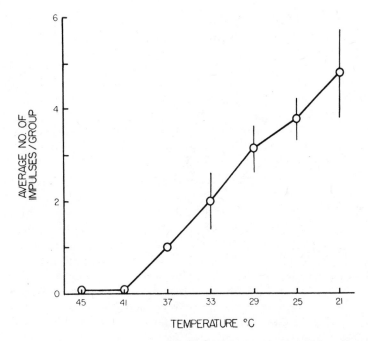

Fig. 9.23. Average number of spikes in grouped discharges of a cold receptor population as a function of steady-state temperature. (From Poulos, 1971.)

Scott, 1966; K. O. Johnson *et al.*, 1973). Adaptation of thermoreceptors occurs within about 30 s (Kenshalo and Duclaux, 1977; Duclaux and Kenshalo, 1978). Steady-state thermal stimuli can be distinguished by human subjects for differences down to about 0.5°C when the stimuli are applied simultaneously (Erikson and Poulos, 1973). However, thermoregulatory responses can be evoked by static temperature changes of less than 1°C (Nadel and Horvath, 1969; Benzinger, 1969). Dykes (1975) suggests that the burst code is utilized in thermoregulatory processing so that the organism can respond appropriately to small temperature changes (see Benzinger, 1969).

The specific thermoreceptors are sensitive not only to static changes in temperature but also to the rate of thermal change. Both cold and warm receptors have dynamic responses resulting in over- and undershoots in the discharge rate when rapid thermal stimuli are applied (Fig. 2-11) (Hensel *et al.*, 1960; Hensel and Kenshalo, 1969; Iggo, 1969; Poulos and Lende, 1970b; Hensel and Iggo, 1971; Darian-Smith *et al.*, 1973; Konietzny and Hensel, 1975; Kenshalo and Duclaux, 1977; Duclaux and Kenshalo, 1978). The sensations of cooling or warming correlate well with the dynamic responses of cold and warm receptors. For example, the threshold for detection of cooling transients is about 0.02–0.05°C in the human (Hardy and Oppel, 1938; Kenshalo et al., 1968), well below the threshold for discrimination of static temperature levels. The thresholds of thermoreceptors in the primate are capable of accounting for psychophysical thresholds in this range (Darian-Smith et al., 1973; K. O. Johnson et al., 1973). Furthermore, at a given adapting temperature, the response of a cold receptor is linearly related to the amplitude of a step or ramp change in temperature (Darian-Smith et al., 1973; Kenshalo and Duclaux, 1977). However, the information conveyed by a single cold receptor to the central nervous system is insufficient to account for the human discriminative capacity (K. O. Johnson et al., 1973), which must therefore depend upon the analysis of the activity of a population of receptors. K. O. Johnson et al. (1973) calculated that the information from at least sixteen cold fibers was required, assuming that all of the fibers operated independently. They estimated that the stimulus activated some fifty to seventy cold fibers, which is a large enough number to account for the human discriminative capacity, even if a part of the population of cold fibers did not discharge independently.

In human psychophysical tests, a decision can be made as to which of two cold stimuli is colder within 2 s (K. O. Johnson et al., 1973). Thus, the decision is made on the basis of the initial neural activity generated at the receptor level. When ramp stimuli are used, a change in the slope of the ramp does not alter the estimate of intensity, but rather the time at which the maximum intensity was experienced (Kenshalo and Duclaux, 1977). Thus, the neural system for judging thermal stimulus intensity acts like an integrator, summing the neural activity during the dynamic response.

The reaction time for the development of a sensation of coolness is distinctly shorter than that for a sensation of warmth; this can be accounted for on the basis of the response latencies of cold and warm fibers (Kenshalo and Duclaux, 1977; Duclaux and Kenshalo, 1978).

Several observations argue against the possibility that the sense of warmth is due to a reduction in the activity of cold receptors by warming. One line of evidence is that cold receptors stop discharging when the skin temperature approaches 40°C, yet the sense of warmth increases in the range between 40–45°C (see Konietzny and Hensel, 1975). Furthermore, warm sensation, but not cold sensation, can be eliminated by local anesthesia, which blocks C fibers before myelinated fibers (Fruhstorfer et al., 1974). A complementary experiment is asphyxial nerve block, which eliminates all sensations except warmth and pain because of blocked conduction in A fibers (D. Clark et al., 1935). Conversely, very little information about cooling can be signaled by a reduction in the discharges of warm receptors, since these cease discharging with cooling. There is a significant change in the discharge rate of warm receptors only when the adapting temperature is 35°C or higher and then only for cooling pulses of up to 2°C (K. O. Johnson et al., 1973). Finally, spinal cord disease can produce a dissociated loss of either cold or warm sensation (Head and Thompson, 1906). The evidence strongly favors independence of the pathways for warm and cold sensations, at least at the levels of the peripheral nervous system and the spinal cord.

Chemical agents can evoke cold or warm sensations. For example, menthol produces a cold sensation, whether applied topically or injected intravenously (Hensel, 1973a), and menthol excites cold receptors (Hensel and Zotterman, 1951d; Dodt et al., 1953).

In addition to actions on specific thermoreceptors, temperature changes affect other kinds of receptors (Werner and Mountcastle, 1965; Iggo, 1969; Duclaux and Kenshalo, 1972; Booth and Hahn, 1974; Burton et al., 1972; Martin and Manning, 1969; 1972; Poulos and Lende, 1970b; Hahn, 1971). For instance, type I and type II slowly adapting cutaneous mechanoreceptors can be excited by cooling. These thermally induced changes may account for Weber's illusion that objects feel heavier if cold (Weber, 1846; Hensel and Zotterman, 1951b; Witt and Hensel, 1959). However, the responses of slowly adapting mechanoreceptors cannot account for thermal sensation. For example, K. O. Johnson et al. (1973) observed that the stimulus-response curves of the slowly adapting mechanoreceptors have a similar form to those of cold receptors, but that the mechanoreceptors are twenty times less sensitive to cold than are the thermoreceptors. Using the same analysis to determine how a population of mechanoreceptors might combine to code for stimulus intensity, it was calculated that it would take more than four thousand receptors to account for the human discriminative capacity, yet there were probably less than one hundred slowly adapting receptors in the area stimulated. Furthermore, the peak of thermal responsiveness and the changes in responses produced by alterations in adapting temperature for type I receptors, at least, do not match psychophysical studies of cold sensation (Kenshalo, 1970; Duclaux and Kenshalo, 1972). Finally, touch can still be felt after local anesthetic has blocked cold and warm sensation, indicating that slowly adapting mechanoreceptors are not sufficient to evoke thermal sensation (Fruhstorfer et al., 1974).

Spinal Pathways

Since the afferent fibers from specific thermoreceptors are Aδ and C fibers, it is likely that they terminate in the most superficial layers of

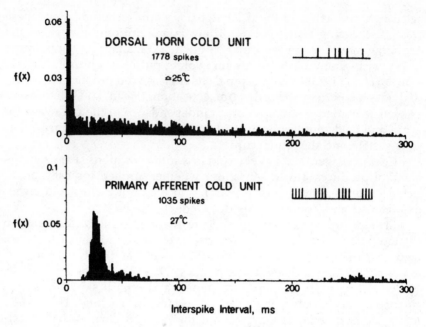

Fig. 9.24. Interspike interval histograms for a second-order neuron transmitting cold information for a cold receptor. Recordings from a monkey. Note the prominence of the burst pattern in the primary afferent and the absence of bursting in the second-order cell. (From Iggo and Ramsey, 1976.)

the dorsal horn (see Chapter 3). Recordings have been made from interneurons in laminae I–III (and also some deeper cells) that behave as if they received input from cold or warm receptors (Christensen and Perl, 1970; Hellon and Misra, 1973a; Kumazawa *et al.*, 1975; Kumazawa and Perl, 1976; Iggo and Ramsey, 1976). The second-order neurons receiving input from cold receptors do not have the pattern of burst discharges that is characteristic of the afferent fibers at certain temperatures, perhaps because the second-order cells receive a convergent input from many receptors that are presumably firing out of phase (Fig. 9.24) (Iggo and Ramsey, 1976). Cold pulses may produce dynamic and then static responses in the second-order cells; these responses are graded with stimulus intensity (Fig. 9.25) (Iggo and Ramsey, 1976). However, some units have only static or only dynamic responses (Hellon and Misra, 1973a). In the few cases tested, a high proportion of these interneurons project to the level of the cervical spinal cord, and the axons appear to be in the anterolateral quadrant contralateral to the cell body of origin (Kumazawa *et al.*, 1975; Iggo and Ramsey, 1976). The destination of the axons in the brain was not determined, but it is possible that the axons terminate in the thalamus.

Many other interneurons of the dorsal horn, including many spinothalamic tract and spinocervical tract neurons, are affected both by mechanical stimuli and by large-amplitude changes in temperature (Wall, 1960; Wall and Cronly-Dillon, 1960; A. G. Brown and Franz, 1969, 1970; Willis *et al.*, 1974; Burton, 1975). However, it seems likely that the thermal effects in these neurons are mediated either by changes in the activity of mechanoreceptors or by thermal nociceptors.

In humans, thermal sensation is lost on the contralateral side following anterolateral cordotomy (Foerster and Gagel 1931; Hyndman and Wolkin, 1943; Kuru, 1949; White and Sweet, 1955, 1969). A single anterolateral quadrant is sufficient to permit thermal sensation on the contralateral side (Noordenbos and Wall, 1976). Furthermore, thermal sensations may be evoked by stimulation in the anterolateral quadrant of the cord (Sweet *et al.*, 1950). Thus, thermal sensation in the human is mediated by a crossed pathway in the anterolateral quadrant, presumably by the spinothalamic tract (Fig. 9.26). There is some evidence that the axons carrying temperature information are at least partially

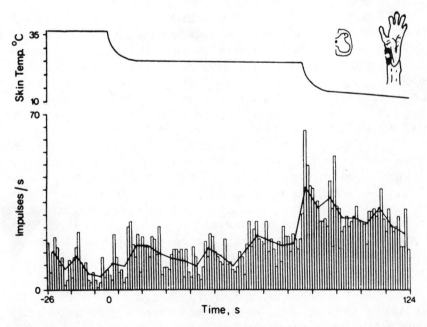

Fig. 9.25. Responses of an interneuron in the dorsal horn (see inset) to two successive cooling steps. Note the dynamic and static responses. (From Iggo and Ramsey, 1976.)

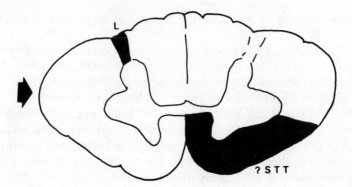

Fig. 9.26. Pathways for thermal information include Lissauer's tract (L) and probably contralateral spinothalamic tract (STT).

segregated from the fibers responsible for pain sensation (Stookey, 1929; Wilson and Fay, 1929; Grant, 1930; Sherman and Arieff, 1948). Lissauer's tract appears to distribute thermal information to several segments up the ipsilateral side of the cord, as it does pain information, since Lissauer tractotomy can alter the level of thermoanesthesia when combined with contralateral cordotomy (Hyndman, 1942).

The destination of the thermal pathway in the brain is thought to be the thalamus. Units have been found in the rat thalamus that respond to warming of scrotal skin (Hellon and Misra, 1973b; Hellon and Mitchell, 1975), and there have been other reports of thalamic units that respond to thermal stimulation of the skin of the extremities or of the tongue (e.g., Landgren, 1960; Poulos and Benjamin, 1968; Burton et al., 1970; Martin and Manning, 1971). It is not known if the pathway to the thalamus is direct or indirect.

An intriguing observation is that many neurons of the spinal cord show alterations of activity when the spinal cord temperature is changed (Wünnenberg and Brück, 1970; Simon and Iriki, 1971; Simon, 1972, 1974; Necker, 1975). Such neurons behave like the hypothalamic neurons, which are thought to act as central thermoreceptors and are believed to help control thermoregulatory processes (Benzinger, 1969; Hensel, 1973b). It seems unlikely that spinal cord neurons showing such behavior participate in thermal sensation.

In summary, there are two thermal sensations—cold and warm—and these are signaled by cold and warm receptors. Cold receptors are supplied by Aδ or C fibers and warm receptors by C fibers. A thermoreceptive afferent may supply one or several spotlike receptive fields. These may correlate with the cold and warm spots that can be mapped in human psycho-

physical studies. The morphology of cold receptors is distinctive; such receptors are found in the basal layer of the epidermis. The structure of warm receptors is unknown. Thermoreceptors have a static discharge at neutral skin temperatures. Lowering the skin temperature increases the discharge of cold receptors and slows the discharge of warm receptors; raising skin temperature does the opposite, except that high skin temperatures may also evoke a paradoxical discharge in cold receptors. The bursting discharges of cold receptors may serve as a code for the lower range of temperatures. Dynamic responses help account for the low thresholds of humans for thermal transients. The coding of temperature appears to depend upon the population response rather than the information carried by individual receptors. The dynamic response is probably responsible for the speed at which the thermal discriminations can be made. Chemical agents like menthol can excite cold receptors and produce a sensation of cold. Mechanoreceptors are unsuited to account for thermal sensation. The sensory pathway carrying thermal information in the human is likely to be the spinothalamic tract; although the evidence from animal experiments is incomplete, there are second-order cells in the marginal zone of the dorsal horn that respond as if they received input from specific thermoreceptors and that project in the contralateral anterolateral white matter at least to the cervical spinal cord. Such neurons show dynamic and static discharges, but not bursting activity. It can be presumed that these cells account for the thermal responses of thalamic neurons, but it is not yet certain if the spinothalamic pathway is a direct one.

POSITION SENSE

Two different sensations can be regarded as submodalities of position sense—static position sense and kinesthesia (Goodwin *et al.*, 1972b; McCloskey, 1973; Horch *et al.*, 1975). Static position sense is a knowledge of the location of a limb in space which depends upon sensory information arising from the limb; kinesthesia is an awareness of movement of a limb.

Receptors

There is a controversy concerning the receptors that are responsible for static position sense and for kinesthesia. The early history of this controversy has been reviewed by Goodwin *et al.* (1972b). Although Sherrington attributed position sense to both joint and muscle receptors, later investigators argued against an involvement of muscle spindles, which were thought not to project to the cerebral cortex and whose operation was complex and perhaps not suited to providing unambiguous signals about joint position. This left the joint receptors, cutaneous receptors, and the "sense of effort" (corollary discharge) as candidate mechanisms to explain position sense.

Joint receptors seemed at first to be a good possibility, since slowly adapting discharges can be recorded from joint nerves at all joint angles, although it is clear that the greatest amount of activity occurs when a joint is held at the extremes of flexion or of extension (Andrew and Dodt, 1953; Boyd and Roberts, 1953; Boyd, 1954; Cohen, 1955; Skoglund, 1956, 1973; McCall et al., 1974). The slowly adapting joint receptors were identified with Ruffini endings (Gardner, 1944; Boyd, 1954; Eklund and Skoglund, 1960; Skoglund, 1956, 1973). However, recently it has been found that Ruffini endings (at least in the knee joint of the cat) only discharge when tension is produced in the joint capsule; therefore, these endings appear to signal joint torque rather than joint position, and they may contribute to a sensation of joint pressure (Burgess and Clark, 1969b; Clark and Burgess, 1975; Clark, 1975; Grigg, 1975, 1976; Grigg and Greenspan, 1977; see also Eklund and Skoglund, 1960). The few slowly adapting receptors with afferents in the posterior articular nerve that do discharge when the knee joint is at an intermediate position are muscle spindle afferents originating in the popliteus muscle (Clark and Burgess, 1975; see also Grigg and Greenspan, 1977).

However, the receptors that signal joint position may vary across joints. For example, there seem to be Ruffini endings in the hip joint that are active at intermediate positions of that joint (Carli et al. 1975; but cf. Grigg et al., 1973). The joints of digits may differ from more proximal joints. The evidence for this is indirect. Slowly adapting cutaneous afferents are not required for static position sense in the knee joint, since the sensation produced by maintained identation of the skin fades within 1–2 minutes, whereas static position sense in the human knee is accurate to within 2–3° even when the position is changed so slowly that there is no sense of an alteration in skin position (Horch et al., 1975). However, static position sense in the toes and fingers is lost within a few minutes, and so it is possible that cutaneous receptors are involved in these distal joints. Type II slowly adapting afferents have been described in recordings from human subjects that discharge at rates proportionate to the amount of finger flexion (Fig. 9.27) (Knibestöl, 1975). Finally, anesthesia of the skin and joints of the digits produces a severe deficit in position sense (Browne et al., 1954; Provins, 1958) that is more likely to be attributable to the absence of input from cutaneous than from joint receptors (Cross and McCloskey, 1973).

Fig. 9.27. Discharges of a type II slowly adapting cutaneous mechano-receptor in the nail region of the human finger. The responses are the flexion of the distal interphalangeal joint (amount indicated in degrees). The graph shows the relationship between firing rate and joint angle. (From Knibestöl, 1975.)

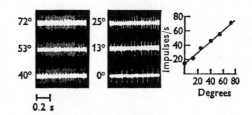

However, muscle spindles cannot be ruled out as contributors to position sense. Information from muscle spindles does in fact reach the cerebral cortex (see discussion of the spinomedullothalamic tract, Chapter 7, and the section below on spinal pathways for position sense). The complexity of operation of muscle spindles does not exclude their participation in position sense, it only requires a complicated mechanism. Evidence in favor of an involvement of muscle spindles in position sense comes from experiments like those of Eklund (1972) and of Goodwin et al. (1972b) in which illusions of movement were produced by vibrating the tendons of various muscles. The illusions were quantitated by asking the blindfolded subjects to track the vibrated arm with the control arm (Fig. 9.28). Such stimulation was thought by Goodwin et al. (1972b) to be relatively specific for activation of muscle spindle afferents, since illusions did not result when the vibrator was applied to the skin over joints or bone.

Anesthesia of a finger was used to determine whether or not muscle afferents contribute to position sense in distal joints (Goodwin et al., 1972a,b). Although position sense was reduced, it was not eliminated. However, the subjects had particular difficulty in detecting slow movements of the anesthetized finger. It was concluded that a number of types of receptors are likely to contribute to position sense, including muscle stretch receptors.

McCloskey (1973) extended these experiments to an analysis of illusions both of movement and of static position of the elbow joint when the biceps brachii tendon was vibrated. Experimental variables included the frequency and amplitude of vibration, the amount of loading of the muscle, and fatigue. Vibration at 100 Hz made the subjects feel that the joint was being extended whether the muscle was loaded or not, although loading reduced the error in matching the vibrated limb with the control limb. Lower-frequency vibration produced an illusion that the arm was positioned as if the muscle had been stretched. If the vibratory rate was low enough, there was no illusion of movement, but rather just one of position. In the case of

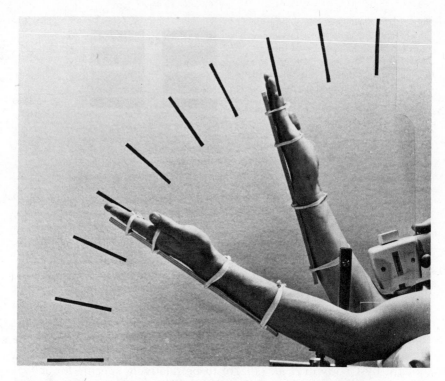

Fig. 9.28. The misalignment in the two arms reflects the extent of the illusion in position sense produced in a subject by vibration of the biceps tendon. The scale markings are 10°. The subject was instructed to align the arms in the absence of visual cues. (From Goodwin *et al.*, 1972b.)

such illusions of position, loading increased the error. Since illusions of movement and of position can be produced independently, there must be separate mechanisms for these sensations. It is speculated that the muscle spindle primary endings might contribute to kinesthesia and the secondary endings to static position sense.

The reduction in position sense in the fingers by local anesthesia could be due to the loss of input from receptors that contribute specifically to position sense, or it may reflect the loss of a more general facilitation of the central pathways activated by muscle afferents. Cross and McCloskey (1973) tried to approach this question by examining patients who had had complete removal and replacement of digital joints (metacarpophalangeal or metatarsophalangeal joints). In all cases studied, position sense was normal despite complete removal of the joint capsule. This was true soon enough after surgery that reinnervation by joint afferents could not have occurred. In one patient, the intrinsic muscles of the foot had been disconnected from a toe. Side-to-side movement of this toe could not be perceived, although flexion and extension movements could. Evidently, the perceptual cues from the long extensor and flexor muscles were more significant for position sense than was cutaneous input.

Further evidence that joint afferents are not required for position sense was obtained by Grigg *et al.* (1973), who found that position sense is almost normal in the hips of patients after total hip joint replacement. The thresholds for detection of abduction were sometimes elevated, and the precision of estimates of small changes in position was reduced by the surgery, but the patients could judge large passive movements normally, and they could position the hip perfectly well. The subjective feeling of abduction was similar to that on the normal side, although the intensity of the sensation was less. It was concluded that hip joint position sense can be mediated by extracapsular receptors.

One difficulty with the suggestion that muscle receptors are important to position sense is the negative results of the study by Gelfan and Carter (1967). They examined patients with tendons exposed at the wrist. When the tendons are pulled so that distal structures in the hand were moved, the subjects perceived the movement in a normal fashion. However, when the tendons were pulled in the opposite direction, stretching the muscles, the subjects did not report any sensations referable to the muscles, although they did notice sensation arising from the skin. This experiment needs to be repeated.

Spinal Pathways

The traditional view is that the main pathway for position sense is the dorsal column–medial lemniscus system (Head and Thompson, 1906). However, diseases that affect dorsal column function may produce a dissociation between vibratory and position sense. For instance, lesions at thoracic or lumbar levels can produce a reduction in vibratory sensation without a deficit in proprioception, whereas cervical lesions may do the opposite (Weinstein and Bender, 1947). Furthermore, experimental interruption of the cervical dorsal columns in monkeys results in a much more severe deficit in proprioception for the forelimbs than for the hind limbs (Ferraro and Barrera, 1934; Gilman and Denny-Brown, 1966). And there is evidence that hindlimb proprioception in monkeys and in the human (except for the toes) can be mediated through the ventral quadrant (Vierck, 1966; Noordenbos and Wall, 1976).

These observations fit the experimental findings in the cat that

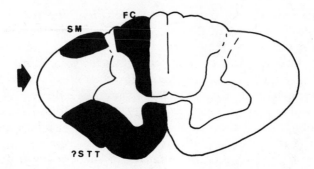

Fig. 9.29. Pathways for position sense include the fasciculus cuneatus (FC), but not the fasciculus gracilis, and the spinomedullothalamic pathway (SM) and a pathway in the ventral quadrant, possibly the spinothalamic tract (STT), all on the side stimulated.

slowly adapting joint and muscle receptors do not ascend to the medulla in the fasciculus gracilis (Lloyd and McIntyre, 1950; Burgess and Clark, 1969a). The pathway used for proprioceptive information from the hindlimbs in the cat is the spinomedullothalamic pathway (Fig. 9.29); this pathway has a relay in the spinal cord and another in nucleus z of the medulla, before crossing to terminate in the boundary area between the ventral posterior lateral and ventral lateral nuclei of the thalamus (Pompeiano and Brodal, 1957; Landgren and Silfvenius, 1971; Grant et al., 1973; Rustioni, 1973; Magherini et al., 1975; Johansson and Silfvenius, 1977a). The pathway is probably, in part, formed by collaterals of the dorsal spinocerebellar tract (Johansson and Silfvenius, 1977a). There is a nucleus z in the human (Sadjapour and Brodal, 1968), suggesting that a similar pathway exists in man.

On the other hand, the pathway for proprioceptive information from the forelimb in the cat involves the fasciculus cuneatus and main cuneate nucleus (Fig. 9.29) (Uddenberg, 1968a; Rosén, 1967, 1969a,b; Rosén and Sjölund, 1973a,b).

It is possible that the spinothalamic tract makes a contribution to position sense in the monkey. Some primate spinothalamic tract neurons respond in a slowly adapting fashion to changes in joint position, and the axons of these cells ascend in a peripheral layer along the ventrolateral aspect of the ventral quadrant (Willis et al., 1974; Applebaum et al., 1975). However, these cells are excited by joint movement on the same side of the body, and the axons decussate at the segmental level. Thus, it is not likely that such neurons can account for the observation of Noordenbos and Wall (1976) that position sense remained intact ipsilaterally to the intact anterolateral quadrant in their patient. A more complete analysis of the pathways mediating position sense must await resolution of the controversy surrounding the nature of the receptors involved.

In summary, position sense can be subdivided into static position sense and kinesthesia. It is likely that the slowly adapting joint receptors (Ruffini endings) signal deep pressure, rather than position, since these only discharge when torque develops in the joint. However, this is controversial. Slowly adapting cutaneous receptors are also unsuitable, since their discharge adapts more quickly that position sense, at least in the human knee. However, cutaneous input may be more significant for position sense in digits. It is possible that muscle spindle afferents contribute to position sense. Other receptors and also a "sense of effort" also need to be considered. The spinal pathways for position sense appear to be different for the hind limbs and the forelimbs. The hindlimb pathway in the cat is the spino-medullothalamic pathway, whereas the forelimb pathway is the fasciculus cuneatus and main cuneate nucleus. Monkeys and humans can utilize a pathway in the ventral quadrant. It is not clear if this is the spinothalamic tract.

VISCERAL SENSE

The most prominent visceral sensation is pain. This has already been discussed. The other visceral sensations mediated by afferents entering the spinal cord include visceral fullness and satiation (for a review, see Leek, 1972). There is apparently no thermal sensation in the viscera, although there may be abdominal thermoreceptors that contribute to thermoregulation (Riedel, 1976).

Receptors

Pacinian corpuscles are abundant in the abdominal cavity, at least in cats, and some of these discharge in phase with cardiovascular pulsations; however, their potential contribution to circulatory regulation has not been completely explored (Gammon and Bronk, 1935; Gernandt and Zotterman, 1946; Leitner and Perl, 1964).

The receptors found in the mesentery and along the serosal surfaces of many visceral organs are activated by movement and by distention of these organs (Paintal, 1957; Todd, 1964; Bessou and Perl, 1966; Ranieri et al., 1973; Morrison, 1973, 1977; Floyd and Morrison, 1974; Floyd et al., 1976). These do not seem to discharge in any precise relationship to changes in intraluminal pressure or volume (Morrison, 1977), but they could contribute to a sense of fullness or, alternatively, to the pain of excessive distention.

Other receptors found in the smooth muscle layers of such organs as the gastrointestinal tract and the bladder can be activated either by distention or by contraction (Iggo, 1955; Winter, 1971; Leek, 1972). Such "in series" receptors may trigger reflex emptying, but it is reasonable to suppose that they also contribute to sensations associated with emptying or to a sense of fullness; in pathological states, they may also produce pain (Leek, 1972). There are also receptors that supply the mucosal linings of visceral organs. Some of these may be nociceptors.

Spinal Pathways

Some large afferents, including those supplying the abdominal Pacinian corpuscles, ascend the cord in the dorsal columns and terminate in the dorsal column nuclei (Fig. 9.30) (Amassian, 1951; Aidar *et al.*, 1952; Perl *et al.*, 1962). Visceral afferents of smaller caliber activate neurons of the spinocervical (Rigamonti and DeMichelle, 1977) and spinothalamic (Hancock *et al.*, 1975) tracts. Furthermore, axons in the ventral quadrant of the cord have been shown to discharge following distention of hollow viscera, such as the gall bladder; these axons may belong to the spinoreticular tract (Fields *et al.*, 1970a,b). However, it is not known what visceral sensations are mediated by the dorsal columns or by pathways in the lateral and ventral funiculi.

In summary, little is known about visceral sensations other than visceral pain. Pacinian corpuscles sometimes discharge in phase with car-

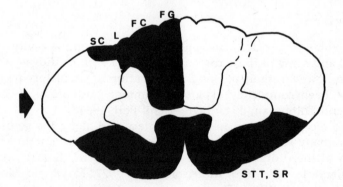

Fig. 9.30. Pathways carrying information from visceral receptors include the fasciculus cuneatus and gracilis (FC, FG), Lissauer's tract (L) and the spinocervical tract (SC) ipsilaterally to the stimulus and ventral quadrant pathways such as the spinothalamic and spinoreticular tract (STT, SR) bilaterally.

diovascular pulsations, but the significance of this is not clear. Receptors that respond to visceral movement or distention may contribute to the sensation of fullness, as may the "in series" receptors in smooth muscle layers that discharge when the muscle is stretched or when it contracts. Alternatively, these receptors could contribute to visceral pain. Visceral receptors are known to activate neurons in the dorsal column pathway, the spinocervical and spinothalamic tracts, and perhaps the spinoreticular tract. However, it is not clear what visceral sensations are mediated by the various ascending tracts.

CENTRIFUGAL CONTROL OF SOMATOVISCERAL SENSATION

The modulation of sensory input by efferent pathways from the brain has received a great deal of attention in recent years. Much of the work has been done on the gamma loop and on pathways of the special senses, especially the auditory system, but there are also a number of studies showing that a similar process occurs in the somatovisceral sensory system. The early studies have been reviewed on several occasions (Livingston, 1959; Granit, 1955; Dawson, 1958; Hagbarth, 1960; Towe, 1973).

Some of the ways in which the descending control of a sensory pathway might be expressed were summarized by Wall and Dubner (1972): a change in gain in the afferent pathway, a change in the degree of selectivity among several kinds of input, a change in receptive field size of central neurons, an alteration in inhibitory surround, the appearance of habituation, and switching of sensory inputs or of the distribution of sensory information to higher centers. Another possibility is that the descending control might serve as a "corollary discharge" by inhibiting the part of the sensory input that would be predicted to result from a voluntary movement (Holst, 1954; Teuber, 1960).

One source of centrifugal control of the somatovisceral sensory pathways is the sensorimotor cortex. Descending commands from the cortex may be transmitted directly to the spinal cord through the corticospinal tract, or they may involve a relay in the brainstem (Nyberg-Hansen and Brodal, 1963; Liu and Chambers, 1964; Petras, 1967; Coulter and Jones, 1977; Carpenter *et al.*, 1963b; Hongo and Jankowska, 1967). Cortical control has been demonstrated for interneurons of the dorsal horn (Wall, 1967; Fetz, 1968), the dorsal column nuclei (Towe and Jabbur, 1961; Jabbur and Towe, 1961; Levitt *et al.*, 1964; Gordon and Jukes, 1964b; Andersen *et al.*, 1964e), the spinocervical tract (A. G. Brown and Short, 1974; A. G. Brown *et al.*, 1977a), the spinothalamic tract (Coulter *et al.*, 1974), and probably the spinoreticular tract (Magni and Oscarsson, 1961; Lundberg *et al.*, 1963).

Another source of descending control is the reticular formation of the brainstem. Stimulation within the reticular formation or cerebellum results in primary afferent depolarization in the lumbar cord (Carpenter *et al.*, 1966; Cangiano *et al.*, 1969). Comparable stimulation affects the discharges of neurons in the dorsal column nuclei either directly or through the generation of primary afferent depolarization (Cesa-Bianchi *et al.*, 1968; Cesa-Bianchi and Sotgiu, 1969); also modulated are the spinocervical tract (Taub, 1964), the spinothalamic tract (McCreery and Bloedel, 1975, 1976), and probably the spinoreticular tract (Holmqvist *et al.*, 1960b; Grillner *et al.*, 1968). It seems likely that the reticular formation serves to integrate information from many sources, which thus have access to the sensory pathways by way of the reticular formation. For example, at least a part of the corticofugal action on the dorsal column nuclei is probably mediated by way of the reticular formation, as is the effect on the same nuclei of stimulation in such diverse structures as the deep cerebellar nuclei, the nonspecific nuclei of the thalamus, and the caudate nucleus (Sotgiu and Cesa-Bianchi, 1970, 1972; Jabbur *et al.*, 1977).

A particularly important descending control system originates near the midline of the caudal brainstem. This is the "dorsal reticulospinal system" of Lundberg's group, which is responsible for a tonic inhibition of the pathways in the spinal cord which are activated by the "flexion reflex afferents" (R. M. Eccles and Lundberg, 1959a,b; Holmqvist and Lundberg, 1959, 1961; Engberg *et al.*, 1968a,b,c,d; see also Job, 1953; Kuno and Perl, 1960; Handwerker *et al.*, 1975; Basbaum *et al.*, 1976; Cervero *et al.*, 1976; Fields *et al.*, 1977a; Guilbaud *et al.* 1977b). This system not only affects spinal cord circuits but also several ascending tracts, including the spinocervical tract (Wall, 1967; A. G. Brown, 1970, 1971; Cervero *et al.*, 1977a), the spinoreticular tract (Beall *et al.*, 1976; Willis *et al.*, 1977), and probably the spinoreticular tract (Holmqvist *et al.*, 1960a). The pathway involves, at least in part, a raphe–spinal projection originating in the nucleus raphe magnus (Kuypers and Maisky, 1975; Basbaum *et al.*, 1976; Basbaum and Fields, 1977; Martin *et al.*, 1978); this portion of the pathway is likely to be serotonergic (Dahlström and Fuxe, 1965; Andén *et al.*, 1966b; Engberg *et al.*, 1968a,b). There may also be a nonserotonergic component of the pathway originating from the reticular formation (Engberg *et al.*, 1968b).

Interest in the "dorsal reticulospinal system" has been heightened recently because of the growing evidence that the analgesia produced by stimulation in the region of the periaqueductal and periventricular gray may depend upon information transmitted to the spinal cord, at least in part, by way of the nucleus raphe magnus (Reynolds, 1969; Akil and Mayer, 1972; Guilbaud *et al.*, 1973a; Mayer and Liebeskind, 1974; Oliveras *et al.*, 1974a, 1975; Akil and Liebeskind, 1975; Proudfit and Anderson, 1975; Ruda, 1975; Giesler and Liebeskind, 1976; Mayer and Price, 1976; Taber-Pierce *et al.*, 1976).

In addition to the possibility that electrical stimulation of certain brain regions may prove useful for therapeutic intervention in cases of chronic pain, there seems to be a relationship between the "intrinsic analgesia" system, the receptors that mediate the actions of the opiate drugs, the encephalins, and the mechanism of acupuncture (Tsou and Jang, 1964; Herz *et al.*, 1970; Samanin *et al.*, 1970; Samanin and Valzelli, 1971; Kuhar *et al.*, 1973; Pert and Snyder, 1973; Pert and Yaksh, 1974; Sharpe *et al.*, 1974; Vogt, 1974; Hughes, 1975; Hughes *et al.*, 1975; Mayer and Hayes, 1975; Adams, 1976; Akil *et al.*, 1976; Simantov *et al.*, 1976; Yaksh *et al.*, 1976a,b; Mayer *et al.*, 1977; Oliveras *et al.*, 1977). In addition to an action in the brainstem, the opiates can also affect neurons in the spinal cord directly (Le Bars *et al.*, 1976a,b; Yaksh and Rudy, 1976; see also LaMotte *et al.*, 1976). This area of research has already proved to be of considerable interest and significance. It is reasonable to expect that a number of other descending pathways will be found to play an important role in the modulation of sensory input from the body and the viscera.

CONCLUSIONS

1. A sensory channel is the mechanism for the transmission of a particular type of sensory information. A sensory channel includes receptors, spinal cord circuits, ascending spinal pathways, and those parts of the brain that process the information and produce perception.

2. Touch–pressure is a sense of maintained contact. The receptors probably include both type I and type II slowly adapting cutaneous mechanoreceptors. Type I receptors activate interneurons in the deeper layers of the dorsal horn; they do not project up the fasciculus gracilis, although axons of type I receptors are found in the fasciculus cuneatus. Type I information from the hind limb is conveyed by a pathway in the dorsolateral fasciculus. Type II receptors project up the dorsal columns. The spinothalamic tract may play a role in touch–pressure in the primate.

3. Flutter–vibration includes two distinct sensations. Flutter is a sense of low-frequency oscillation, while vibration is a sense of high-frequency oscillation.

4. Flutter is detected by Meissner's corpuscles in the glabrous skin and by G2 hair-follicle receptors in the hairy skin. The receptor for vibration is the Pacinian corpuscle. The receptors for flutter activate neurons in the dorsal horn, whereas Pacinian corpuscles may not. The ascending pathways involved in flutter include the dorsal columns, the spinocervical tract, and the spinothalamic tract. Vibration is conveyed just through the dorsal column.

5. There are several kinds of pain. Superficial pain can be subdivided into bright (or first) pain and burning (or second) pain. Deep pain includes that arising in the muscles, tendons, and joints and that originating in viscera.

6. In addition to the sensory experience of pain, noxious (potentially damaging) stimuli evoke autonomic and somatic motor responses, arousal, and aversive behavior.

7. The receptors for pain include a variety of cutaneous, muscle, visceral, and other nociceptors. Some of these are activated just by mechanical stimuli, while others can also be excited by thermal or chemical noxious stimuli. It seems unlikely that there is a common chemical mediator that activates all nociceptors, but chemical agents released in areas of damage probably do play a role in sensitization of nociceptors. The afferents of the nociceptors terminate in the upper layers of the dorsal horn and in lamina V. The ascending pathways include the spinothalamic tract, the spinocervical tract, the second-order dorsal column pathway, the spinoreticular tract, and the spinotectal tract. The most important spinal pathway for pain sensation in man is the spinothalamic tract.

8. Referred pain is best explained by the convergence–projection theory of Ruch. Both somatic and visceral afferents converge upon spinal neurons, including cells giving rise to ascending tracts. Activation of these tracts is more commonly associated with somatic inputs than with visceral ones, and so through learning it is likely that information evoked in the same pathways by visceral input will be attributed to a somatic input.

9. The mechanism of "counterirritation" is not yet understood in detail.

10. Thermal sensations include cold and warm.

11. Cold and warm receptors are responsible for the thermal sensations. They also contribute to thermoregulation. The activity of some mechanoreceptors can be affected by thermal changes, but mechanoreceptors cannot account for thermal sensation. The afferents from ther-

moreceptors terminate in the upper layers of the dorsal horn. The ascending pathway is probably the spinothalamic tract.

12. Position sense includes the sensations of static position and of kinesthesia (the sense of movement of a limb).

13. There is a controversy concerning the receptors that are responsible for position sense. The slowly adapting joint receptors may not prove to be involved as was once thought. Instead, muscle spindle afferents may signal both static position sense and kinesthesia. However, several joint and cutaneous receptors may contribute, along with the "sense of effort" that accompanies muscular exertion. The proprioceptors of the hindlimb synapse upon neurons in the deeper layers of the dorsal horn and in Clarke's column. The ascending pathways, from the hind limb include the spinomedullothalamic pathway and perhaps the spinothalamic tract, but not the dorsal column. Proprioceptors of the forelimb project both to the lateral cuneate and to the main cuneate nuclei. The dorsal column pathway thus may be responsible for position sense in the forelimb.

14. In addition to visceral pain, the visceral sensations that are mediated by spinal nerves include visceral fullness and satiation.

15. Visceral receptors include Pacinian corpuscles, but their sensory role is unclear. Receptors located in the mesentery and along the serosal surfaces of abdominal viscera may contribute to a sense of fullness, as may receptors located "in series" with the smooth muscle within the walls of the hollow organs. The ascending pathway for the large visceral afferents is the dorsal columns, while those for the small afferents are the spinothalamic, spinocervical, and spinoreticular tracts.

16. Sensory channels are controlled by pathways descending from the brain. These pathways can regulate the gain, select inputs, alter receptive field size, affect inhibitory inputs, redistribute information at the level of the brain, or serve as a "corollary discharge."

17. The sensorimotor cortex exerts an important control on interneurons, the dorsal column nuclei, the spinocervical tract, the spinothalamic tract, and probably also the spinoreticular tract.

18. The reticular formation is another source of descending control. It undoubtedly serves as an integrative center through which many brain structures can affect sensory transmission. Among the sensory pathways known to be influenced by the reticular formation are the dorsal column–medial lemniscus pathway, the spinocervical tract, the spinothalamic tract, and probably the spinoreticular tract.

19. The "dorsal reticulospinal system" of Lundberg not only provides a tonic descending inhibition of spinal cord interneurons in the flexion reflex pathways, but it also controls the information carried by

ascending pathways, including the spinocervical tract, the spinothalamic tract, and probably the spinoreticular tract. Of considerable recent interest is the probable involvement of this pathway in the "intrinsic analgesia system," which is thought to mediate "stimulus-produced analgesia" and the effects of the opiates, both exogenous and endogenous.

20. It is likely that a number of other descending pathways will be found to exert significant effects upon ascending pathways of the somatovisceral sensory system.

References

Abrahams, V. C., and Rose, P. K. (1975a). The spinal course and distribution of fore and hind limb muscle afferent projections to the superior colliculus of the cat. *J. Physiol.* **247**, 117–130.

Abrahams, V. C., and Rose, P. K. (1975b). Projections of extraocular, neck muscle and retinal afferents to superior colliculus in the cat: their connections to cells of origin of tectospinal tract. *J. Neurophysiol.* **38**, 10–18.

Adair, E. R., Stevens, J. C., and Marks, L. E. (1968). Thermally induced pain: the dol scale and the psychophysical power law. *Amer. J. Psychol.* **81**, 147–164.

Adams, J. E. (1976). Naloxone reversal of analgesia produced by brain stimulation in the human. *Pain* **2**, 161–166.

Adrian, E. D. (1928). *The Basis of Sensation.* Reprinted by Hafner Publishing Co., New York, 1964.

Adrian, E. D., and Zotterman, Y. (1926a). The impulses produced by sensory nerve-endings. Part 2. The response of a single end-organ. *J. Physiol.* **61**, 151–171.

Adrian, E. D., and Zotterman, Y. (1926b). The impulses produced by sensory nerve endings. Part 3. Impulses set up by touch and pressure. *J. Physiol.* **61**, 465–483.

Aidar, O., Geohegan, W. A., and Ungewitter, L. H. (1952). Splanchnic afferent pathways in the central nervous system. *J. Neurophysiol.* **15**, 131–138.

Akil, H., and Liebeskind, J. C. (1975). Monoaminergic mechanisms of stimulation-produced analgesia. *Brain Res.* **94**, 279–296.

Akil, H., and Mayer, D. J. (1972). Antagonism of stimulation-produced analgesia by p-CPA, a serotonin synthesis inhibitor. *Brain Res.* **44**, 692–697.

Akil, H., Mayer, D. J., and Liebeskind, J. C. (1976). Antagonism of stimulation-produced analgesia by naloxone, a narcotic antagonist. *Science* **191**, 961–962.

Albe-Fessard, D., Levante, A., and Lamour, Y. (1974). Origin of spino-thalamic tract in monkeys. *Brain Res.* **65**, 503–509.

Albe-Fessard, D., Boivie, J., Grant, G., and Levante, A. (1975). Labelling of cells in the medulla oblongata and the spinal cord of the monkey after injections of horseradish peroxidase in the thalamus. *Neurosci. Lett.* **1**, 75–80.

Amassian, V. E. (1951). Fiber groups and spinal pathways of cortically represented visceral afferents. *J. Neurophysiol.* **14**, 445–460.

Amassian, V. E. (1952). Interaction in the somatovisceral projection system. *Res. Publ. Assoc. Res. Nerv. Mental Dis.* **30**, 371–402.

Amassian, V. E., and DeVito, R. V. (1954). Unit activity in reticular formation and nearby structures. *J. Neurophysiol.* **17**, 575–603.

Amassian, V. E., and DeVito, J. L. (1957). La transmission dans le noyau de Burdach (nucleus cuneatus). Étude analytique par unités isolées d'un relais somato-sensoriel primaire. *Colloq. Int. Cent. Nat. Rech. Sci., Paris* **67**, 353–393.

Amassian, V. E., and Giblin, D. (1974). Periodic components in steady-state activity of cuneate neurones and their possible role in sensory coding. *J. Physiol.* **243**, 353–385.

Andén, N. E., Jukes, M. G. M., Lundberg, A., and Vyklický, L. (1966a). The effects of DOPA on the spinal cord. 1. Influence on transmission from primary afferents. *Acta Physiol. Scand.* **67**, 373–386.

Andén, N. E., Jukes, M. G. M., Lundberg, A., and Vyklický, L. (1966b). The effect of DOPA on the spinal cord. 3. Depolarization evoked in the central terminals of ipsilateral Ia afferents by volleys in the flexor reflex afferents. *Acta Physiol. Scand.* **68**, 322–336.

Andersen, P., Eccles, J. C., Oshima, T., and Schmidt, R. F. (1964a). Mechanisms of synaptic transmission in the cuneate nucleus. *J. Neurophysiol.* **27**, 1096–1116.

Andersen, P., Eccles, J. C., Schmidt, R. F., and Yokota, T. (1964b). Slow potential waves produced in the cuneate nucleus by cutaneous volleys and by cortical stimulation. *J. Neurophysiol.* **27**, 78–91.

Andersen, P., Eccles, J. C., Schmidt, R. F., and Yokota, T. (1964c). Depolarization of presynaptic fibers in the cuneate nucleus. *J. Neurophysiol.* **27**, 92–106.

Andersen, P., Eccles, J. C., Schmidt, R. F., and Yokota, T. (1964d). Identification of relay cells and interneurons in the cuneate nucleus. *J. Neurophysiol.* **27**, 1080–1095.

Andersen, P., Eccles, J. C., and Sears, T. A. (1964e). Cortically evoked depolarization of primary afferent fibers in the spinal cord. *J. Neurophysiol.* **27**, 63–77.

Andersen, P., Andersson, S. A., and Landgren, S. (1966). Some properties of the thalamic relay cells in the spino-cervico-lemniscal path. *Acta Physiol. Scand.* **68**, 72–83.

Andersen, P., Etholm, B., and Gordon, G. (1970). Presynaptic and post-synaptic inhibition elicited in the cat's dorsal column nuclei by mechanical stimulation of skin. *J. Physiol.* **210**, 433–455.

Andersen, P., Gjerstad, L., and Pasztor, E. (1972a). Effect of cooling on synaptic transmission through the cuneate nucleus. *Acta Physiol. Scand.* **84**, 433–447.

Andersen, P., Gjerstad, L., and Pasztor, E. (1972b). Effects of cooling on inhibitory processes in the cuneate nucleus. *Acta Physiol. Scand.* **84**, 448–461.

Anderson, F. D., and Berry, C. M. (1959). Degeneration studies of long ascending fiber systems in the cat brain stem. *J. Compar. Neurol.* **111**, 195–229.

Anderson, S. D., Basbaum, A. I., and Fields, H. L. (1977). Response of medullary raphe neurons to peripheral stimulation and to systemic opiates. *Brain Res.* **123**, 363–368.

Andersson, S. A. (1962). Projection of different spinal pathways to the second somatic sensory area in cat. *Acta Physiol. Scand.* **56** (Suppl. 194), 1–74.

Andersson, S. A., and Leissner, P. E. (1975). Does the spinocervical pathway exist? *Brain Res.* **98**, 359–363.

Andersson, S. A., Norrsell, K., and Norrsell, U. (1972). Spinal pathways projecting to the cerebral first somatosensory area in the monkey. *J. Physiol.* **225**, 589–597.

Andersson, S. A., Finger, S., and Norrsell, U. (1975). Cerebral units activated by tactile stimuli via a ventral spinal pathway in monkeys. *Acta Physiol. Scand.* **93**, 119–128.

Andres, K. H., and Düring, M. von (1973). Morphology of cutaneous receptors. In: *Handbook of Sensory Physiology*. Vol. II, *Somatosensory System*, pp. 3–28 (A. Iggo, ed.). Springer, New York.

Andres-Trelles, F., Cowan, C. M., and Simmonds, M. A. (1976). The negative potential wave evoked in cuneate nucleus by stimulation of afferent pathways: its origins and susceptibility to inhibition. *J. Physiol.* **258**, 173–186.

Andrew, B. L., and Dodt, E. (1953). The deployment of sensory nerve endings at the knee joint of the cat. *Acta Physiol. Scand.* **28**, 287–296.

Angaut-Petit, D. (1975a). The dorsal column system: I. Existence of long ascending post-synaptic fibres in the cat's fasciculus gracilis. *Exp. Brain Res.* **22**, 457–470.

Angaut-Petit, D. (1975b). The dorsal column system: II. Functional properties and bulbar relay of the postsynaptic fibres of the cat's fasciculus gracilis. *Exp. Brain Res.* **22**, 471–493.

Antonetty, C. M., and Webster, K. E. (1975). The organization of the spinotectal projection. An experimental study in the rat. *J. Compar. Neurol.* **163**, 449–466.

Aoyama, M., Hongo, T., and Kudo, N. (1973). An uncrossed ascending tract originating from below Clarke's column and conveying group I impulses from the hindlimb muscles in the cat. *Brain Res.* **62**, 237–241.

Appelberg, B., Bessou, P., and Laporte, Y. (1966). Action of static and dynamic fusimotor fibres on secondary endings of cat's spindles. *J. Physiol.* **185**, 160–171.

Applebaum, A. E., Beall, J. E., Foreman, R. D., and Willis, W. D. (1975). Organization and receptive fields of primate spinothalamic tract neurons. *J. Neurophysiol.* **38**, 572–586.

Applebaum, M. L., Clifton, G. L., Coggeshall, R. E., Coulter, J. D., Vance, W. H., and Willis, W. D. (1976). Unmyelinated fibres in the sacral 3 and caudal 1 ventral roots of the cat. *J. Physiol.* **256**, 557–572.

Arbuthnott, E. R., Boyd, I. A., and Kalu, K. U. (1975). Ultrastructure and conduction velocity of small, myelinated peripheral nerve fibers. In: *The Somatosensory System*, pp. 168–175 (H. H. Kornhuber, ed.). Thieme, Stuttgart.

Armett, C. J., Gray, J. A. B., and Palmer, J. F. (1961). A group of neurones in the dorsal horn associated with cutaneous mechanoreceptors. *J. Physiol.* **156**, 611–622.

Armett, C. J., Gray, J. A. B., Hunsperger, R. W., and Lal, S. (1962). The transmission of information in primary receptor neurones and second-order neurones of a phasic system. *J. Physiol.* **164**, 395–421.

Atweh, S. F., Banna, N. R., Jabbur, S. J., and To'mey, G. F. (1974). Polysensory interactions in the cuneate nucleus. *J. Physiol.* **238**, 343–355.

Austin, G. M., and McCouch, G. P. (1955). Presynaptic component of intermediary cord potential. *J. Neurophysiol.* **18**, 441–451.

Avanzino, G. L., Hösli, L., and Wolstencroft, J. H. (1966). Identification of cerebellar projecting neurones in nucleus reticularis gigantocellularis. *Brain Res.* **3**, 201–203.

Azulay, A., and Schwartz, A. S. (1975). The role of the dorsal funiculus of the primate in tactile discrimination. *Exp. Neurol.* **46**, 315–332.

Balagura, S., and Ralph, T. (1973). The analgesic effect of electrical stimulation of the diencephalon and mesencephalon. *Brain Res.* **60**, 369–379.

Banna, N. R., and Jabbur, S. J. (1969). Pharmacological studies on inhibition in the cuneate nucleus of the cat. *Int. J. Neuropharmacol.* **8**, 299–307.

Banna, N. R., and Jabbur, S. J. (1971). The effects of depleting GABA on cuneate presynaptic inhibition. *Brain Res.* **33**, 530–532.

Banna, N. R., Naccache, A., and Jabbur, S. J. (1972). Picrotoxin-like action of bicuculline. *Eur. J. Pharmacol.* **17**, 301–302.

Barker, D. (1962). The structure and distribution of muscle receptors. In: *Symposium on Muscle Receptors*, pp. 227–240 (D. Barker, ed.). Hong Kong Univ. Press, Hong Kong.

Barker, J. L., and Nicoll, R. A. (1973). The pharmacology and ionic dependency of amino acid responses in the frog spinal cord. *J. Physiol.* **228**, 259–277.

Barnes, C. D., and Pompeiano, O. (1971). Effects of muscle afferents on brain stem reticular and vestibular units. *Brain Res.* **25**, 179–183.

Barron, D. H., and Matthews, B. H. C. (1938). The interpretation of potential changes in the spinal cord. *J. Physiol.* **92**, 276–321.

Basbaum, A. I. (1973). Conduction of the effects of noxious stimulation by short-fiber multisynaptic systems of the spinal cord in the rat. *Exp. Neurol.* **40**, 699–716.

Basbaum, A. I., and Fields, H. L. (1977). The dorsolateral funiculus of the spinal cord: a major route for descending brainstem control. *Soc. Neurosci. Abstr.* **3**, 499.

Basbaum, A. I., and Hand, P. J. (1973). Projections of cervicothoracic dorsal roots to the cuneate nucleus of the rat, with observations on cellular "bricks." *J. Compar. Neurol.* **148**, 347–360.

Basbaum, A. I., Clanton, C. H., and Fields, H. L. (1976). Opiate and stimulus-produced analgesia: functional anatomy of a medullospinal pathway. *Proc. Natl. Acad. Sci.* **73**, 4685–4688.

Basbaum, A. I., Marley, N. J. E., O'Keefe, J., and Clanton, C. H. (1977). Reversal of morphine and stimulus-produced analgesia by subtotal spinal cord lesions. *Pain* **3**, 43–56.

Bazett, H. C., and McGlone, B. (1930). Experiments on the mechanism of stimulation of end-organs for cold. *Amer. J. Physiol.* **93**, 632.

Bazett, H. C., McGlone, B., and Brocklehurst, R. J. (1930). The temperatures in the tissues which accompany temperature sensations. *J. Physiol.* **69**, 88–112.

Beal, J. A., and Fox, C. A. (1976). Afferent fibers in the substantia gelatinosa of the adult monkey (*Macaca mulatta*): A Golgi study. *J. Compar. Neurol.* **168**, 113–144.

Beall, J. E., Martin, R. F., Applebaum, A. E., and Willis, W. D. (1976). Inhibition of primate spinothalamic tract neurons by stimulation in the region of the nucleus raphe magnus. *Brain Res.* **114**, 328–333.

Beall, J. E., Applebaum, A. E., Foreman, R. D., and Willis, W. D. (1977). Spinal cord potentials evoked by cutaneous afferents in the monkey. *J. Neurophysiol.* **40**, 199–211.

Beck, P. W., and Handwerker, H. O. (1974). Bradykinin and serotonin effects on various types of cutaneous nerve fibres. *Pfluegers Arch.* **347**, 209–222.

Beck, P. W., Handwerker, H. O., and Zimmermann, M. (1974). Nervous outflow from the cat's foot during noxious radiant heat stimulation. *Brain Res.* **67**, 373–386.

Békésy, G. von (1967). *Sensory Inhibition.* Princeton Univ. Press, Princeton, New Jersey.

Bell, C. (1811). *Idea of a New Anatomy of the Brain.* Strahan and Preston, London. Reprinted in Cranefield, P. F. (ed.) (1974). *The way in and the way out: Francois Magendie, Charles Bell and the roots of the spinal nerves.* Futura Publ. Co., New York.

Bell, C., Sierra, G. Buendia, N., and Segundo, J. P. (1964). Sensory properties of neurons in the mesencephalic reticular formation. *J. Neurophysiol.* **27**, 961–987.

Benjamin, R. M. (1970). Single neurons in the rat medulla responsive to nociceptive stimulation. *Brain Res.* **24**, 525–529.

Benoist, J. M., Besson, J. M., Conseiller, C., and Le Bars, D. (1972). Action of bicuculline on presynaptic inhibition of various origins in the cat's spinal cord. *Brain Res.* **43**, 672–676.

Benoist, J. M., Besson, J. M., and Boissier, J. R. (1974). Modifications of presynaptic inhibition of various origins by local application of convulsant drugs on cat's spinal cord. *Brain Res.* **71**, 172–177.

Benzinger, T. H. (1969). Heat regulation: homeostasis of central temperature in man. *Physiol. Rev.* **49**, 671–759.

Berkley, K. J. (1975). Different targets of different neurons in nucleus gracilis of the cat. *J. Comp. Neurol.* **163**, 285–304.

Berman, A. L. (1968). The brain stem of the cat. A cytoarchitectonic atlas with stereotaxic coordinates. Univ. Wisconsin Press, Madison, Wisconsin.

Bernard, C. (1858). Leçons sur la physiologie et la pathologie du système nerveux. Vol. 1, pp. 20–112. J. B. Baillière et Fils, Paris.

Bernhard, C. G. (1953). The spinal cord potentials in leads from the cord dorsum in relation to peripheral source of afferent stimulation. *Acta Physiol. Scand.* **29** (Suppl. 106), 1–29.

Bernhard, C. G., and Widen, L. (1953). On the origin of the negative and positive cord potentials evoked by stimulation of low threshold cutaneous fibers. *Acta Physiol. Scand.* **29** (Suppl. 106), 42–54.

Berry, C. M., Karl, R. C., and Hinsey, J. C. (1950). Course of spinothalamic and medial lemniscus pathways in cat and rhesus monkey. *J. Neurophysiol.* **13**, 149–156.

Besson, J. M., Conseiller, C., Hamann, K. F., and Maillard, M. C. (1972). Modifications of dorsal horn cell activities in the spinal cord, after intra-arterial injection of bradykinin. *J. Physiol.* **221**, 189–205.

Besson, J. M., Guilbaud, G., and LeBars, D. (1975). Descending inhibitory influences exerted by the brain stem upon the activities of dorsal horn lamina V cells induced by intra-arterial injection of bradykinin into the limbs. *J. Physiol.* **248**, 725–739.

Bessou, P., and Laporte, Y. (1961). Étude des récepteurs musculaires innervés par les fibres afférentes du groupe III (fibres myelinisées fines), chez le chat. *Arch. Ital. Biol.* **99**, 293–321.

Bessou, P., and Perl, E. R. (1966). A movement receptor of the small intestine. *J. Physiol.* **182**, 404–426.

Bessou, P., and Perl, E. R. (1969). Response of cutaneous sensory units with unmyelinated fibers to noxious stimuli. *J. Neurophysiol.* **32**, 1025–1043.

Bessou, P., Laporte, Y., and Pagès, B. (1968). Frequencygrams of spindle primary endings elicited by stimulation of static and dynamic fusimotor fibres. *J. Physiol.* **196**, 47–63.

Bessou, P., Burgess, P. R., Perl, E. R., and Taylor, C. B. (1971). Dynamic properties of mechanoreceptors with unmyelinated (C) fibers. *J. Neurophysiol.* **34**, 116–131.

Beusekom, G. T. van (1955). *Fiber Analysis of the Anterior and Lateral Funiculi of the Cord in the Cat.* Eduard Ijdo, Leiden, N.V.

Bianconi, R., and van der Meulen, J. P. (1963). The responses to vibration of the end organs of mammalian muscle spindles. *J. Neurophysiol.* **26**, 177–190.

Biedenbach, M. A. (1972). Cell density and regional distribution of cell types in the cuneate nucleus of the rhesus monkey. *Brain Res.* **45**, 1–14.

Biedenbach, M. A., Jabbur, S. J., and Towe, A. L. (1971). Afferent inhibition in the cuneate nucleus of the rhesus monkey. *Brain Res.* **27**, 179–183.

Bishop, P. O., Burke, W., and Davis, R. (1962). Single-unit recording from antidromically activated optic radiation neurones. *J. Physiol.* **162**, 432–450.

Blix, M. (1884). Experimentelle Beiträge zur Losung der Frage über die specifische Energie der Hautnerven. *Z. Biol.* **20**, 141–156.

Blomqvist, A., and Westman, J. (1975). Combined HRP and Fink–Heimer staining applied on the gracile nucleus in the cat. *Brain Res.* **99**, 339–342.

Blomqvist, A., and Westman, J. (1976). Interneurons and initial axon collaterals in the feline gracile nucleus demonstrated with the rapid Golgi technique. *Brain Res.* **111**, 407–410.

Blum, P., Bromberg, M. B., and Whitehorn, D. (1975). Population analysis of single units in the cuneate nucleus of the cat. *Exp. Neurol.* **48**, 57–78.

Bobillier, P., Seguin, S., Petitjean, F., Salvert, D., Touret, M., and Jouvet, M. (1976). The raphe nuclei of the cat brain stem: a topographical atlas of their efferent projections as revealed by autoradiography. *Brain Res.* **113**, 449–486.

Boesten, A. J. P., and Voogd, J. (1975). Projections of the dorsal column nuclei and the spinal cord on the inferior olive in the cat. *J. Compar. Neurol.* **161**, 215–238.

Bohm, E. (1953). An electro-physiological study of the ascending spinal anterolateral fibre system connected to coarse cutaneous afferents. *Acta Physiol. Scand.* **29** (Suppl. 106), 106–137.

Boivie, J. (1970). The termination of the cervicothalamic tract in the cat. An experimental study with silver impregnation methods. *Brain Res.* **19**, 333–360.

Boivie, J. (1971a). The termination in the thalamus and the zona incerta of fibres from the dorsal column nuclei (DCN) in the cat. An experimental study with silver impregnation methods. *Brain Res.* **28**, 459–490.

Boivie, J. (1971b). The termination of the spinothalamic tract in the cat. An experimental study with silver impregnation methods. *Exper. Brain Res.* **12**, 331–353.

Boivie, J., and Perl, E. R. (1975). Neural substrates of somatic sensation. In: *MTP International Review of Science, Physiology Series One.* Vol. 3, *Neurophysiology,* p. 303–411 (C. C. Hunt, ed.). University Park Press, Baltimore.

Boivie, J., Grant, G., Albe-Fessard, D., and Levante, A. (1975). Evidence for a projection to the thalamus from the external cuneate nucleus in the monkey. *Neurosci. Lett.* **1**, 3–8.

Bok, S. T. (1928). Das Rückenmark. In: *Von Mollendorff's Handbuch d. micr. Anat. d. Menschen.* Vol. 4, pp. 478–578.

Booth, C. S., and Hahn, J. F. (1974). Thermal and mechanical stimulation of type II receptors and field receptors in cat. *Exp. Neurol.* **44**, 49–59.

Boring, E. G. (1916). Cutaneous sensation after nerve-division. *Quart. J. Exp. Physiol.* **10**, 1–95.

Boring, E. G. (1942). *Sensation and Perception in the History of Experimental Psychology.* Appleton-Century-Crofts, New York.

Bowsher, D. (1957). Termination of the central pain pathway in man: The conscious appreciation of pain. *Brain* **80**, 606–622.

Bowsher, D. (1958). Projection of the gracile and cuneate nuclei in *Macaca mulatta:* An experimental degeneration study. *J. Compar. Neurol.* **110,** 135–155.

Bowsher, D. (1961). The termination of secondary somatosensory neurons within the thalamus of *Macaca mulatta:* An experimental degeneration study. *J. Compar. Neurol.* **117**, 213–227.

Bowsher, D. (1970). Place and modality analysis in caudal reticular formation. *J. Physiol.* **209**, 473–486.

Bowsher, D., and Westman, J. (1970). The gigantocellular reticular region and its spinal afferents: a light and electron microscope study in the cat. *J. Anat.* **106**, 23–36.

Bowsher, D., Mallart, A., Petit, D., and Albe-Fessard, D. (1968). A bulbar relay to the centre median. *J. Neurophysiol.* **31**, 288–300.

Boyd, E. S., Meritt, D. A., and Gardner, L. C. (1966). The effect of convulsant drugs on transmission through the cuneate nucleus. *J. Pharmacol. Exp. Therap.* **154**, 398–409.

Boyd, I. A. (1954). The histological structure of the receptors in the knee-joint of the cat correlated with their physiological response. *J. Physiol.* **124**, 476–488.

Boyd, I. A., and Roberts, T. D. M. (1953). Proprioceptive discharges from stretch-receptors in the knee-joint of the cat. *J. Physiol.* **122**, 38–58.

Bradley, K., and Eccles, J. C. (1953). Analysis of the fast afferent impulses from thigh muscles. *J. Physiol.* **122**, 462–473.

Breazile, J. E., and Kitchell, R. L. (1968). Ventrolateral spinal cord afferents to the brain stem in the domestic pig. *J. Compar. Neurol.* **133,** 363–372.

Brodal, A. (1957). *The Reticular Formation of the Brain Stem. Anatomical Aspects and Functional Correlations.* Oliver and Boyd, Edinburgh and London.

Brodal, A., and Pompeiano, O. (1957). The vestibular nuclei in the cat. *J. Anat.* **91**, 438–454.

Brodal, A., and Rexed, B. (1953). Spinal afferents to the lateral cervical nucleus in the cat. *J. Compar. Neurol.* **98**, 179–211.

Brodal, A., and Rossi, G. F. (1955). Ascending fibers in brain stem reticular formation of cat. *Arch. Neurol. Psychiat.* **74**, 68–87.

Brodal, A., Taber, E., and Walberg, F. (1960a). The raphe nuclei of the brain stem in the cat. II. Efferent connections. *J. Compar. Neurol.* **114**, 239–260.

Brodal, A., Walberg, F., and Taber, E. (1960b). The raphe nuclei of the brain stem in the cat. III. Afferent connections. *J. Compar. Neurol.* **114**, 261–279.

Bromberg, M. B., and Fetz, E. E. (1977). Responses of single units in cervical spinal cord of alert monkeys. *Exp. Neurol.* **55**, 469–482.

Bromberg, M. B., and Towe, A. L. (1977). Rostrally and caudally projecting neurons in the dorsal column nuclei of the domestic cat. *Soc. Neurosci. Abstr.* **3**, 477.

Bromberg, M. B., and Whitehorn, D. (1974). Myelinated fiber types in the superficial radial nerve of the cat and their central projections. *Brain Res.* **78**, 157–163.

Bromberg, M. B., Blum, P., and Whitehorn, D. (1975). Quantitative characteristics of inhibition in the cuneate nucleus of the cat. *Exp. Neurol.* **48**, 37–56.

Browder, J., and Gallagher, J. P. (1948). Dorsal cordotomy for painful phantom limb. *Ann. Surg.* **128**, 456–469.

Brown, A. G. (1968). Cutaneous afferent fibre collaterals in the dorsal columns of the cat. *Exp. Brain Res.* **5**, 293–305.

Brown, A. G. (1970). Descending control of the spinocervical tract in decerebrate cats. *Brain Res.* **17**, 152–155.

Brown, A. G. (1971). Effects of descending impulses on transmission through the spinocervical tract. *J. Physiol.* **219**, 103–125.

Brown, A. G. (1973). Ascending and long spinal pathways: dorsal columns, spinocervical tract and spinothalamic tract. In: *Handbook of Sensory Physiology.* Vol. II, *Somatosensory System*, pp. 315–338 (A. Iggo, ed.). Springer, New York.

Brown, A. G. (1977). Cutaneous axons and sensory neurones in the spinal cord. *Brit. Med. Bull.* **33**, 109–112.

Brown, A. G., and Franz, D. N. (1969). Responses of spinocervical tract neurones to natural stimulation of identified cutaneous receptors. *Exp. Brain Res.* **7**, 231–249.

Brown, A. G., and Franz, D. N. (1970). Patterns of response in spinocervical neurones to different stimuli of long duration. *Brain Res.* **17**, 156–160.

Brown, A. G., and Hayden, R. E. (1971). The distribution of cutaneous receptors in the rabbit's hind limb and differential electrical stimulation of their axons. *J. Physiol.* **213**, 495–506.

Brown, A. G., and Iggo, A. (1967). A quantitative study of cutaneous receptors and afferent fibres in the cat and rabbit. *J. Physiol.* **193**, 707–733.

Brown, A. G., and Kirk, E. J. (1972). Ipsilateral and contralateral inhibitory actions on transmission through the spinocervical tract. *Brain Res.* **43**, 268–271.

Brown, A. G., and Martin, H. F. (1973). Activation of descending control of the spinocervical tract by impulses ascending the dorsal columns and relaying through the dorsal column nuclei. *J. Physiol.* **235**, 535–550.

Brown, A. G., and Short, A. D. (1974). Effects from the somatic sensory cortex on transmission through the spinocervical tract. *Brain Res.* **74**, 338–341.

Brown, A. G., Hamann, W. C., and Martin, H. F. (1973a). Interactions of cutaneous myelinated (A) and non-myelinated (C) fibres on transmission through the spinocervical tract. *Brain Res.* **53**, 222–226.

Brown, A. G., Hamann, W. C., and Martin, H. F. (1973b). Descending influences on spinocervical tract cell discharges evoked by non-myelinated cutaneous afferent nerve fibres. *Brain Res.* **53**, 218–221.

Brown, A. G., Kirk, E. J., and Martin, H. F. (1973c). Descending and segmental inhibition of transmission through the spinocervical tract. *J. Physiol.* **230**, 689–705.

Brown, A. G., Gordon, G., and Kay, R. H. (1974). A study of single axons in the cat's medial lemniscus. *J. Physiol.* **236**, 225–246.

Brown, A. G., Hamann, W. C., and Martin, H. F. (1975). Effects of activity in non-myelinated afferent fibres on the spinocervical tract. *Brain Res.* **98**, 243–259.

Brown, A. G., House, C. R., Rose, P. K., and Snow, P. J. (1976). The morphology of spinocervical tract neurones in the cat. *J. Physiol.* **260**, 719–738.

Brown, A. G., Coulter, J. D., Rose, P. K., Short, A. D., and Snow, P. J. (1977a). Inhibition of spinocervical tract discharges from localized areas of the sensorimotor cortex in the cat. *J. Physiol.* **264**, 1–16.

Brown, A. G., Rose, P. K., and Snow, P. J. (1977b). The morphology of spinocervical tract neurones revealed by intracellular injection of horseradish peroxidase. *J. Physiol.* **270**, 747–764.

Brown, A. G., Rose, P. K., and Snow, P. J. (1977c). The morphology of hair follicle afferent fibre collaterals in the spinal cord of the cat. *J. Physiol.* **272**, 779–797.

Brown, A. M. (1967). Excitation of afferent cardiac sympathetic nerve fibres during myocardial ischaemia. *J. Physiol.* **190**, 35–53.

Brown, M. C., Engberg, I., and Matthews, P. B. C. (1967). The relative sensitivity to vibration of muscle receptors of the cat. *J. Physiol.* **192**, 773–800.

Brown, P. B. (1969). Response of cat dorsal horn cells to variations of intensity, location, and area of cutaneous stimuli. *Exp. Neurol.* **23**, 249–265.

Brown, P. B., and Fuchs, J. L. (1975). Somatotopic representation of hindlimb skin in cat dorsal horn. *J. Neurophysiol.* **38**, 1–9.

Brown, P. B., Moraff, H., and Tapper, D. N. (1973). Functional organization of the cat's dorsal horn: spontaneous activity and central cell response to single impulses in single type I fibers. *J. Neurophysiol.* **36**, 827–839.

Brown, P. B., Fuchs, J. L., and Tapper, D. N. (1975). Parametric studies of dorsal horn neurons responding to tactile stimulation. *J. Neurophysiol.* **38**, 19–25.

Browne, K., Lee, J., and Ring, P. A. (1954). The sensation of passive movement at the metatarso-phalangeal joint of the great toe in man. *J. Physiol.* **126**, 448–458.

Bruggencate, G. ten, and Engberg, I. (1968). Analysis of glycine actions on spinal interneurones by intracellular recording. *Brain Res.* **11**, 446–450.

Bruggencate, G. ten, Lux, H. D., and Liebl, L. (1974). Possible relationships between extracellular potassium activity and presynaptic inhibition in the spinal cord of the cat. *Pflügers Arch.* **349**, 301–317.

Bryan, R. N., Trevino, D. L., Coulter, J. D., and Willis, W. D. (1973). Location and somatotopic organization of the cells of origin of the spinocervical tract. *Exp. Brain Res.* **17**, 177–189.

Bryan, R. N., Coulter, J. D., and Willis, W. D. (1974). Cells of origin of the spinocervical tract in the monkey. *Exp. Neurol.* **42**, 574–586.

Burch, G. E., and DePasquale, N. P. (1962). Bradykinin, digital blood flow, and the arteriovenous anastomoses. *Circulation Res.* **10**, 105–115.

Burgess, P. R., and Clark, F. J. (1969a). Dorsal column projection of fibres from the cat knee joint. *J. Physiol.* **203**, 301–315.

Burgess, P. R., and Clark, F. J. (1969b). Characteristics of knee joint receptors in the cat. *J. Physiol.* **203**, 317–335.

Burgess, P. R., and Perl, E. R. (1967). Myelinated afferent fibres responding specifically to noxious stimulation of the skin. *J. Physiol.* **190**, 541–562.

Burgess, P. R., and Perl, E. R. (1973). Cutaneous mechanoreceptors and nociceptors. In: *Handbook of Sensory Physiology*. Vol. II, *Somatosensory System*, pp. 29–78 (A. Iggo, ed.). Springer, New York.

Burgess, P. R., Petit, D., and Warren, R. M. (1968). Receptor types in cat hairy skin supplied by myelinated fibers. *J. Neurophysiol.* **31**, 833–848.

Burgess, P. R., Howe, J. F., Lessler, M. J., and Whitehorn, D. (1974). Cutaneous receptors supplied by myelinated fibers in the cat. II. Number of mechanoreceptors excited by a local stimulus. *J. Neurophysiol.* **37**, 1373–1386.

Burke, R. E., Rudomín, P., Vyklický, L., and Zajac, F. E. (1971). Primary afferent depolarization and flexion reflexes produced by radiant heat stimulation of the skin. *J. Physiol.* **213**, 185–214.

Burr, H. S. (1928). The central nervous system of *Orthagoriscus mola*. *J. Compar. Neurol.* **45**, 33–128.

Burton, H. (1968). Somatic sensory properties of caudal bulbar reticular neurons in the cat (*Felis domestica*). *Brain Res.* **11**, 357–372.

Burton, H. (1975). Responses of spinal cord neurons to systematic changes in hindlimb skin temperatures in cats and primates. *J. Neurophysiol.* **38**, 1060–1079.

Burton, H., and Jones, E. G. (1976). The posterior thalamic region and its cortical projection in new world and old world monkeys. *J. Compar. Neurol.* **168**, 249–302.

Burton, H., and Loewy, A. D. (1976). Descending projections from the marginal cell layer and other regions of the monkey spinal cord. *Brain Res.* **116**, 485–491.

Burton, H., and Loewy, A. D. (1977). Projections to the spinal cord from medullary somatosensory relay nuclei. *J. Compar. Neurol.* **173**, 773–792.

Burton, H., Forbes, D. J., and Benjamin, R. M. (1970). Thalamic neurons responsive to temperature changes of glabrous hand and foot skin in squirrel monkey. *Brain Res.* **24**, 179–190.

Burton, H., Terashima, S., and Clark, J. (1972). Response properties of slowly adapting mechanoreceptors to temperature stimulation in cats. *Brain Res.* **45**, 401–416.

Busch, H. F. M. (1961). *An Anatomical Analysis of the White Matter in the Brain Stem of the Cat.* Van Gorcum and Co., Assen, N.V.

Bystrzycka, E., Nail, B. S., and Rowe, M. (1977). Inhibition of cuneate neurones: its afferent source and influence on dynamically sensitive 'tactile' neurones. *J. Physiol.* **268**, 251–270.

Cadwalader, W. B., and Sweet, J. E. (1912). Experimental work on the function of the anterolateral column of the spinal cord. *JAMA.*, **58**, 1490–1493.

Calne, D. B., and Pallis, C. A. (1966). Vibratory sense: a critical review. *Brain* **89**, 723–746.

Calvin, W. H., and Loeser, J. D. (1975). Doublet and burst firing patterns within the dorsal column nuclei of cat and man. *Exp. Neurol.* **48**, 406–426.

Cangiano, A., Cook, W. A., and Pompeiano, O. (1969). Primary afferent depolarization in the lumbar cord evoked from the fastigial nucleus. *Arch. Ital. Biol.* **107**, 321–340.

Carli, G., Diete-Spiff, K., and Pompeiano, O. (1967a). Transmission of sensory information through the lemniscal pathway during sleep. *Arch. Ital. Biol.* **105**, 31–51.

Carli, G., Diete-Spiff, K., and Pompeiano, O. (1967b). Presynaptic and postsynaptic inhibition of transmission of somatic afferent volleys through the cuneate nucleus during sleep. *Arch. Ital. Biol.* **105**, 52–82.

Carli, G., Diete-Spiff, K., and Pompeiano, O. (1967c). Vestibular influences during sleep. V. Vestibular control on somatic afferent transmission in the cuneate nucleus during desynchronized sleep. *Arch. Ital. Biol.* **105**, 83–103.

Carli, G., Farabollini, F., and Fontani, G. (1975). Static characteristics of slowly adapting hip joint receptors in the cat. *Exp. Brain Res.* Suppl. **23**, 36.

Carlsson, A., Falck, B., Fuxe, K., and Hillarp, N. A. (1964). Cellular localization of monoamines in the spinal cord. *Acta Physiol. Scand.* **60**, 112–119.

Carpenter, D., Engberg, I., Funkenstein, H., and Lundberg, A. (1963a). Decerebrate control of reflexes to primary afferents. *Acta Physiol. Scand.* **59**, 424–437.

Carpenter, D., Lundberg, A., and Norrsell, U. (1963b). Primary afferent depolarization evoked from the sensorimotor cortex. *Acta Physiol. Scand.* **59**, 126–142.

Carpenter, D., Engberg, I., and Lundberg, A. (1965). Differential supraspinal control of inhibitory and excitatory actions from the FRA to ascending spinal pathways. *Acta Physiol. Scand.* **63**, 103–110.

Carpenter, D., Engberg, I., and Lundberg, A. (1966). Primary afferent depolarization evoked from the brain stem and the cerebellum. *Arch. Ital. Biol.* **104**, 73–85.

Carpenter, M. B., Stein, B. M., and Shriver, J. E. (1968). Central projections of spinal dorsal roots in the monkey. II. Lower thoracic, lumbosacral and coccygeal dorsal roots. *Amer. J. Anat.* **123**, 75–118.

Casey, K. L. (1966). Unit analysis of nociceptive mechanisms in the thalamus of the awake squirrel monkey. *J. Neurophysiol.* **29**, 727–750.

Casey, K. L. (1969). Somatic stimuli, spinal pathways, and size of cutaneous fibers influencing unit activity in the medical medullary reticular formation. *Exp. Neurol.* **25**, 35–56.

Casey, K. L. (1971a). Responses of bulboreticular units to somatic stimuli eliciting escape behavior in the cat. *Internat. J. Neurosci.* **2**, 15–28.

Casey, K. L. (1971b). Escape elicited by bulboreticular stimulation in the cat. *Internat. J. Neurosci.* **2**, 29–34.

Catalano, J. V., and Lamarche, G. (1957). Central pathway for cutaneous impulses in the cat. *Amer. J. Physiol.* **189**, 141–144.

Cauna, N. (1956). Nerve supply and nerve endings in Meissner's corpuscles. *Amer. J. Anat.* **99**, 315–350.

Cauna, N., and Mannan, G. (1958). The structure of human digital Pacinian corpuscles (corpuscula lamellosa) and its functional significance. *J. Anat.* **92**, 1–24.

Cauna, N., and Ross, L. L. (1960). The fine structure of Meissner's touch corpuscles of human fingers. *J. Biophys. Biochem. Cytol.* **8**, 467–482.

Cervero, F., Iggo, A., and Ogawa, H. (1976). Nociceptor-driven dorsal horn neurones in the lumbar spinal cord of the cat. *Pain* **2**, 5–24.

Cervero, F., Iggo, A., and Molony, V. (1977a). Responses of spinocervical tract neurones to noxious stimulation of the skin. *J. Physiol.* **267**, 537–558.

Cervero, F., Molony, V., and Iggo, A. (1977b). Extracellular and intracellular recordings from neurones in the substantia gelatinosa Rolandi. *Brain Res.* **136**, 565–569.

Cesa-Bianchi, M. G., and Sotgiu, M. L. (1969). Control by brain stem reticular formation of sensory transmission in Burdach nucleus. Analysis of single units. *Brain Res.* **13**, 129–139.

Cesa-Bianchi, M. G., Mancia, M., and Sotgiu, M. L. (1968). Depolarization of afferent fibers to the Goll and Burdach nuclei induced by stimulation of the brain-stem. *Exp. Brain Res.* **5**, 1–15.

Chambers, M. R., Andres, K. H., Duering, M. von, and Iggo, A. (1972). The structure and function of the slowly adapting type II mechanoreceptor in hairy skin. *Quart. J. Exp. Physiol.* **57**, 417–445.

Chambers, W. W., and Liu, C. N. (1957). Cortico-spinal tract of the cat. An attempt to correlate the pattern of degeneration with deficits in reflex activity following neocortical lesions. *J. Compar. Neurol.* **108**, 23–56.

Chambers, W. W., Liu, C. N., and McCouch, G. P. (1970). Cutaneous reflexes and pathways affecting them in the monkey, *Macaca mulatta*. *Exp. Neurol.* **28**, 243–256.

Chang, H. T., and Ruch, T. C. (1947a). Organization of the dorsal columns of the spinal cord and their nuclei in the spider monkey. *J. Anat.* **81**, 140–149.

Chang, H. T., and Ruch, T. C. (1947b). Topographical distribution of spinothalamic fibres in the thalamus of the spider monkey. *J. Anat.* **81**, 150–164.

Cheek, M. D., Rustioni, A., and Trevino, D. L. (1975). Dorsal column nuclei projections to the cerebellar cortex in cats as revealed by the use of the retrograde transport of horseradish peroxidase. *J. Compar. Neurol.* **164**, 31–46.

Chouchkov, C. N. (1973). The fine structure of small encapsulated receptors in human digital glabrous skin. *J. Anat.* **114**, 25–33.

Christiansen, J. (1966). Neurological observations of macaques with spinal cord lesions. *Anat. Rec.* **154**, 330.

Christensen, B. N., and Perl, E. R. (1970). Spinal neurons specifically excited by noxious or thermal stimuli: marginal zone of the dorsal horn. *J. Neurophysiol.* **33**, 293–307.

Clark, D., Hughes, J., and Gasser, H. S. (1935). Afferent function in the group of nerve fibers of slowest conduction velocity. *Amer. J. Physiol.* **114**, 69–76.

Clark, F. J. (1972). Central projection of sensory fibers from the cat knee joint. *J. Neurobiol.* **3**, 101–110.

Clark, F. J. (1975). Information signaled by sensory fibers in medial articular nerve. *J. Neurophysiol.* **38**, 1464–1472.

Clark, F. J., and Burgess, P. R. (1975). Slowly adapting receptors in cat knee joint: can they signal joint angle? *J. Neurophysiol.* **38**, 1448–1463.

Clark, F. J., Landgren, S., and Silfvenius, H. (1973). Projections to the cat's cerebral cortex from low threshold joint afferents. *Acta Physiol. Scand.* **89**, 504–521.

Clark, W. E. L. (1936). The termination of ascending tracts in the thalamus of the macaque monkey. *J. Anat.* **71**, 7–40.

Clarke, J. L. (1859). Further researches on the grey substance of the spinal cord. *Philos. Trans. Roy. Soc. London.* **149**, 437–467.

Clezy, J. K. A., Dennis, B. J., and Kerr, D. I. B. (1961). A degeneration study of the somaesthetic afferent systems in the marsupial phalanger *Trichosurus vulpecula*. *Austral. J. Exp. Biol.* **39**, 19–28.

Clifton, G. L., Coggeshall, R. E., Vance, W. H., and Willis, W. D. (1976). Receptive fields of unmyelinated ventral root afferent fibres in the cat. *J. Physiol.* **256**, 573–600.

Coffman, J. D. (1966). The effect of aspirin on pain and hand blood flow responses to intra-arterial injection of bradykinin in man. *Clin. Pharmacol. Ther.* **7**, 26–37.

Coggeshall, R. E., and Ito, H. (1977). Sensory fibres in ventral roots L7 and S1 in the cat. *J. Physiol.* **267**, 215–235.

Coggeshall, R. E., Coulter, J. D., and Willis, W. D. (1974). Unmyelinated axons in the ventral roots of the cat lumbosacral enlargement. *J. Compar. Neurol.* **153**, 39–58.

Cohen, L. A. (1955). Activity of knee joint proprioceptors recorded from the posterior articular nerve. *Yale J. Biol. Med.* **28**, 225–232.

Coimbra, A., Sodré-Borges, B. P., and Magalhães, M. M. (1974). The substantia gelatinosa Rolandi of the rat. Fine structure, cytochemistry (acid phosphatase) and changes after dorsal root section. *J. Neurocytol.* **3**, 199–217.

Collier, J., and Buzzard, E. F. (1903). The degenerations resulting from lesions of posterior nerve roots and from transverse lesions of the spinal cord in man. A study of twenty cases. *Brain* **26**, 559–591.

Collins, W. F., and O'Leary, J. L. (1954). Study of a somatic evoked response of midbrain reticular substance. *E.E.G. Clin. Neurophysiol.* **6**, 619–628.

Collins, W. F., and Randt, C. T. (1956). An electrophysiological study of small myelinated axons in anterolateral column in cat. *J. Neurophysiol.* **19**, 438–445.

Collins, W. F., and Randt, C. T. (1960). Midbrain evoked responses relating to peripheral unmyelinated or "C" fibers in cat. *J. Neurophysiol.* **23,** 47–53.

Collins, W. F., Nulsen, F. E., and Randt, C. T. (1960). Relation of peripheral nerve fiber size and sensation in man. *Arch. Neurol. Psychiat.* **3,** 381–385.

Conradi, S. (1969). On motoneuron synaptology in adult cats. *Acta Physiol. Scand.* Suppl. 332, 1–115.

Cook, A. W., and Browder, E. J. (1965). Function of posterior columns in man. *Arch. Neurol. Psychiat.* **12,** 72–79.

Cook, W. A., Cangiano, A., and Pompeiano, O. (1969a). Dorsal root potentials in the lumbar cord evoked from the vestibular system. *Arch. Ital. Biol.* **107,** 275–295.

Cook, W. A., Cangiano, A. and Pompeiano, O. (1969b). Vestibular control of transmission in primary afferents to the lumbar spinal cord. *Arch. Ital. Biol.* **107,** 296–320.

Cooke, J. D., Larson, B., Oscarsson, O., and Sjölund, B. (1971). Origin and termination of cuneocerebellar tract. *Exp. Brain Res.* **13,** 339–358.

Coombs, J. S., Curtis, D. R., and Landgren, S. (1956). Spinal cord potentials generated by impulses in muscle and cutaneous afferent fibres. *J. Neurophysiol.* **19,** 452–467.

Cooper, S., Daniel, P. M., and Whitteridge, D. (1953). Nerve impulses in the brainstem and cortex of the goat. Spontaneous discharges and responses to visual and other afferent stimuli. *J. Physiol.* **120,** 514–527.

Coquery, J. M., Malcuit, G., and Coulmance, M. (1971). Altérations de la perception d'un stimulus somesthésique durant un mouvement volontaire. *C. R. Acad. Sci. Paris* **165,** 1946–1951.

Corvaja, N., Grofová, I., Pompeiano, O., and Walberg, F. (1977). The lateral reticular nucleus in the cat. I. An experimental anatomical study of its spinal and supraspinal afferent connections. *Neuroscience* **2,** 537–553.

Coulter, J. D. (1974). Sensory transmission through lemniscal pathway during voluntary movement in the cat. *J. Neurophysiol.* **37,** 831–845.

Coulter, J. D., and Jones, E. G. (1977). Differential distribution of corticospinal projections from individual cytoarchitectonic fields in the monkey. *Brain Res.* **129,** 335–340.

Coulter, J. D., Maunz, R. A., and Willis, W. D. (1974). Effects of stimulation of sensorimotor cortex on primate spinothalamic neurons. *Brain Res.* **65,** 351–356.

Coulter, J. D., Foreman, R. D., Beall, J. E., and Willis, W. D. (1976a). Cerebral cortical modulation of primate spinothalamic neurons. In: *Advances in Pain Research and Therapy.* Vol. 1, pp. 271–277 (J. J. Bonica and D. Albe-Fessard, eds.) Raven Press, New York.

Coulter, J. D., Mergner, T., and Pompeiano, O. (1976b). Effects of static tilt on cervical spinoreticular tract neurons. *J. Neurophysiol.* **39,** 45–62.

Courtney, K. R., and Fetz, E. E. (1973). Unit responses recorded from cervical spinal cord of awake monkey. *Brain Res.* **53,** 445–450.

Craig, A. D. (1976). Spinocervical tract cells in cat and dog, labeled by the retrograde transport of horseradish peroxidase. *Neurosci. Lett.* **3,** 173–177.

Craigie, E. H. (1928). Observations of the brain of the humming bird (*Chrysolampis mosquitus* Linn. and *Chlorostilbon caribaeus* Lawr.). *J. Compar. Neurol.* **45,** 377–481.

Cranfield, P. F. (ed.) (1974). *The Way In and the Way Out.* Futura Publishing Co., Mount Kisco, New York.

Cross, M. J., and McCloskey, D. I. (1973). Position sense following surgical removal of joints in man. *Brain Res.* **55,** 443–445.

Croze, S., Duclaux, R., and Kenshalo, D. R. (1976). The thermal sensitivity of the polymodal nociceptors in the monkey. *J. Physiol.* **263,** 539–562.

Curry, M. J. (1972). The exteroceptive properties of neurones in the somatic part of the posterior group (PO). *Brain Res.* **44,** 439–462.

Curry, M. J., and Gordon, G. (1972). The spinal input to the posterior group in the cat. An electrophysiological investigation. *Brain Res.* **44**, 417–437.

Curtis, D. R., Phillis, J. W., and Watkins, J. C. (1960). The chemical excitation of spinal neurones by certain acidic amino acids. *J. Physiol.* **150**, 656–682.

Curtis, D. R., and Ryall, R. W. (1966). Pharmacological studies upon spinal presynaptic fibres. *Exp. Brain Res.* **1**, 195–204.

Curtis, D. R., Hösli, L., and Johnston, G. A. R. (1968). A pharmacological study of the depression of spinal neurones by glycine and related amino acids. *Exp. Brain Res.* **6**, 1–18.

Curtis, D. R., Duggan, A. W., Felix, D., and Johnston, G. A. R. (1971a). Bicuculline, an antagonist of GABA and synaptic inhibition in the spinal cord of the cat. *Brain Res.* **32**, 69–96.

Curtis, D. R., Duggan, A. W., and Johnston, G. A. R. (1971b). The specificity of strychnine as a glycine antagonist in the mammalian spinal cord. *Exp. Brain Res.* **12**, 547–565.

Curtis, D. R., Lodge, D., and Brand, S. J. (1977). GABA and spinal afferent terminal excitability in the cat. *Brain Res.* **130**, 360–363.

Czarkowska, J., Jankowska, E., and Sybirska, E. (1976). Axonal projections of spinal interneurones excited by group I afferents in the cat, revealed by intracellular straining with horseradish peroxidase. *Brain Res.* **118**, 115–118.

Dahlström, A., and Fuxe, K. (1965). Evidence for the existence of monoamine neurons in the central nervous system. *Acta Physiol. Scand.* **64** (Suppl. 247), 1–36.

Dallenbach, K. M. (1927). The temperature spots and end-organs. *Amer. J. Psychol.* **39**, 402–427.

Darian-Smith, I., Phillips, G., and Ryan, R. D. (1963). Functional organization in the trigeminal main sensory and rostral spinal nuclei of the cat. *J. Physiol.* **168**, 129–146.

Darian-Smith, I., Johnson, K. O., and Dykes, R. (1973). "Cold" fiber population innervating palmar and digital skin of the monkey: response to cooling pulses. *J. Neurophysiol.* **36**, 325–346.

Dart, A. M. (1971). Cells of the dorsal column nuclei projecting down into the spinal cord. *J. Physiol.* **219**, 29–30P.

Dart, A. M., and Gordon, G. (1970). Excitatory and inhibitory afferent inputs to the dorsal column nuclei not involving the dorsal columns. *J. Physiol.* **211**, 36–37P.

Dart, A. M., and Gordon, G. (1973). Some properties of spinal connections of the cat's dorsal column nuclei which do not involve the dorsal columns. *Brain Res.* **58**, 61–68.

Davidoff, R. A. (1972). The effects of bicuculline on the isolated spinal cord of the frog. *Exp. Neurol.* **35**, 179–193.

Davidoff, R. A., Aprison, M. H., and Werman, R. 1969. The effects of strychnine on the inhibition of interneurons by glycine and γ-aminobutyric acid. *Internat. J. Neuropharmacol.* **8**, 191–194.

Davidson, N., and Smith, C. A. (1972). A recurrent collateral pathway for presynaptic inhibition in the rat cuneate nucleus. *Brain Res.* **44**, 63–71.

Davidson, N., and Southwick, C. A. P. (1971). Amino acids and presynaptic inhibition in the rat cuneate nucleus. *J. Physiol.* **219**, 689–708.

Davies, J., and Watkins, J. C. (1973). Microelectrophoretic studies on the depressant action of HA-966 on chemically and synaptically excited neurones in the cat cerebral cortex and cuneate nucleus. *Brain Res.* **59**, 311–322.

Davison, C., and Wechsler, I. S. (1936). Amyotrophic lateral sclerosis with involvement of posterior column and sensory disturbances. *Arch. Neurol. Psychiat.* **35**, 229–239.

Dawson, G. D. (1958). The central control of sensory inflow. *Proc. Roy. Soc. Med.* **51**, 531–535.

Dawson, G. D., Merrill, E. G., and Wall, P. D. (1970). Dorsal root potentials produced by stimulation of fine afferents. *Science* **167**, 1385–1387.

DeGroat, W. C., Lalley, P. M., and Saum, W. R. (1972). Depolarization of dorsal root ganglia in the cat by GABA and related amino acids: antagonism by picrotoxin and bicuculline. *Brain Res.* **44**, 273–277.

Denny-Brown, D., Kirk, E. J., and Yanagisawa, N. (1973). The tract of Lissauer in relation to sensory transmission in the dorsal horn of spinal cord in the macaque monkey. *J. Compar. Neurol.* **151**, 175–200.

Deschenes, M., and Feltz, P. (1976). GABA-induced rise of extracellular potassium in rat dorsal root ganglia: an electrophysiological study *in vivo*. *Brain Res.* **118**, 494–499.

Deschenes, M., Feltz, P. and Lamour, Y. (1976). A model for an estimate *in vivo* of the ionic basis of presynaptic inhibition: an intracellular analysis of the GABA-induced depolarization in rat dorsal root ganglia. *Brain Res.* **118**, 486–493.

De Vito, J. L., and Ruch, T. C. (1956). Central pathways subserving weight discrimination in monkey. *Federation Proc.* **15**, 48–49.

De Vito, J. L., Ruch, T. C., and Patton, H. D. (1964). Analysis of residual weight discriminatory ability and evoked cortical potentials following section of dorsal columns in monkeys. *Indian J. Physiol. Pharmacol.* **8**, 117–126.

Devor, M., and Wall, P. D. (1976). Dorsal horn cells with proximal cutaneous receptive fields. *Brain Res.* **118**, 325–328.

Diamond, I. T., Randall, W., and Springer, L. (1964). Tactual localization in cats deprived of cortical areas SI and SII and the dorsal columns. *Psychon. Sci.* **1**, 261–262.

Dilly, P. N., Wall, P. D., and Webster, K. E. (1968). Cells of origin of the spinothalamic tract in the cat and rat. *Exp. Neurol.* **21**, 550–562.

Dimsdale, J. A., and Kemp, J. M. (1966). Afferent fibres in ventral nerve roots in the rat. *J. Physiol. (London)* **187**, 25–26P.

Dobry, P. J. K., and Casey, K. L. (1972a). Roughness discrimination in cats with dorsal column lesions. *Brain Res.* **44**, 385–397.

Dobry, P. J. K., and Casey, K. L. (1972b). Coronal somatosensory unit responses in cats with dorsal column lesions. *Brain Res.* **44**, 399–416.

Dodt, E. (1952). The behaviour of thermoreceptors at low and high temperatures with special reference to Ebbecke's temperature phenomena. *Acta Physiol. Scand.* **27**, 295–314.

Dodt, E., and Zotterman, Y. (1952a). Mode of action of warm receptors. *Acta Physiol. Scand.* **26**, 345–357.

Dodt, E., and Zotterman, Y. (1952b). The discharge of specific cold fibres at high temperatures. *Acta Physiol. Scand.* **26**, 358–365.

Dodt, E., Skouby, A. P., and Zotterman, Y. (1953). The effect of cholinergic substances on the discharges from thermal receptors. *Acta Physiol. Scand.* **28**, 101–114.

Dogiel, A. S. 1896. Der Bau der Spinalganglien bei den Säugetieren. *Anat. Anz.* **12**, 140–152.

Donaldson, H. H. (1885). On the temperature sense. *Mind* **10**, 399–416.

Dong, W. K., and Wagman, I. H. (1976). Modulation of nociceptive responses in the thalamic posterior group of nuclei. In *Advances in Pain Research and Therapy*. Vol. 1, pp. 455–460 (J. J. Bonica and D. Albe-Fessard eds.). Raven Press, New York.

Dostrovsky, J. O., Millar, J., and Wall, P. D. (1976). The immediate shift of afferent drive of dorsal column nucleus cells following deafferentation: A comparison of acute and chronic deafferentation in gracile nucleus and spinal cord. *Exp. Neurol.* **52**, 480–495.

Douglas, W. W., and Ritchie, J. M. (1957). Non-medullated fibres in the saphenous nerve which signal touch. *J. Physiol.* **139**, 385–399.

Dreyer, D. A., Schneider, R. J., Metz, C. B., and Whitsel, B. L. (1974). Differential contributions of spinal pathways to body representation in postcentral gyrus of *Macaca mulatta*. *J. Neurophysiol.* **37**, 119–145.

Dubner, R., Sumino, R., and Wood, W. I. (1975). A peripheral "cold" fiber population responsive to innocuous and noxious thermal stimuli applied to monkey's face. *J. Neurophysiol.* **38**, 1373–1389.

Dubrovsky, B., and Garcia-Rill, E. (1973). Role of dorsal columns in sequential motor acts requiring precise forelimb projection. *Exp. Brain Res.* **18**, 165–177.

Dubrovsky, B., Davelaar, E., and Garcia-Rill, E. (1971). The role of dorsal columns in serial order acts. *Exp. Neurol.* **33**, 93–102.

Duclaux, R., and Kenshalo, D. R. (1972). The temperature sensitivity of the type I slowly adapting mechanoreceptors in cats and monkeys. *J. Physiol.* **224**, 647–664.

Duclaux, R., and Kenshalo, D. R. (1973). Cutaneous receptive fields of primate cold fibers. *Brain Res.* **55**, 437–442.

Duclaux, R., and Kenshalo, D. R. (1978). Response characteristics of cutaneous warm receptors in the monkey. *J. Neurophysiol.* (in press).

Duggan, A. W., and Johnston, G. A. R. (1970). Glutamate and related amino acids in cat spinal roots, dorsal root ganglia and peripheral nerves. *J. Neurochem.* **17**, 1205–1208.

Duncan, D., and Morales, R. (1973a). Location of nerve cells producing the synaptic vesicles situated in the substantia gelatinosa of the spinal cord. *Amer. J. Anat.* **138**, 139–144.

Duncan, D., and Morales, R. (1973b). Location of large cored synaptic vesicles in the dorsal gray matter of the cat and dog spinal cord. *Amer. J. Anat.* **136**, 123–127.

Dyhre-Poulsen, P. (1975). Increased vibration threshold before movements in human subjects. *Exp. Neurol.* **47**, 516–522.

Dykes, R. W. (1975). Coding of steady and transient temperatures by cutaneous "cold" fibers serving the hand of monkeys. *Brain Res.* **98**, 485–500.

Earle, K. M. (1952). The tract of Lissauer and its possible relation to the pain pathway. *J. Compar. Neurol.* **96**, 93–109.

Ebbesson, S. O. E. (1967). Ascending axon degeneration following hemisection of the spinal cord in the Tegu lizard (*Tupinambis nigropunctatus*). *Brain Res.* **5**, 178–206.

Ebbesson, S. O. E. (1968). A connection between the dorsal column nuclei and the dorsal accessory olive. *Brain Res.* **8**, 393–397.

Ebbesson, S. O. E. (1969). Brainstem afferents from the spinal cord in a sample of reptilian and amphibian species. *Ann. N.Y. Acad. Sci.* **167**, 80–101.

Eccles, J. C. (1964). *The Physiology of Synapses*. Springer, New York.

Eccles, J. C., and Krnjević, K. (1959). Potential changes recorded inside primary afferent fibres within the spinal cord. *J. Physiol.* **149**, 250–273.

Eccles, J. C. Fatt, P., Landgren, S., and Winsbury, G. J. (1954). Spinal cord potentials generated by volley in the large muscle afferents. *J. Physiol.* **125**, 590–606.

Eccles, J. C., Fatt, P., and Landgren, S. (1956). Central pathway for direct inhibitory action of impulses in largest afferent nerve fibres to muscle. *J. Neurophysiol.* **19**, 75–98.

Eccles, J. C., Eccles, R. M., and Lundberg, A. (1957). Synaptic actions on motoneurones in relation to the two components of the group I muscle afferent volley. *J. Physiol.* **136**, 527–546.

Eccles, J. C., Eccles, R. M., and Lundberg, A. (1960). Types of neurone in and around the intermediate nucleus of the lumbosacral cord. *J. Physiol.* **154**, 89–114.

Eccles, J. C., Kozak, W., and Magni, F. (1961). Dorsal root reflexes of muscle group I afferent fibres. *J. Physiol.* **159**, 128–146.

Eccles, J. C., Kostyuk, P. G., and Schmidt, R. F. (1962a). Central pathways responsible for depolarization of primary afferent fibres. *J. Physiol.* **161**, 237–257.

Eccles, J. C. Kostyuk, P. G., and Schmidt, R. F. (1962b). Presynaptic inhibition of the central actions of flexor reflex afferents. *J. Physiol.* **161**, 258–281.

Eccles, J. C., Magni, F., and Willis, W. D. (1962c). Depolarization of central terminals of group I afferent fibres from muscle. *J. Physiol.* **160**, 62–93.

Eccles, J. C., Schmidt, R. F., and Willis, W. D. (1963a). Depolarization of the central terminals of cutaneous afferent fibers. *J. Neurophysiol.* **26**, 646–661.

Eccles, J. C., Schmidt, R. F., and Willis, W. D. (1963b). Pharmacological studies on presynaptic inhibition. *J. Physiol.* **168**, 500–530.

Eccles, R. M. (1965). Interneurones activated by higher threshold group I muscle afferents. In: *Studies in Physiology*, pp. 59–64 (D. R. Curtis and A. K. McIntyre, eds.). New York, Springer.

Eccles, R. M., and Lundberg, A. (1959a). Synaptic actions in motoneurones by afferents which may evoke the flexion reflex. *Arch. Ital. Biol.* **97**, 199–221.

Eccles, R. M., and Lundberg, A. (1959b). Supraspinal control of interneurones mediating spinal reflexes. *J. Physiol.* **147**, 565–584.

Edinger, L. (1889). Vergleichend-entwicklungsgeschichtliche und anatomische Studien im Bereiche des Centralnervensystems. 2. Über die Fortsetzung der hinteren Rückenmarkswurzeln zum Gehirn. *Anat. Anz.* **4**, 121–128.

Edinger, L. (1890). Einiges vom verlauf der gefühlsbahnen im centralen Nervensysteme. *Deut. Med. Woch.* **16**, 421–426.

Edwards, S. B. (1972). The ascending and descending projections of the red nucleus in the cat: An experimental study using an autoradiographic tracing method. *Brain Res.* **48**, 45–63.

Eidelberg, E., and Woodbury, C. M. (1972). Apparent redundancy in the somatosensory system in monkeys. *Exp. Neurol.* **37**, 573–581.

Eidelberg, E., Kreinick, C. J., and Langescheid, C. (1975). On the possible functional role of afferent pathways in skin sensation. *Exp. Neurol.* **47**, 419–432.

Eidelberg, E., Woolf, B., Kreinick, C. J., and Davis. F. (1976). Role of the dorsal funiculi in movement control. *Brain Res.* **114**, 427–438.

Eklund, G. (1972). Position sense and state of contraction; the effects of vibration. *J. Neurol. Neurosurg. Psychiat.* **35**, 606–611.

Eklund, G. and Skoglund, S. (1960). On the specificity of the Ruffini like joint receptors. *Acta Physiol. Scand.* **49**, 184–191.

Eldred, E., Yellin, H., DeSantis, M., and Smith, C. M. (1977). Supplement to bibliography on muscle receptors: their morphology, pathology, physiology, and pharmacology. *Exp. Neurol.* **55** (no. 3, part 2), 1–118.

Emery, D. G., Ito, H., and Coggeshall, R. E. (1977). Unmyelinated axons in thoracic ventral roots of the cat. *J. Compar. Neurol.* **172**, 37–48.

Engberg, I., and Ryall, R. W. (1966). The inhibitory action of noradrenaline and other monoamines on spinal neurones. *J. Physiol.* **185**, 298–322.

Engberg, I., Lundberg, A. and Ryall, R. W. (1968a). The effect of reserpine on transmission in the spinal cord. *Acta Physiol. Scand.* **72**, 115–122.

Engberg, I., Lundberg, A., and Ryall, R. W. (1968b). Is the tonic decerebrate inhibition of reflex paths mediated by monoaminergic pathways? *Acta Physiol. Scand.* **72**, 123–133.

Engberg, I., Lundberg, A., and Ryall, R. W. (1968c). Reticulospinal inhibition of transmission in reflex pathways. *J. Physiol.* **194**, 201–223.

Engberg, I., Lundberg, A., and Ryall, R. W. (1968d). Reticulospinal inhibition of interneurones. *J. Physiol.* **194**, 225–236.

Ennever, J. A., and Towe, A. L. (1974). Response of somatosensory cerebral neurons to stimulation of dorsal and dorsolateral spinal funiculi. *Exp. Neurol.* **43**, 124–142.

Erickson, R. P., and Poulos, D. A. (1973). On the qualitative aspect of the temperature sense. *Brain Res.* **61**, 107–112.

Erlanger, J., and Gasser, H. S. (1937). *Electrical Signs of Nervous Activity.* Univ. Pennsylvania Press, Philadelphia.

Erulkar, S. D., Sprague, J. M., Whitsel, B. L., Dogan, S., and Jannetta, P. J. (1966). Organization of the vestibular projection to the spinal cord of the cat. *J. Neurophysiol.* **29**, 626–664.

Escolar, J. (1948). The afferent connections of the 1st, 2nd, and 3rd cervical nerves in the cat. *J. Compar. Neurol.* **89**, 79–92.

Evarts, E. V. (1971). Feedback and corollary discharge: a merging of the concepts. *Neurosci. Res. Progr. Bull.* **9**, 86–112.

Falconer, M. A., and Lindsay, J. S. B. (1946). Painful phantom limb treated by high cervical chordotomy. Report of two cases. *Brit. J. Surg.* **33**, 301–306.

Favale, E., Loeb, C., Manfredi, M., and Sacco, G. (1965). Somatic afferent transmission and cortical responsiveness during natural sleep and arousal in the cat. *EEG Clin. Neurophysiol.* **18**, 354–368.

Fedina, L., Gordon, G., and Lundberg, A. (1968). The source and mechanisms of inhibition in the lateral cervical nucleus of the cat. *Brain Res.* **11**, 694–696.

Felten, D. L., Laties, A. M., and Carpenter, M. B. (1974). Monoamine-containing cell bodies in the squirrel monkey brain. *Amer. J. Anat.* **139**, 153–166.

Fernandez de Molina, A., and Gray, J. A. B. (1957). Activity in the dorsal spinal grey matter after stimulation of cutaneous nerves. *J. Physiol.* **137**, 126–140.

Ferraro, A., and Barrera, S. E. (1934). Effects of experimental lesions of the posterior columns in *Macacus rhesus* monkeys. *Brain* **57**, 307–332.

Ferraro, A., and Barrera, S. E. (1935a). The nuclei of the posterior funiculi in the *Macacus rhesus.* An anatomic and experimental investigation. *Arch. Neurol. Psychiat.* **33**, 262–275.

Ferraro, A., and Barrera, S. E. (1935b). Posterior column fibers and their termination in *Macacus rhesus. J. Compar. Neurol.* **62**, 507–530.

Fetz, E. E. (1968). Pyramidal tract effects on interneurons in the cat lumbar dorsal horn. *J. Neurophysiol.* **31**, 69–80.

Fields, H. L., Meyer, G. A., and Partridge, L. D. (1970a). Convergence of visceral and somatic input onto cat spinal neurons. *Exp. Neurol.* **26**, 36–52.

Fields, H. L., Partridge, L. D., and Winter, D. L. (1970b). Somatic and visceral receptive field properties of fibers in ventral quadrant white matter of the cat spinal cord. *J. Neurophysiol.* **33**, 827–837.

Fields, H. L., Wagner, G. M., and Anderson, S. D. (1975). Some properties of spinal neurons projecting to the medial brain-stem reticular formation. *Exp. Neurol.* **47**, 118–134.

Fields, H. L., Basbaum, A. I., Clanton, C. H., and Anderson, S. D. (1977a). Nucleus raphe magnus inhibition of spinal cord dorsal horn neurons. *Brain Res.* **126**, 441–453.

Fields, H. L., Clanton, C. H., and Anderson, S. D. (1977b). Somatosensory properties of spinoreticular neurons in the cat. *Brain Res.* **120**, 49–66.

Fitzgerald, M., and Lynn, B. (1977). The sensitization of high threshold mechanoreceptors with myelinated axons by repeated heating. *J. Physiol.* **265**, 549–563.

Fjällbrant, N., and Iggo, A. (1961). The effect of histamine, 5-hydroxytryptamine and acetylcholine on cutaneous afferent fibres. *J. Physiol.* **156**, 578–590.

Floyd, K., and Morrison, J. F. B. (1974). Splanchnic mechanoreceptors in the dog. *Quart. J. Exp. Physiol.* **59**, 361–366.

Floyd, K., Hick, V. E., and Morrison, J. F. B. (1976). Mechanosensitive afferent units in the hypogastric nerve of the cat. *J. Physiol.* **259**, 457–471.

Fock, S., and Mense, S. (1976). Excitatory effects of 5-hydroxytryptamine, histamine and potassium ions on muscular group IV afferent units: a comparison with bradykinin. *Brain Res.* **105**, 459–469.

Foerster, O., and Gagel, O. (1931). Die Vorderseitenstrangdurchschneidung beim Menschen. Eine klinisch-patho-physiologisch-anatomische Studie. *Z. Ges. Neurol. Psychiat.* **138**, 1–92.

Foreman, R. D., Applebaum, A. E., Beall, J. E., Trevino, D. L., and Willis, W. D. (1975a). Responses of primate spinothalamic tract neurons to electrical stimulation of hindlimb peripheral nerves. *J. Neurophysiol.* **38**, 132–145.

Foreman, R. D., Hancock, M. B., and Willis, W. D. (1975b). Convergence of visceral and cutaneous input onto spinothalamic tract neurons in the thoracic spinal cord of the Rhesus monkey. *Soc. Neurosci. Abstr.* **1**, 148.

Foreman, R. D., Beall, J. E., Applebaum, A. E., Coulter, J. D., and Willis, W. D. (1976a). Effects of dorsal column stimulation on primate spinothalamic tract neurons. *J. Neurophysiol.* **39**, 534–546.

Foreman, R. D., Beall, J. E., Applebaum, A. E., Coulter, J. D., and Willis, W. D. (1976b). Inhibition of primate spinothalamic tract neurons by electrical stimulation of dorsal column or peripheral nerve. In: *Advances in Pain Research and Therapy.* Vol. 1, pp. 405–410. (J. J. Bonica and D. Albe-Fessard, eds.) Raven Press, New York.

Foreman, R. D., Schmidt, R. F., and Willis, W. D. (1977). Convergence of muscle and cutaneous input onto primate spinothalamic tract neurons. *Brain Res.* **124**, 555–560.

Fox, J. C., and Klemperer, W. W. (1942). Vibratory sensibility: A quantitative study of its thresholds in nervous disorders. *Arch. Neurol. Psychiat.* **48**, 622–645.

Fox, J. L. (1974). Dorsal column stimulation for relief of intractable pain: problems encountered with neuropacemakers. *Surg. Neurol.* **2**, 59–64.

Frank, K., and Fuortes, M. G. F. (1956). Unitary activity of spinal interneurones of cats. *J. Physiol.* **131**, 425–435.

Frankenhaeuser, B. (1949). Impulses from a cutaneous receptor with slow adaptation and low mechanical threshold. *Acta Physiol. Scand.* **18**, 68–74.

Franz, D. N., and Iggo, A. (1968). Dorsal root potentials and ventral root reflexes evoked by nonmyelinated fibers. *Science* **162**, 1140–1142.

Franz, M., and Mense, S. (1975). Muscle receptors with group IV afferent fibres responding to application of bradykinin. *Brain Res.* **92**, 369–383.

Frazier, C. H. (1920). Section of the anterolateral columns of the spinal cord for the relief of pain. A report of six cases. *Arch. Neurol. Psychiat.* **4**, 137–147.

French, L. A., and Peyton, W. T. (1948). Ipsilateral sensory loss following cordotomy. *J. Neurosurg.* **5**, 403–404.

Frey, M. von (1906). The distribution of afferent nerves in the skin. *J.A.M.A.* **47**, 645–648.

Frey, M. von (1910). Physiologie der Sinnesorgane der Menschlichen Haut. *Ergenbnisse Physiol.* **9**, 351–368.

Frommer, G. P., Trefz, B. R., and Casey, K. L. (1977). Somatosensory function and cortical unit activity in cats with only dorsal column fibers. *Exp. Brain Res.* **27**, 113–129.

Fruhstorfer, H., Zenz, M., Nolte, H., and Hensel, H. (1974). Dissociated loss of cold and warm sensibility during regional anaesthesia. *Pflügers Arch.* **349**, 73–82.

Frykholm, R. (1951). Cervical root compression resulting from disc degeneration and root-sleeve fibrosis. A clinical investigation. *Acta Chir. Scand.* (*Suppl.*), p. 160.

Frykholm, R., Hyde, J., Norlen, G., and Skoglund, C. R. (1953). On pain sensations produced by stimulation of ventral roots in man. *Acta Physiol. Scand.* **29** (Suppl. 106), 455–469.

Fuller, J. H., and Schlag, J. D. (1976). Determination of antidromic excitation by the collision test: problems of interpretation. *Brain Res.* **112**, 283–298.

Galindo, A., Krnjević, K., and Schwartz, S. (1967). Micro-iontophoretic studies on neurones in the cuneate nucleus. *J. Physiol.* **192**, 359–377.

Galindo, A., Krnjević, K., and Schwartz, S. (1968). Patterns of firing in cuneate neurones and some effects of flaxedil. *Exp. Brain Res.* **5**, 87–101.

Gambarian, L. S. (1960). Spinal paths for the cortical projection of proprioceptive signals. *Fiziol. Zh. SSSR* **46**, 1098–1104. Eng. Trans.: *Sechenov. Physiol. J. USSR* **46**, 1283–1290 (1960).

Game, C. J. A. and Lodge, D. (1975) The pharmacology of the inhibition of dorsal horn neurones by impulses in myelinated cutaneous afferents in the cat. *Exp. Brain Res.* **23**, 75–84.

Gammon, G. D., and Bronk, D. M. (1935). The discharge of impulses from Pacinian corpuscles in the mesentery and its relation to vascular changes. *Amer. J. Physiol.* **114**, 77–84.

Gardner, E. (1944). The distribution and termination of nerves in the knee joint of the cat. *J. Compar. Neurol.* **80**, 11–32.

Gardner, E., and Cuneo, H. M. (1945). Lateral spinothalamic tract and associated tracts in man. *Arch. Neurol. Psychiat.* **53**, 423–430.

Gardner, E., and Haddad, B. (1953). Pathways to the cerebral cortex for afferent fibers from the hindleg of the cat. *Amer. J. Physiol.* **172**, 475–482.

Gardner, E. D., and Morin, F. (1953). Spinal pathways for projection of cutaneous and muscular afferents to the sensory and motor cortex of the monkey (*Macaca mulatta*). *Amer. J. Physiol.* **174**, 149–154.

Gardner, E., and Morin, F. (1957). Projection of fast afferents to the cerebral cortex of monkey. *Amer. J. Physiol.* **189**, 152–158.

Gardner, E., and Noer, R. (1952). Projection of afferent fibers from muscles and joints to the cerebral cortex of the cat. *Amer. J. Physiol.* **168**, 437–441.

Gardner, E. Thomas, L. M., and Morin, F. (1955). Cortical projections of fast visceral afferents in the cat and monkey. *Amer. J. Physiol.* **183**, 438–444.

Gasser, H. S. (1950). Unmedullated fibers originating in dorsal root ganglia. *J. Gen. Physiol.* **33**, 651–690.

Gasser, H. S., and Graham, H. T. (1933). Potentials produced in the spinal cord by stimulation of dorsal roots. *Amer. J. Physiol.* **103**, 303–320.

Gaze, R. M., and Gordon, G. 1955. Some observations on the central pathway for cutaneous impulses in the cat. *Quart. J. Exp. Physiol.* **40**, 187–194.

Geldard, F. A. (1953). *The Human Senses.* John Wiley and Sons, Inc., c., New York.

Gelfan, S., and Carter, S. (1967). Muscle sense in man. *Exp. Neurol.* **18**, 469–473.

Georgopoulos, A. P. (1976). Functional properties of primary afferent units probably related to pain mechanisms in primate glabrous skin. *J. Neurophysiol.* **39**, 71–83.

Georgopoulos, A. P. (1977). Stimulus–response relations in high-threshold mechanothermal fibers innervating primate glabrous skin. *Brain Res.* **128**, 547–552.

Gerard, R. W. (1951). The physiology of pain: abnormal neuron states in causalgia and related phenomena. *Anesthesiology* **12**, 1–13.

Gernandt, B., and Zotterman, Y. (1946). Intestinal pain: an electrophysiological investigation on mesenteric nerves. *Acta Physiol. Scand.* **12**, 56–72.

Getz, B. (1952). The termination of spinothalamic fibres in the cat as studied by the method of terminal degeneration. *Acta Anat.* **16**, 271–290.

Ghelarducci, B., Pisa, M., and Pompeiano, O. (1970). Transformation of somatic afferent volleys across the prethalamic and thalamic components of the lemniscal system during the rapid eye movements of sleep. *EEG Clin. Neurophysiol.* **29**, 348–357.

Ghez, C., and Lenzi, G. L. (1971). Modulation of sensory transmission in cat lemniscal system during voluntary movement. *Pflügers Arch.* **323**, 273–278.

Ghez, C., and Pisa, M. (1972). Inhibition of afferent transmission in cuneate nucleus during voluntary movement in the cat. *Brain Res.* **40**, 145–151.

Giesler, G. J., and Liebeskind, J. C. (1976). Inhibition of visceral pain by electrical stimulation of the periaqueductal gray matter. *Pain* **2**, 43–48.

Giesler, G. J., Menétrey, D., Guilbaud, G., and Besson, J. M. (1976). Lumbar cord neurons at the origin of the spinothalamic tract in the rat. *Brain Res.* **118**, 320–324.

Giesler, G. J., Basbaum, A. I., and Menétrey, D. (1977). Projections and origins of the spinothalamic tract in the rat. *Soc. Neurosci. Abstr.* **3**, 500.

Gilman, S., and Denny-Brown, D. (1966). Disorders of movement and behaviour following dorsal column lesions. *Brain* **89**, 397–418.

Glees, P., and Soler, J. (1951). Fibre content of the posterior column and synaptic connections of nucleus gracilis. *Z. Zellforsch.* **36**, 381–400.

Gobel, S. (1974). Synaptic organization of the substantia gelatinosa glomeruli in the spinal trigeminal nucleus of the adult cat. *J. Neurocytol.* **3**, 219–243.

Gobel, S. (1976). Dendroaxonic synapses in the substantia gelatinosa glomeruli of the spinal trigeminal nucleus of the cat. *J. Compar. Neurol.* **167**, 165–176.

Goldby, F., and Robinson, L. R. (1962). The central connexions of dorsal spinal nerve roots and the ascending tracts in the spinal cord of *Lacerta viridis*. *J. Anat.* **96**, 153–170.

Goldman, P. L., Collins, W. F., Taub, A., and Fitzmartin, J. (1972). Evoked bulbar reticular unit activity following delta fiber stimulation of peripheral somatosensory nerve in cat. *Exp. Neurol.* **37**, 597–606.

Goldstein, K. (1910). Über die aufsteigende Degeneration nach Querschnittsunterbrechung des Rückenmarks (Tractus spino-cerebellaris posterior, Tractus spino-olivaris, Tractus spino-thalamicus). *Neurol. Centr.* **29**, 898–911.

Goodwin, G. M., McCloskey, D. I., and Matthews, P. B. C. (1972a). The persistence of appreciable kinesthesia after paralysing joint afferents but preserving muscle afferents. *Brain Res.* **37**, 326–329.

Goodwin, G. M., McCloskey, D. I., and Matthews, P. B. C. (1972b). The contribution of muscle afferents to kinaesthesia shown by vibration induced illusions of movement and by the effects of paralysing joint afferents. *Brain* **95**, 705–748.

Gordon, B. (1973). Receptive fields in deep layers of cat superior colliculus. *J. Neurophysiol.* **36**, 157–178.

Gordon, G. (1973). The concept of relay nuclei. In: *Handbook of Sensory Physiology.* Vol. II, *Somatosensory System*, pp. 137–50. A. Iggo (ed.). Springer-Verlag, New York.

Gordon, G., and Grant, G. (1972). Afferents to the dorsal column nuclei from the dorsolateral funiculus of the spinal cord. *Acta Physiol. Scand.* **84**, 30–31A.

Gordon, G., and Horrobin, D. (1967). Antidromic and synaptic responses in the cat's gracile nucleus to cerebellar stimulation. *Brain Res.* **5**, 419–421.

Gordon, G., and Jukes, M. G. M. (1963). An investigation of cells in the lateral cervical nucleus of the cat which respond to stimulation of the skin. *J. Physiol.* **169**, 28–29P.

Gordon, G., and Jukes, M. G. M. (1964a). Dual organization of the exteroceptive components of the cat's gracile nucleus. *J. Physiol.* **173**, 263–290.

Gordon, G., and Jukes, M. G. M. (1964b). Descending influences on the exteroceptive organizations of the cat's gracile nucleus. *J. Physiol.* **173**, 291–319.

Gordon, G., and Miller, R. (1969). Identification of cortical cells projecting to the dorsal column nuclei of the cat. *Quart. J. Exp. Physiol.* **54**, 85–98.

Gordon, G., and Paine, C. H. (1960). Functional organization in nucleus gracilis of the cat. *J. Physiol.* **153**, 331–349.

Gordon, G., and Seed, W. A. (1961). An investigation of the nucleus gracilis of the cat by antidromic stimulation. *J. Physiol.* **155**, 589–601.

Gowers, W. R. (1878). A case of unilateral gunshot injury to the spinal cord. *Trans. Clin. London* **11**, 24–32.

Graham, L. T., Shank, R. P., Werman, R., and Aprison, M. H. (1967). Distribution of some synaptic transmitter suspects in cat spinal cord: glutamic acid, aspartic acid, γ-aminobutric acid, glycine, and glutamine. *J. Neurochem.* **14**, 465–472.

Granit, R. (1955). *Receptors and Sensory Perception.* Yale Univ. Press, New Haven, Connecticut.

Grant, F. C. (1930). Value of cordotomy for the relief of pain. *Ann. Surg.* **92**, 998–1006.

Grant, F. C. (1932). Results with cordotomy for relief of intractable pain due to carcinoma of the pelvic organs. *Amer. J. Obstet. Gynecol.* **24**, 620–625.

Grant, G. (1962). Spinal course and somatotopically localized termination of the spinocerebellar tracts. An experimental study in the cat. *Acta Physiol. Scand.* **56** (Suppl. 193), 1–45.

Grant, G., and Westman, J. (1969). The lateral cervical nucleus in the cat. IV. A light and electron microscopical study after midbrain lesions with demonstration of indirect Wallerian degeneration at the ultra-structural level. *Exp. Brain Res.* **7**, 51–67.

Grant, G., Boivie, J. and Brodal, A. (1968). The question of a cerebellar projection from the lateral cervical nucleus re-examined. *Brain Res.* **9**, 95–102.

Grant, G., Boivie, J., and Silfvenius, H. (1973). Course and termination of fibres from the nucleus Z of the medulla oblongata. An experimental light microscopical study in the cat. *Brain Res.* **55**, 55–70.

Gray, E. G. (1963). Electron microscopy of presynaptic organelles of the spinal cord. *J. Anat.* **97**, 101–106.

Gray, E. G., and Guillery, R. W. (1966). Synaptic morphology in the normal and degenerating nervous system. *Internat. Rev. Cytol.* **19**, 111–182.

Gregor, M., and Zimmermann, M. (1972). Characteristics of spinal neurones responding to cutaneous myelinated and unmyelinated fibres. *J. Physiol.* **221**, 555–576.

Gregor, M., and Zimmermann, M. (1973). Dorsal root potentials produced by afferent volleys in cutaneous group III fibres. *J. Physiol.* **232**, 413–425.

Grigg, P. (1975). Mechanical factors influencing response of joint afferent neurons from cat knee. *J. Neurophysiol.* **38**, 1473–1484.

Grigg, P. (1976). Response of joint afferent neurons in cat medial articular nerve to active and passive movements of the knee. *Brain Res.* **118**, 482–485.

Grigg, P., and Greenspan, B. J. (1977). Response of primate joint afferent neurons to mechanical stimulation of knee joint. *J. Neurophysiol.* **40**, 1–8.

Grigg, P., Finerman, G. A., and Riley, L. H. (1973). Joint-position sense after total hip replacement. *J. Bone Joint Surg.* **55A**, 1016–1025.

Grillner, S., Hongo, T., and Lund, S. (1968). The origin of descending fibres monosynaptically activating spinoreticular neurones. *Brain Res.* **10**, 259–262.

Groenewegen, H. J., Boesten, A. J. P., and Voogd, J. (1975). The dorsal column nuclear projections to the nucleus ventralis posterior lateralis thalami and the inferior olive in the cat: an autoradiographic study. *J. Compar. Neurol* **162**, 505–518.

Guilbaud, G., Besson, J. M., Oliveras, J. L., and Liebeskind, J. C. (1973a). Suppression by LSD of the inhibitory effect exerted by dorsal raphe stimulation on certain spinal cord interneurons in the cat. *Brain Res.* **61**, 417–422.

Guilbaud, G., Besson, J. M., Oliveras, J. L., and Wyon-Maillard, M. C. (1973b). Modifications of the firing rate of bulbar reticular units (nucleus gigantocellularis) after intra-arterial injection of bradykinin into the limbs. *Brain Res.* **63**, 131–140.

Guilbaud, G., Benelli, G., and Besson, J. M. (1977a). Responses of thoracic dorsal horn interneurons to cutaneous stimulation and to the administration of algogenic substances into the mesenteric artery in the spinal cat. *Brain Res.* **124**, 437–448.

Guilbaud, G., Oliveras, J. L., Giesler, G., and Besson, J. M. (1977b). Effects induced by stimulation of the centralis inferior nucleus of the raphe on dorsal horn interneurons in cat's spinal cord. *Brain Res.* **126**, 355–360.

Gulley, R. L. (1973). Golgi studies of the nucleus gracilis in the rat. *Anat. Rec.* **177**, 325–342.

Guzman, F., Braun, C., and Lim, R. K. S. (1962). Visceral pain and the pseudoaffective response to intra-arterial injection of bradykinin and other algesic agents. *Arch. Internat. Pharmacodynam. Ther.* **136**, 353–384.

Guzmán-Flores, C., Buendía, N., Anderson, C., and Lindsley, D. B. (1962). Cortical and reticular influences upon evoked responses in dorsal column nuclei. *Exp. Neurol.* **5**, 37–46.

Gwyn, D. G., and Waldron, H. A. (1968). A nucleus in the dorsolateral funiculus of the spinal cord of the rat. *Brain Res.* **10**, 342–351.

Gwyn, D. G., and Waldron, H. A. (1969). Observations on the morphology of a nucleus in the dorsolateral funiculus of the spinal cord of the guinea pig, rabbit, ferrit and cat. *J. Compar. Neurol.* **136**, 233–236.

Ha, H. (1971). Cervicothalamic tract in the Rhesus monkey. *Exp. Neurol.* **33**, 205–212.

Ha, H., and Liu, C. N. (1961). An anatomical investigation on the lateral cervical nucleus of the cat. *Anat. Rec.* **139**, 234.

Ha, H., and Liu, C. N. (1963). Synaptology of spinal afferents in the lateral cervical nucleus of the cat. *Exp. Neurol.* **8**, 318–327.

Ha, H., and Liu, C. N. (1966). Organization of the spino-cervico-thalamic system. *J. Compar. Neurol.* **127**, 445–470.

Ha, H., and Morin, F. (1964). Comparative anatomical observations of the cervical nucleus, N. cervicalis lateralis, of some primates. *Anat. Rec.* **148**, 374–375.

Ha, H. Kitai, S. T., and Morin, F. (1965). The lateral cervical nucleus of the raccoon. *Exp. Neurol.* **11**, 441–450.

Haapanen, L., Kolmodin, G. M., and Skoglund, C. R. (1958). Membrane and action potentials of spinal interneurons in the cat. *Acta Physiol. Scand.* **43**, 315–348.

Hagbarth, K. E. (1960). Centrifugal mechanisms of sensory control. *Ergebn. Biol.* **22**, 47–66.

Hagbarth, K. E., and Kerr, D. I. B. (1954). Central influences on spinal afferent conduction. *J. Neurophysiol.* **17**, 295–307.

Hagbarth, K. E., Hongell, A., Hallin, R. G., and Torebjörk, H. E. (1970). Afferent impulses in median nerve fascicles evoked by tactile stimuli of the human hand. *Brain Res.* **24**, 423–442.

Hagg, S., and Ha, H. (1970). Cervicothalamic tract in the dog. *J. Compar. Neurol.* **139**, 357–374.

Hahn, J. F. (1971). Thermal-mechanical stimulus interactions in low-threshold C-fiber mechanoreceptors of cat. *Exp. Neurol.* **33**, 607–617.

Haldeman, S., and McLennan, H. (1972). The antagonistic action of glutamic acid diethylester towards amino acid-induced and synaptic excitations of central neurones. *Brain Res.* **45**, 393–400.

Hallin, R. G., and Torebjörk, H. E. (1976). Studies on cutaneous A and C fibre afferents, skin nerve blocks and perception. In: *Sensory Functions of the Skin in Primates, with Special Reference to Man*, pp. 137–148 (Y. Zotterman, ed.). Pergamon Press, New York.

Hamilton, T. C., and Johnson, J. I. (1973). Somatotopic organization related to nuclear morphology in the cuneate–gracile complex of opossums *Didelphis marsupialis virginiana. Brain Res.* **51**, 125–140.

Hancock, M. B., Willis, W. D., and Harrison, F. (1970). Viscerosomatic interactions in lumbar spinal cord of the cat. *J. Neurophysiol.* **33**, 46–58.

Hancock, M. B., Rigamonti, D. D., and Bryan, R. N. (1973). Convergence in the lumbar spinal cord pathways activated by splanchnic nerve and hind limb cutaneous nerve stimulation. *Exp. Neurol.* **38**, 337–348.

Hancock, M. B., Foreman, R. D., and Willis, W. D. (1975). Convergence of visceral and cutaneous input onto spinothalamic tract cells in the thoracic spinal cord of the cat. *Exp. Neurol.* **47**, 240–248.

Hand, P. J. (1966). Lumbosacral dorsal root terminations in the nucleus gracilis of the cat: some observations on terminal degenerations in other medullary sensory nuclei. *J. Compar. Neurol.* **126**, 137–156.

Hand, P., and Liu, C. N. (1966). Efferent projections of the nucleus gracilis. *Anat. Rec.* **154**, 353–354.

Hand, P. J., and van Winkle, T. (1977). The efferent connections of the feline nucleus cuneatus. *J. Compar. Neurol.* **171**, 83–110.

Handwerker, H. O., and Neher, K. D. (1976). Characteristics of C-fibre receptors in the cat's foot responding to stepwise increase of skin temperature to noxious levels. *Pflügers Arch.* **365**, 221–229.

Handwerker, H. O., Iggo, A., and Zimmermann, M. (1975). Segmental and supraspinal actions on dorsal horn neurons responding to noxious and non-noxious skin stimuli. *Pain* **1**, 147–165.

Hardy, J. D., Goodell, H., and Wolff, H. G. (1951). The influence of skin temperature upon the pain threshold as evoked by thermal radiation. *Science* **114**, 149–150.

Hardy, J. D., and Oppel, T. W. (1938). Studies in temperature sensation. IV. The stimulation of cold sensation by radiation. *J. Clin. Invest.* **17**, 771–778.

Harrington, T., and Merzenich, M. M. (1970). Neural coding in the sense of touch: human sensations of skin indentation compared with the responses of slowly adapting mechanoreceptive afferents innervating the hairy skin of monkeys. *Exp. Brain Res.* **10**, 251–264.

Hartline, P. H. (1974). Thermoreception in snakes. In: *Handbook of Sensory Physiology.* Vol. III/3, *Electroreceptors and Other Specialized Receptors in Lower Vertebrates,* pp. 297–312 (A. Fessard, ed.). Springer, New York.

Hayes, R. L., Newlon, P. G., Rosecrans, J. A., and Mayer, D. J. (1977). Reduction of stimulation-produced analgesia by lysergic acid diethylamide, a depressor of serotonergic neural activity. *Brain Res.* **122**, 367–372.

Hayle, T. H. (1973). A comparative study of spinal projections to the brain (except cerebellum) in three classes of poikilothermic vertebrates. *J. Compar. Neurol.* **149**, 463–476.

Hazlett, J. C., Dom, R., and Martin, G. F. (1972). Spino-bulbar, spino-thalamic and medial lemniscal connections in the American opossum, *Didelphis marsupialis virginiana. J. Compar. Neurol.* **146**, 95–118.

Head, H. (1893). On disturbances of sensation with especial reference to the pain of visceral disease. *Brain* **16**, 1–132.

Head, H. (1920). *Studies in Neurology.* Vol. I. pp. 55–65 and 225–329. Oxford Univer. Press, London.

Head, H., and Thompson, T. (1906). The grouping of afferent impulses within the spinal cord. *Brain* **29**, 537–741.

Heavner, J. E., and DeJong, R. H. (1973). Spinal cord neuron response to natural stimuli. A microelectrode study. *Exp. Neurol.* **39**, 293–306.

Hebb, D. O. (1949). *The Organization of Behavior.* John Wiley and Sons, New York.

Heimer, L., and Wall, P. D. (1968). The dorsal root distribution to the substantia gelatinosa of the rat with a note on the distribution in the cat. *Exp. Brain Res.* **6**, 89–99.

Heinbecker, P., Bishop, G. H., and O'Leary, J. (1933). Pain and touch fibers in peripheral nerves. *Arch. Neurol. Psychiat.* **29**, 771–789.

Heinbecker, P., Bishop, G. H., and O'Leary, J. (1934). Analysis of sensation in terms of the nerve impulse. *Arch. Neurol. Psychiat.* **31**, 34–53.

Hellon, R. F., and Misra, N. K. (1973a). Neurones in the dorsal horn of the rat responding to scrotal skin temperature changes. *J. Physiol.* **232**, 375–388.

Hellon, R. F., and Misra, N. K. (1973b). Neurones in the ventrobasal complex of the rat thalamus responding to scrotal skin temperature changes. *J. Physiol.* **232**, 389–399.

Hellon, R. F., and Mitchell, D. (1975). Convergence in a thermal afferent pathway in the rat. *J. Physiol.* **248**, 359–376.

Hellon, R. F., Hensel, H., and Schäfer, K. (1975). Thermal receptors in the scrotum of the rat. *J. Physiol.* **248**, 349–357.

Henry, J. L. (1976). Effects of substance P on functionally identified units in cat spinal cord. *Brain Res.* **114**, 439–451.

Hensel, H. (1973a). Cutaneous thermoreceptors. In: *Handbook of Sensory Physiology.* Vol. II. *Somatosensory System*, pp. 79–110 (A. Iggo, ed.). Springer, New York.

Hensel, H. (1973b). Neural processes in thermoregulation. *Physiol. Rev.* **53**, 948–1017.

Hensel, H. (1974). Thermoreceptors. *Ann. Rev. Physiol.* **36**, 233–249.

Hensel, H., and Boman, K. K. A. (1960). Afferent impulses in cutaneous sensory nerves in human subjects. *J. Neurophysiol.* **23**, 564–578.

Hensel, H., and Iggo, A. (1971). Analysis of cutaneous warm and cold fibres in primates. *Pflüg Arch.* **329**, 1–8.

Hensel, H., and Kenshalo, D. R. (1969). Warm receptors in the nasal region of cats. *J. Physiol.* **204**, 99–112.

Hensel, H., and Zotterman, Y. (1951a). The response of the cold receptors to constant cooling. *Acta Physiol. Scand.* **22**, 96–105.

Hensel, H., and Zotterman, Y. (1951b). The persisting cold sensation. *Acta Physiol. Scand.* **22**, 106–113.

Hensel, H., and Zotterman, Y. (1951c). Action potentials of cold fibres and intracutaneous temperature gradient. *J. Neurophysiol.* **14**, 377–385.

Hensel, H., and Zotterman, Y. (1951d). The effect of menthol on the thermoreceptors. *Acta Physiol. Scand.* **24**, 27–34.

Hensel, H., Ström, L., and Zotterman, Y. (1951). Electrophysiological measurements of depth of thermoreceptors. *J. Neurophysiol.* **14**, 423–429.

Hensel, H., Iggo, A., and Witt, I. (1960). A quantitative study of sensitive cutaneous thermoreceptors with C afferent fibres. *J. Physiol.* **153**, 113–126.

Hensel, H., Andres, K. H., and Düring, M. von (1974). Structure and function of cold receptors. *Pflüg Arch.* **352**, 1–10.

Hentall, I. (1977). Delayed "off-responses" in the substantia gelatinosa. *Soc. Neurosci. Abstr.* **3**, 502.

Hernández-Peón, R., Scherrer, H., and Velasco, M. (1956). Central influences on afferent conduction in the somatic and visual pathways. *Acta. Neurol. Latinoamer.* **2**, 8–22.

Herrick, C. J. (1939). Cerebral fiber tracts of *Amblystoma tigrinum* in midlarval stages. *J. Compar. Neurol.* **71**, 511–612.

Hertel, H. C., Howaldt, B., and Mense, S. (1976). Responses of group IV and group III muscle afferents to thermal stimuli. *Brain Res.* **113**, 201–205.

Herz, A., Albus, K., Metyš, J., Schubert, P., and Teschemacher, H. (1970). On the central sites for the antinociceptive action of morphine and fentanyl. *Neuropharmacol.* **9**, 539–551.

Hill, R. G., Simmonds, M. A., and Straughan, D. W. (1976). Antagonism of γ-aminobutyric acid and glycine by convulsants in the cuneate nucleus of cat. *Brit. J. Pharmacol.* **56**, 9–19.

Hillman, P., and Wall, P. D. (1969). Inhibitory and excitatory factors influencing the receptive fields of lamina 5 spinal cord cells. *Exp. Brain Res.* **9**, 284–306.

Hiss, E., and Mense, S. (1976). Evidence for the existence of different receptor sites for algesic agents at the endings of muscular group IV afferent units. *Pflüger. Arch.* **362**, 141–146.

Hník, P., Hudlická, O., Kučera, J., and Payne, R. (1969). Activation of muscle afferents by nonproprioceptive stimuli. *Amer. J. Physiol.* **217**, 1451–1458.

Hodge, C. J. (1972). Potential changes inside central afferent terminals secondary to stimulation of large- and small-diameter peripheral nerve fibers. *J. Neurophysiol.* **35**, 30–43.

Hökfelt, T., Kellerth, J. O., Nilsson, C., and Pernow, B. (1975). Experimental immunohistochemical studies on the localization and distribution of substance P in cat primary sensory neurons. *Brain Res.* **100**, 235–252.

Hökfelt, T., Elde, R., Johansson, O., Luft, R., Nilsson, G., and Arimura, A. (1976). Immunohistochemical evidence for separate populations of somatostatin-containing and substance P-containing primary afferent neurons in the rat. *Neuroscience* **1**, 131–136.

Holmqvist, B., and Lundberg, A. (1959). On the organization of the supraspinal inhibitory control of interneurones of various spinal reflex arcs. *Arch. Ital. Biol.* **97**, 340–356.

Holmqvist, B., and Lundberg, A. (1961). Differential supraspinal control of synaptic actions evoked by volleys in the flexion reflex afferents in alpha motoneurones. *Acta Physiol. Scand.* **54** (Suppl. 186), 1–51.

Holmqvist, B., Lundberg, A., and Oscarsson, O. (1960a). Supraspinal inhibitory control of transmission to three ascending spinal pathways influenced by the flexion reflex afferents. *Arch. Ital. Biol.* **98**, 60–80.

Holmqvist, B., Lundberg, A., and Oscarsson, O. (1960b). A supraspinal control system monosynaptically connected with an ascending spinal pathway. *Arch. Ital. Biol.* **98**, 402–422.

Holmqvist, B., Oscarsson, O., and Rosén, I. (1963). Functional organization of the cuneocerebellar tract in the cat. *Acta Physiol. Scand.* **58**, 216–235.

Holst, E. von (1954). Relations between the central nervous system and the peripheral organs. *Brit. J. Animal Behav.* **2**, 89–94.

Hongo, T., and Jankowska, E. (1967). Effects from the sensorimotor cortex on the spinal cord in cats with transected pyramids. *Exp. Brain Res.* **3**, 117–134.

Hongo, T., and Okada, Y. (1967). Cortically evoked pre- and postsynaptic inhibition of impulse transmission to the dorsal spinocerebellar tract. *Exp. Brain Res.* **3**, 163–177.

Hongo, T., Jankowska, E., and Lundberg, A. (1966). Convergence of excitatory and inhibitory action on interneurones in the lumbosacral cord. *Exp. Brain Res.* **1**, 338–358.

Hongo, T., Okada, Y., and Sato, M. (1967). Corticofugal influences on transmission to the dorsal spinocerebellar tract from hindlimb primary afferents. *Exp. Brain Res.* **3**, 135–149.

Hongo, T., Jankowska, E., and Lundberg, A. (1968). Post-synaptic excitation and inhibition from primary afferents in neurones of the spinocervical tract. *J. Physiol.* **199**, 569–592.

Horch, K. W., Whitehorn, D., and Burgess, P. R. (1974). Impulse generation in type I cutaneous mechanoreceptors. *J. Neurophysiol.* **37**, 267–281.

Horch, K. W., Clark, F. J., and Burgess, P. R. (1975). Awareness of knee joint angle under static conditions. *J. Neurophysiol.* **38**, 1436–1447.

Horch, K. W., Burgess, P. R., and Whitehorn, D. (1976). Ascending collaterals of cutaneous neurons in the fasciculus gracilis of the cat. *Brain Res.* **117**, 1–17.

Hore, J., Preston, J. B., Durkovic, R. G., and Cheney, P. D. (1976). Responses of cortical neurons (areas 3a and 4) to ramp stretch of hindlimb muscles in the baboon. *J. Neurophysiol.* **39**, 484–500.

Horn, G., and Hill, R. M. (1966). Responsiveness to sensory stimulation of units in the superior colliculus and subjacent tectotegmental regions of the rabbit. *Exp. Neurol.* **14**, 199–223.

Horrax, G. (1929). Experiences with cordotomy. *Arch. Surg.* **18**, 1140–1164.

Horrobin, D. F. (1966). The lateral cervical nucleus of the cat; an electrophysiological study. *Quart. J. Exp. Physiol.* **51**, 351–371.

Houk, J., and Henneman, E. (1967). Responses of Golgi tendon organs to active contractions of the soleus muscle of the cat. *J. Neurophysiol.* **30**, 466–481.

Howland, B., Lettvin, J. Y., McCulloch, W. S., Pitts, W., and Wall, P. D. (1955). Reflex inhibition by dorsal root interaction. *J. Neurophysiol.* **18**, 1–17.

Hubbard, J. E., and DiCarlo, V. (1974). Fluorescence histochemistry of monoamine-containing cell bodies in the brain stem of the squirrel monkey (*Saimiri sciureus*). III. Serotonin-containing groups. *J. Compar. Neurol.* **153**, 385–398.

Hubbard, S. J. (1958). A study of rapid mechanical events in a mechanoreceptor. *J. Physiol.* **141**, 198–218.

Hughes, A. (1976). The development of the dorsal funiculus in the human spinal cord. *J. Anat.* **122**, 169–175.

Hughes, J. (1975). Isolation of an endogenous compound from the brain with pharmacological properties similar to morphine. *Brain Res.* **88**, 295–308.

Hughes, J., Smith, T. W., Kosterlitz, H. W., Fothergill, L. A., Morgan, B. A., and Morris, H. R. (1975). Identification of two related pentapeptides from the brain with potent opiate agonist activity. *Nature* **258**, 577–579.

Hunt, C. C. (1954). Relation of function to diameter in afferent fibers of muscle nerves. *J. Gen. Physiol.* **38**, 117–131.

Hunt, C. C. (1961). On the nature of vibration receptors in the hind limb of the cat. *J. Physiol.* **155**, 175–186.

Hunt, C. C., and Kuno, M. (1959a). Properties of spinal interneurones. *J. Physiol.* **147**, 346–363.

Hunt, C. C., and Kuno, M. (1959b). Background discharge and evoked responses of spinal interneurones. *J. Physiol.* **147**, 364–384.

Hunt, C. C., and McIntyre, A. K. (1960a). Properties of cutaneous touch receptors in cat. *J. Physiol.* **153**, 88–98.

Hunt, C. C., and McIntyre, A. K. (1960b). Characteristics of responses from receptors from the flexor longus digitorum muscle and the adjoining interosseous region of the cat. *J. Physiol.* **153**, 74–87.

Hursh, J. B. (1939). Conduction velocity and diameter of nerve fibers. *Amer. J. Physiol.* **127**, 131–139.

Hursh, J. B. (1940). Relayed impulses in ascending branches of dorsal root fibers. *J. Neurophysiol.* **3**, 166–174.

Hwang, Y. C., Hinsman, E. J., and Roesel, O. F. (1975). Caliber spectra of fibers in the fasciculus gracilis of the cat cervical spinal cord: a quantitative electron microscopic study. *J. Compar. Neurol.* **162**, 195–204.

Hyndman, O. R. (1942). Lissauer's tract section. A contribution to chordotomy for the relief of pain (preliminary report). *J. Internat. Coll. Surgeons* **5**, 394–400.

Hyndman, O. R., and Van Epps, C. (1939). Possibility of differential section of the spinothalamic tract. *Arch. Surg.* **38**, 1036–1053.

Hyndman, O. R., and Wolkin, J. (1943). Anterior chordotomy. Further observations on physiologic results and optimum manner of performance. *Arch. Neurol. Psychiat.* **50**, 129–148.

Iggo, A. (1955). Tension receptors in the stomach and the urinary bladder. *J. Physiol.* **128**, 593–607.

Iggo, A. (1959). Cutaneous heat and cold receptors with slowly conducting (C) afferent fibres. *Quart. J. Exp. Physiol.* **44**, 362–370.

Iggo, A. (1960). Cutaneous mechanoreceptors with afferent C fibres. *J. Physiol.* **152**, 337–353.

Iggo, A. (1961). Non-myelinated afferent fibres from mammalian skeletal muscle. *J. Physiol.* **155**, 52–53P.

Iggo, A. (1962). Non-myelinated visceral, muscular and cutaneous afferent fibres and pain. In: *The Assessment of Pain in Man and Animals*, pp. 74–87. C. A. Keele, and R. Smith (eds.). Livingstone, London.

Iggo, A. (1969). Cutaneous thermoreceptors in primates and sub-primates. *J. Physiol.* **200**, 403–430.

Iggo, A., and Kornhuber, H. H. (1977). A quantitative study of C-mechanoreceptors in hairy skin of the cat. *J. Physiol.* **271**, 549–565.

Iggo, A., and Muir, A. R. (1969). The structure and function of a slowly adapting touch corpuscle in hairy skin. *J. Physiol.* **200**, 763–796.

Iggo, A., and Ogawa, H. (1971). Primate cutaneous thermal nociceptors. *J. Physiol.* **216**, 77–78P.

Iggo, A., and Ogawa, H. (1977). Correlative physiological and morphological studies of rapidly adapting mechanoreceptors in cat's glabrous skin. *J. Physiol.* **266**, 275–296.

Iggo, A., and Ramsey, R. L. (1976). Thermosensory mechanisms in the spinal cord of monkeys. In: *Sensory Functions of the Skin in Primates, with Special Reference to Man*, pp. 285–302. Y. Zotterman (ed.). Pergamon Press, New York.

Imai, Y., and Kusama, T. (1969). Distribution of the dorsal root fibers in the cat. An experimental study with the Nauta method. *Brain Res.* **13**, 338–359.

Ingvar, S. (1927). Zur Morphogenese der Tabes. *Acta Med. Scand.* **65**, 645–674.

Iriuchijima, J., and Zotterman, Y. (1960). The specificity of afferent cutaneous C fibres in mammals. *Acta Physiol. Scand.* **49**, 267–278.

Ito, M. (1957). The electrical activity of spinal ganglion cells investigated with intracellular microelectrodes. *Jpn. J. Physiol.* **7**, 297–323.

Ito, M., Udo, M., and Mano, N. (1970). Long inhibitory and excitatory pathways converging onto cat reticular and Deiters' neurons and their relevance to the reticulofugal axons. *J. Neurophysiol.* **33**, 210–226.

Jabbur, S. J., and Banna, N. R. (1968). Presynaptic inhibition of cuneate transmission by widespread cutaneous inputs. *Brain Res.* **10**, 273–276.

Jabbur, S. J., and Banna, N. R. (1970). Widespread cutaneous inhibition in dorsal column nuclei. *J. Neurophysiol.* **33**, 616–624.

Jabbur, S. J., and Towe, A. L. (1961). Cortical excitation of neurons in dorsal column nuclei of cat, including an analysis of pathways. *J. Neurophysiol.* **24**, 499–509.

Jabbur, S. J., Harik, S. I., and Hush, J. A. (1977). Caudate influence on transmission in the cuneate nucleus. *Brain Res.* **120**, 559–563.

Jacquet, Y. F., and Lajtha, A. (1976). The periaqueductal gray: site of morphine analgesia and tolerance as shown by 2-way cross tolerance between systemic and intracerebral injections. *Brain Res.* **103**, 501–513.

Jänig, W. (1971a). The afferent innervation of the central pad of the cat's hind foot. *Brain Res.* **28**, 203–216.

Jänig, W. (1971b). Morphology of rapidly and slowly adapting mechanoreceptors in the hairless skin of the cat's hind foot. *Brain Res.* **28**, 217–231.

Jänig, W., and Zimmermann, M. (1971). Presynaptic depolarization of myelinated afferent fibres evoked by stimulation of cutaneous C fibres. *J. Physiol.* **214**, 29–50.

Jänig, W., Schmidt, R. F., and Zimmermann, M. (1968a). Single unit responses and the total afferent outflow from the cat's foot pad upon mechanical stimulation. *Exp. Brain Res.* **6**, 100–115.

Jänig, W., Schmidt, R. F., and Zimmermann, M. (1968b). Two specific feedback pathways to the central afferent terminals of phasic and tonic mechanoreceptors. *Exp. Brain Res.* **6**, 116–129.

Jane, J. A., and Schroeder, D. M. (1971). A comparison of dorsal column nuclei and spinal afferents in the European hedgehog (*Erinaceus europeaus*). *Exp. Neurol.* **30**, 1–17.

Jankowska, E. (1975). Identification of interneurons interposed in different spinal reflex pathways. In: *Golgi Centennial Symposium*, pp. 235–246. M. Santini (ed.). Raven Press, New York.

Jankowska, E., Rastad, J., and Westman, J. (1976). Intracellular application of horseradish peroxidase and its light and electron microscopical appearance in spinocervical tract cells. *Brain Res.* **105**, 557–562.

Järvilehto, T., Hämäläinen, H., and Laurinen, P. (1976). Characteristics of single mechanoreceptive fibres innervating hairy skin of the human hand. *Exp. Brain Res.* **25**, 45–61.

Jassik-Gerschenfeld, D. (1966). Activity of somatic origin evoked in the superior colliculus of the cat. *Exp. Neurol.* **16**, 104–118.

Job, C. (1953). Über autogene Inhibition und Reflexumkehr bei spinalisierten und decerebrierten Katzen. *Pflügers. Arch.* **256**, 406–418.

Johansson, H., and Silfvenius, H. (1977a). Axon-collateral activation by dorsal spinocerebellar tract fibres of group I relay cells of nucleus Z in the cat medulla oblongata. *J. Physiol.* **265**, 341–369.

Johansson, H., and Silfvenius, H. (1977b). Input from ipsilateral proprio- and exteroceptive hind limb afferents to nucleus Z of the cat medulla oblongata. *J. Physiol.* **265**, 371–393.

Johansson, H., and Silfvenius, H. (1977c). Connexions from large, ipsilateral hind limb muscle and skin afferents to the rostral main cuneate nucleus and to the nucleus X region in the cat. *J. Physiol.* **265**, 395–428.

Johansson, R. S. (1976). Receptive field sensitivity profile of mechanosensitive units innervating the glabrous skin of the human hand. *Brain Res.* **104**, 330–334.

Johnson, F. H. (1952). Microelectrode studies on the cuneate and gracile nuclei of the cat. *Amer. J. Physiol.* **171**, 737.

Johnson, F. H. (1954). Experimental study of spino-reticular connections in the cat. *Anat. Rec.* **118**, 316.

Johnson, J. I., Welker, W. I., and Pubols, B. H. (1968). Somatotopic organization of raccoon dorsal column nuclei. *J. Compar. Neurol.* **132**, 1–44.

Johnson, J. I., Hamilton, T. C., Hsung, J. C., and Ulinski, P. S. (1972). Gracile nucleus absent in adult opossums after leg removal in infancy. *Brain Res.* **38**, 421–424.

Johnson, J. L. (1972). Glutamic acid as a synaptic transmitter in the nervous system. A review. *Brain Res.* **37**, 1–19.

Johnson, J. L., and Aprison, M. H. (1970). The distribution of glutamic acid, a transmitter candidate, and other amino acids in the dorsal sensory neuron of the cat. *Brain Res.* **24**, 285–292.

Johnson, K. O. (1974). Reconstruction of population response to a vibratory stimulus in quickly adapting mechanoreceptive afferent fiber population innervating glabrous skin of the monkey. *J. Neurophysiol.* **37**, 48–72.

Johnson, K. O., Darian-Smith, I., and LaMotte, C. (1973). Peripheral neural determinants of temperature discrimination in man: A correlative study of responses to cooling skin. *J. Neurophysiol.* **36**, 347–370.

Jones, E. G., and Burton, H. (1974). Cytoarchitecture and somatic sensory connectivity of thalamic nuclei other than the ventrobasal complex in the cat. *J. Compar. Neurol.* **154**, 395–431.

Jones, E. G., and Leavitt, R. Y. (1974). Retrograde axonal transport and the demonstration of non-specific projections to the cerebral cortex and striatum from thalamic intralaminar nuclei in the rat, cat and monkey. *J. Compar. Neurol.* **154**, 349–378.

Jones, F. N. (1960). Some subjective magnitude functions for touch. In: *Symposium on Cutaneous Sensibility* (G. R. Hawkins, ed.). Report No. 424, U.S. Army Med. Res. Lab., Ft. Knox, Kentucky.

Jordan, L. M., Kenshalo, D. R., Martin, R. F., Haber, L. H., and Willis, W. D. (1978). Depression of primate spinothalamic tract neurons by iontophoretic application of 5-hydroxyltryptamine. *Pain* (in press).

Kahn, E. A. (1933). Anterolateral chordotomy for intractable pain. *J.A.M.A.* **100**, 1925–1928.

Kahn, E. A., and Peet, M. M. (1948). The technique of anterolateral cordotomy. *J. Neurosurg.* **5**, 276–283.

Kane, K., and Taub, A. (1975). A history of local electrical analgesia. *Pain* **1**, 125–138.

Kappers, C. U. A., Huber, G. C., and Crosby, E. C. (1936) (reprinted in 1960). *The Comparative Anatomy of the Nervous System of Vertebrates, Including Man.* Hafner, New York.

Karten, H. J. (1963). Ascending pathways from the spinal cord in the pigeon (*Columba livia*). *Proc. 16th Internat. Congr. Zool., Washington, D.C.* **2**, 23.

Kato, M., and Hirata, Y. (1968). Sensory neurons in the spinal ventral roots of the cat. *Brain Res.* **7**, 479–482.

Kato, M., and Tanji, J. (1971). Physiological properties of sensory fibers in the spinal ventral roots in the cat. *Jpn. J. Physiol.* **21**, 71–77.

Keegan, J. J., and Garrett, F. D. (1948). The segmental distribution of the cutaneous nerves in the limbs of man. *Anat. Rec.* **102**, 409–437.

Keller, J. H., and Hand, P. J. (1970). Dorsal root projections to nucleus cuneatus of the cat. *Brain Res.* **20**, 1–17.

Kelly, D. D., and Glusman, M. (1968). Aversive thresholds following midbrain lesions. *J. Compar. Physiol. Psychol.* **66**, 25–34.

Kelly, J. S., and Renaud, L. P. (1973a). On the pharmacology of the γ-aminobutyric acid receptors on the cuneo-thalamic relay cells of the cat. *Brit. J. Pharmacol.* **48**, 369–386.

Kelly, J. S., and Renaud, L. P. (1973b). On the pharmacology of the glycine receptors on the cuneo-thalamic relay cells in the cat. *Brit. J. Pharmacol.* **48**, 387–395.

Kelly, J. S., and Renaud, L. P. (1973c). On the pharmacology of ascending, descending and recurrent postsynaptic inhibition of the cuneo-thalamic relay cells in the cat. *Brit. J. Pharmacol.* **48**, 396–408.

Kennard, M. A. (1954). The course of ascending fibers in the spinal cord of the cat essential to the recognition of painful stimuli. *J. Compar. Neurol.* **100**, 511–524.

Kenshalo, D. R. (1970). Psychophysical studies of temperature sensitivity. In: *Contribu-*

tion to Sensory Physiology. Vol. 4, pp. 19–74 (W. D. Neff, ed.). Academic Press, New York.

Kenshalo, D. R., and Duclaux, R. (1977). Response characteristics of cutaneous cold receptors in the monkey. *J. Neurophysiol.* **40**, 319–332.

Kenshalo, D. R., and Scott, H. A. (1966). Temporal course of thermal adaptation. *Science* **151**, 1095–1096.

Kenshalo, D. R., and Scott, H. A. (1966). Temporal course of thermal adaptation. *Science* function of rate of stimulus temperature change. *Percept. Psychophys.* **3**, 81–84.

Kerr, F. W. L. (1966). The ultrastructure of the spinal tract of the trigeminal nerve and the substantia gelatinosa. *Exp. Neuro.* **16**, 359–376.

Kerr, F. W. L. (1968). The descending pathway to the lateral cuneate nucleus, the nucleus of Clarke and the ventral horn. *Anat. Rec.* **160**, 375.

Kerr, F. W. L. (1970a). The fine structure of the subnucleus caudalis of the trigeminal nerve. *Brain Res.* **23**, 129–145.

Kerr, F. W. L. (1970b). The organization of primary afferents in the subnucleus caudalis of the trigeminal: a light and electron microscopic study of degeneration. *Brain Res.* **23**, 147–165.

Kerr, F. W. L. (1975a). Neuroanatomical substrates of nociception in the spinal cord. *Pain* **1**, 325–356.

Kerr, F. W. L. (1975b). The ventral spinothalamic tract and other ascending systems of the ventral funiculus of the spinal cord. *J. Compar. Neurol.* **159**, 335–356.

Kerr, F. W. L. (1975c). Pain, a new central inhibitory balance theory. *Mayo Clin. Proc.* **50**, 685–690.

Kerr, F. W. L., and Lippman, H. H. (1974). The primate spinothalamic tract as demonstrated by anterolateral cordotomy and commissural myelotomy. In: *Advances in Neurology.* Vol. 4. *International Symposium on Pain,* pp. 147–156 (J. J. Bonica, ed.). Raven, New York.

Khattab, F. I. (1968). A complex synaptic apparatus in spinal cords of cats. *Experientia* **24**, 690–691.

Kircher, C., and Ha, H. (1968). The nucleus cervicalis lateralis in primates, including the human. *Anat. Rec.* **160**, 376.

Kirk, E. J., and Denny-Brown, D. (1970). Functional variation in dermatomes in the macaque monkey following dorsal root lesions. *J. Compar. Neurol.* **139**, 307–320.

Kitai, S. T., and Weinberg, J. (1968). Tactile discrimination study of the dorsal column–medial lemniscal system and spinocervico-thalamic tract in cat. *Exp. Brain Res.* **6**, 234–246.

Kitai, S. T., Ha, H., and Morin, F. (1965). Lateral cervical nucleus of the dog: anatomical and microelectrode studies. *Amer. J. Physiol.* **209**, 307–312.

Knibestöl, M. (1973). Stimulus–response functions of rapidly adapting mechanoreceptors in the human glabrous skin area. *J. Physiol.* **232**, 427–452.

Knibestöl, M. (1975). Stimulus–response functions of slowly adapting mechanoreceptors in the human glabrous skin area. *J. Physiol.* **245**, 63–80.

Knibestöl, M., and Vallbo, A. B. (1970). Single unit analysis of mechanoreceptor activity from the human glabrous skin. *Acta Physiol. Scand.* **80**, 178–195.

Knibestöl, M., and Vallbo, A. B. (1976). Stimulus–response functions of primary afferents and psychophysical intensity estimation on mechanical skin stimulation in the human hand. In: *Sensory Functions of the Skin in Primates, with Special Reference to Man,* pp. 201–213 (Y. Zotterman, ed.). Pergamon Press, New York.

Kniffki, K. D., Mense, S., and Schmidt, R. F. (1977). Activation of neurones of the spinocervical tract by painful stimulation of skeletal muscle. *Proc. Internat. Union Physiol. Sci.* **13**, 393.

Knyihár, E., and Gerebtzoff, M. A. (1973). Extra-lysosomal localization of acid phosphatase in the spinal cord of the rat. *Exp. Brain Res.* **18**, 383–395.

Knyihár, E., László, I., and Tornyos, S. (1974). Fine structure and fluoride resistant acid phosphatase activity of electron dense sinusoid terminals in the substantia gelatinosa Rolandi of the rat after dorsal root transection. *Exp. Brain Res.* **19**, 529–544.

Koizumi, K., Ushiyama, J., and Brooks, C. McC. (1959). A study of reticular formation action on spinal interneurons and motoneurons. *Jpn. J. Physiol.* **9**, 282–303.

Koketsu, K. (1956). Intracellular potential changes of primary afferent nerve fibers in spinal cords of cats. *J. Neurophysiol.* **19**, 375–392.

Kolmodin, G. M., and Skoglund, C. R. (1958). Slow membrane potential changes accompanying excitation and inhibition in spinal moto- and interneurons in the cat during natural activation. *Acta Physiol. Scand.* **44**, 11–54.

Kolmodin, G. M., and Skoglund, C. R. (1960). Analysis of spinal interneurons activated by tactile and nociceptive stimulation. *Acta Physiol. Scand.* **50**, 337–355.

Konietzny, F., and Hensel, H. (1975). Warm fiber activity in human skin nerves. *Pflügers. Arch.* **359**, 265–267.

Konishi, S., and Otsuka, M. (1974). The effects of substance P and other peptides on spinal neurons of the frog. *Brain Res.* **65**, 397–410.

Kostiuk, P. G. (1960). Electrophysiological characteristics of individual spinal cord neurons. *Sechenov Physiol. J. USSR* **46**, 10–22.

Krause, W. (1859). Über Nervenendigungen. *Z. Rat. Med.* **5**, 28–43.

Kříž, N., Syková, E., Ujec, E., and Vyklický, L. (1974). Changes of extracellular potassium concentration induced by neuronal activity in the spinal cord of the cat. *J. Physiol.* **238**, 1–15.

Kříž, N., Syková, E., and Vyklický, L. (1975). Extracellular potassium changes in the spinal cord of the cat and their relation to slow potentials, active transport and impulse transmission. *J. Physiol.* **249**, 167–182.

Krnjević, K., and Morris, M. E. (1974). Extracellular accumulation of K^+ evoked by activity of primary afferent fibers in the cuneate nucleus and dorsal horn of cats. *Can. J. Physiol. Pharmacol.* **52**, 852–871.

Krnjević, K., and Morris, M. E. (1976). Input–output relation of transmission through cuneate nucleus. *J. Physiol.* **257**, 791–815.

Kruger, L., and Witkovsky, P. (1961). A functional analysis of neurons in the dorsal column nuclei and spinal nucleus of the trigeminal in the reptile (*Alligator mississippiensis*). *J. Compar. Neurol.* **117**, 97–105.

Kruger, L., and Kenton, B. (1973). Quantitative neural and psychophysical data for cutaneous mechanoreceptor function. *Brain Res.* **49**, 1–24.

Kruger, L., Siminoff, R., and Witkovsky, P. (1961). Single neuron analysis of dorsal column nuclei and spinal nucleus of trigeminal in cat. *J. Neurophysiol.* **24**, 333–349.

Kuhar, M. J., Pert, C. B., and Snyder, S. H. (1973). Regional distribution of opiate receptor binding in monkey and human brain. *Nature* **245**, 447–450.

Kuhn, R. A. (1949). Topographical pattern of cutaneous sensibility in the dorsal column nuclei of the cat. *Trans. Amer. Neurol. Assoc.* **74**, 227–230.

Kumazawa, T., and Mizumura, K. (1977a). The polymodal receptors in the testis of dog. *Brain Res.* **136**, 553–558.

Kumazawa, T., and Mizumura, K. (1977b). Thin-fibre receptors responding to mechanical, chemical, and thermal stimulation in the skeletal muscle of the dog. *J. Physiol.* **273**, 179–194.

Kumazawa, T., and Perl, E. R. (1976). Differential excitation of dorsal horn and substantia gelatinosa marginal neurons by primary afferent units with fine (Aδ and C) fibers.

In: *Sensory Functions of the Skin in Primates, with Special Reference to Man*, pp. 67–88. (Y. Zotterman, ed.), Pergamon, New York.

Kumazawa, T., and Perl, E. R. (1978). Excitation of marginal and substantia gelatinosa neurons in the primate spinal cord: indications of their place in dorsal horn functional organization. *J. Compar. Neurol.* **177**, 417–434.

Kumazawa, T., Perl, E. R., Burgess, P. R., and Whitehorn, D. (1975). Ascending projections from marginal zone (lamina I) neurons of the spinal dorsal horn. *J. Compar. Neurol.* **162**, 1–12.

Kuno, M., and Perl, E. R. (1960). Alteration of spinal reflexes by interaction with suprasegmental and dorsal root activity. *J. Physiol.* **151**, 103–122.

Kuno, M., Muñoz-Martinez, E. J., and Randić, M. (1973). Sensory inputs to neurones in Clarke's column from muscle, cutaneous and joint receptors. *J. Physiol.* **228**, 327–342.

Kuru, M. (1949). *Sensory Paths in the Spinal Cord and Brain Stem of Man*. Sogensya, Tokyo.

Kuypers, H. G. J. M. (1958). An anatomical analysis of cortico-bulbar connexions to the pons and lower brain stem in the cat. *J. Anat.* **92**, 198–218.

Kuypers, H. G. J. M., and Maisky, V. A. (1975). Retrograde axonal transport of horseradish peroxidase from spinal cord to brain stem cell groups in the cat. *Neurosci. Lett.* **1**, 9–14.

Kuypers, H. G. J. M., and Tuerk, J. D. (1964). The distribution of the cortical fibres within the nuclei cuneatus and gracilis in the cat. *J. Anat.* **98**, 143–162.

LaMotte, C. (1977). Distribution of the tract of Lissauer and the dorsal root fibers in the primate spinal cord. *J. Compar Neurol.* **172**, 529–562.

LaMotte, C., Pert, C. B., and Snyder, S. H. (1976). Opiate receptor binding in primate spinal cord: distribution and changes after dorsal root section. *Brain Res.* **112**, 407–412.

LaMotte, R. H., and Mountcastle, V. B. (1975). Capacities of humans and monkeys to discriminate between vibratory stimuli of different frequency and amplitude: a correlation between neural events and psychophysical measurements. *J. Neurophysiol.* **38**, 539–559.

Landgren, S. (1960). Thalamic neurones responding to cooling of the cat's tongue. *Acta Physiol. Scand.* **48**, 255–267.

Landgren, S., and Silfvenius, H. (1971) Nucleus Z, the medullary relay in the projection path to the cerebral cortex of group I muscle afferents from the cat's hind limb. *J. Physiol.* **218**, 551–571.

Landgren, S., Nordwall, A., and Wengström, C. (1965). The location of the thalamic relay in the spino-cervico-lemniscal path. *Acta Physiol. Scand.* **65**, 164–175.

Landgren, S., Silfvenius, H., and Wolsk, D. (1967). Somato-sensory paths to the second cortical projection area of the group I muscle afferents. *J. Physiol.* **191**, 543–559.

Landon, D. N. (ed.) (1976). *The Peripheral Nerve*. John Wiley and Sons, New York.

Lasek, R., Joseph, B. S., and Whitlock, D. G. (1968). Evaluation of a radioautographic neuroanatomical tracing method. *Brain Res.* **8**, 319–336.

Le Bars, D., Guilbaud, G., Jurna, I., and Besson, J. M. (1976a). Differential effects of morphine on responses of dorsal horn lamina V type cells elicited by A and C fibre stimulation in the spinal cat. *Brain Res.* **115**, 518–524.

Le Bars, D., Menétrey, D., and Besson, J. M. (1976b). Effects of morphine upon the lamina V type cells activities in the dorsal horn of the decerebrate cat. *Brain Res.* **113**, 293–310.

LeBlanc, H. J., and Gatipon, G. B. (1974). Medial bulboreticular response to peripherally applied noxious stimuli. *Exp. Neurol.* **42**, 264–273.

Mayer, D. J., and Price, D. D. (1976). Central nervous system mechanisms of analgesia. *Pain* 2, 379–404.

Mayer, D. J., Wolfle, T. L., Akil, H., Carder, B., and Liebeskind, J. C. (1971). Analgesia from electrical stimulation in the brainstem of the rat. *Science* 174, 1351–1354.

Mayer, D. J., Price, D. D., and Becker, D. P. (1975). Neurophysiological characterization of the anterolateral spinal cord neurons contributing to pain perception in man. *Pain* 1, 51–58.

Mayer, D. J., Price, D. D., and Rafii, A. (1977). Antagonism of acupuncture analgesia in man by the narcotic antagonist naloxone. *Brain Res.* 121, 368–372.

Maynard, C. W., Leonard, R. B., Coulter, J. D., and Coggeshall, R. E. (1977). Central connections of ventral root afferents as demonstrated by the HRP method. *J. Compar. Neurol.* 172, 601–608.

McCall, W. D., Farias, M. C., Williams, W. J., and Bement, S. L. (1974). Static and dynamic responses of slowly adapting joint receptors. *Brain Res.* 70, 221–243.

McCloskey, D. I. (1973). Differences between the senses of movement and position shown by the effects of loading and vibration of muscles in man *Brain Res.* 63, 119–131.

McComas, A. J. (1963). Responses of the rat dorsal column system to mechanical stimulation of the hind paw. *J. Physiol.* 166, 435–448.

McComas, A. J., and Wilson, P. (1968). An investigation of pyramidal tract cells in the somatosensory cortex of the rat. *J. Physiol.* 194, 271–288.

McCreery, D. B., and Bloedel, J. R. (1975). Reduction of the response of cat spinothalamic neurons to graded mechanical stimuli by electrical stimulation of the lower brain stem. *Brain Res.* 97, 151–156.

McCreery, D. B., and Bloedel, J. R. (1976). Effect of trigeminal stimulation on the excitability of cat spinothalamic neurons. *Brain Res.* 117, 136–140.

McIntyre, A. K. (1962). Cortical projection of impulses in the interosseous nerve of the cat's hind limb. *J. Physiol.* 163, 46–60.

McIntyre, A. K., Holman, M. E., and Veale, J. L. (1967). Cortical responses to impulses from single Pacinian corpuscles in the cat's hind limb. *Exp. Brain Res.* 4, 243–255.

McLaughlin, B. J. (1972). Dorsal root projections to the motor nuclei in the cat spinal cord. *J. Compar. Neurol.* 144, 461–474.

McLaughlin, B. J., Barber, R., Saito, K., Roberts, E., and Wu, J. Y. (1975). Immunocytochemical localization of glutamate decarboxylase in rat spinal cord. *J. Compar. Neurol.* 164, 305–322.

Meessen, H., and Olszewski, J. (1949). A cytoarchitectonic atlas of the rhombencephalon of the rabbit. Karger, New York.

Mehler, W. R. (1962). The anatomy of the so-called "pain tract" in man: An analysis of the course and distribution of the ascending fibers of the fasciculus anterolateralis. In: *Basic Research in Paraplegia*, pp. 26–55 (J. D. French and R. W. Porter, eds.). Springfield, Thomas.

Mehler, W. R. (1966). Some observations on secondary ascending afferent systems in the central nervous system. In: *Pain*, pp. 11–32 (R. S. Knighton and P. R. Dumke, eds.). Little, Brown, Boston.

Mehler, W. R. (1969). Some neurological species differences—a posteriori. *Ann. N.Y. Acad. Sci.* 167, 424–468.

Mehler, W. R. (1974). Central pain and the spinothalamic tract. In: *Advances in Neurology*. Vol. 4. *International Symposium on Pain*, pp. 127–146 (J. J. Bonica, ed.). Raven, New York.

Mehler, W. R., Feferman, M. E., and Nauta, W. J. H. (1960). Ascending axon degeneration following anterolateral cordotomy. An experimental study in the monkey. *Brain* **83**, 718–750.

Meissner, G. (1859). Untersuchungen über den Tastsinn. *Z. Rat. Med.* **7**, 92–118.

Melzack, R. (1973). *The Puzzle of Pain*. Basic Books, New York.

Melzack, R., and Bridges, J. A. (1971). Dorsal column contributions to motor behavior. *Exp. Neurol.* **33**, 53–68.

Melzack, R., and Casey, K. L. (1968). Sensory, motivational and central control determinants of pain. In: *The Skin Senses*, pp. 423–443 (D. R. Kenshalo, ed.). Thomas, Springfield.

Melzack, R., and Melinkoff, D. F. (1974). Analgesia produced by brain stimulation: evidence of a prolonged onset period. *Exp. Neurol.* **43**, 369–374.

Melzack, R., and Southmayd, S. E. (1974). Dorsal column contributions to anticipatory motor behavior. *Exp. Neurol.* **42**, 274–281.

Melzack, R., and Wall, P. D. (1962). On the nature of cutaneous sensory mechanisms. *Brain* **85**, 331–356.

Melzack, R., and Wall, P. D. (1965). Pain mechanisms: A new theory. *Science* **150**, 971–979.

Melzack, R., Stotler, W. A., and Livingston, W. K. (1958). Effects of discrete brainstem lesions in cats on perception of noxious stimulation. *J. Neurophysiol.* **21**, 353–367.

Melzack, R., Weisz, A. Z., and Sprague, L. T. (1963). Stratagems for controlling pain: contributions of auditory stimulation and suggestion. *Exp. Neurol.* **8**, 239–247.

Mendell, L. M. (1966). Physiological properties of unmyelinated fiber projection to the spinal cord. *Exp. Neurol.* **16**, 316–332.

Mendell, L. (1970). Positive dorsal root potentials produced by stimulation of small diameter muscle afferents. *Brain Res.* **18**, 375–379.

Mendell, L. (1972). Properties and distribution of peripherally evoked presynaptic hyperpolarization in cat lumbar spinal cord. *J. Physiol.* **226**, 769–792.

Mendell, L. (1973). Two negative dorsal root potentials evoke a positive dorsal root potential. *Brain Res.* **55**, 198–202.

Mendell, L. M., and Wall, P. D. (1964). Presynaptic hyperpolarization: a role for fine afferent fibres. *J. Physiol.* **172**, 274–294.

Mendell, L. M., and Wall, P. D. (1965). Responses of single dorsal cord cells to peripheral cutaneous unmyelinated fibres. *Nature* **206**, 97–99.

Menétrey, D., Giesler, G. J., and Besson, J. M. (1977). An analysis of response properties of spinal cord dorsal horn neurones to nonnoxious and noxious stimuli in the spinal rat. *Exp. Brain Res.* **27**, 15–33.

Mense, S. (1977). Nervous outflow from skeletal muscle following chemical noxious stimulation. *J. Physiol.* **267**, 75–88.

Mense, S., and Schmidt, R. F., (1974). Activation of group IV afferent units from muscle by algesic agents. *Brain Res.* **72**, 305–310.

Menzies, J. E. (1976). Histochemical and electrophysiological studies on the origins and sites of termination of the spinal serotonergic pathway. Masters thesis, Univ. of Manitoba, Winnipeg, Canada.

Merkel, F. (1875). Tastzellen und Tastkörperchen bei den Hausthieren und beim Menschen. *Arch. Mikroskop. Anat.* **11**, 636–652.

Merzenich, M. M. and Harrington, T. (1969). The sense of flutter–vibration evoked by stimulation of the hairy skin of primates: comparison of human sensory capacity with the responses of mechanoreceptive afferents innervating the hairy skin of monkeys. *Exp. Brain Res.* **9**, 236–260.

Messing, R. B., and Lytle, L. D. (1977) Serotonin-containing neurons: their possible role in pain and analgesia. *Pain* **4**, 1–21.

Millar, J. (1973a). Joint afferent fibres responding to muscle stretch, vibration and contraction. *Brain Res* **63**, 380–383.

Millar, J. (1973b). The topography and receptive fields of ventroposterolateral thalamic
neurons excited by afferents projecting through the dorsolateral funiculus of the
spinal cord. *Exp. Neurol.* **41**, 303–313.

Millar, J., and Basbaum, A. I. (1975). Topography of the projection of the body surface of
the cat to cuneate and gracile nuclei. *Exp. Neurol.* **49**, 281–290.

Millar, J., Basbaum, A. I., and Wall, P. D. (1976). Restructuring of the somatotopic map
and appearance of abnormal neuronal activity in the gracile nucleus after partial
deafferentation. *Exp. Neurol.* **50**, 658–672.

Miller, G. A. (1956). The magical number seven, plus or minus two: some limits on our
capacity for processing information. *Psychol. Rev.* **63**, 81–97.

Mizuno, N. (1966). An experimental study of the spino-olivary fibers in the rabbit and
the cat. *J. Compar. Neurol.* **127**, 267–292.

Mizuno, N., Nakano, K., Imaizumi, M., and Okamoto, M. (1967). The lateral cervical
nucleus of the Japanese monkey (*Macaca fuscata*). *J. Compar. Neurol.* **129**, 375–384.

Molenaar, I., Rustioni, A., and Kuypers, H. G. J. M. (1974). The location of cells of origin of the fibers in the ventral and the lateral funiculus of the cat's lumbo-sacral
cord. *Brain Res.* **78**, 239–254.

Moolenaar, G. M., Holloway, J. A., and Trouth, C. O. (1976). Responses of caudal raphe
neurons to peripheral somatic stimulation. *Exp. Neurol.* **53**, 304–313.

Morest, D. K. (1967). Experimental study of the projections of the nucleus of the tractus
solitarius and the area postrema in the cat. *J. Compar. Neurol.* **130**, 277–300.

Morin, F. (1953). Afferent projections to the midbrain tegmentum and their spinal
course. *Amer. J. Physiol.* **172**, 483–496.

Morin, F. (1955). A new spinal pathway for cutaneous impulses. *Amer. J. Physiol.* **183**,
245–252.

Morin, F., and Catalano, J. V. (1955). Central connections of a cervical nucleus (nucleus
cervicalis lateralis of the cat). *J. Compar. Neurol.* **103**, 17–32.

Morin, F., and Thomas, L. M. (1955). Spinothalamic fibers and tactile pathways in cat.
Anat. Rec. **121**, 344.

Morin, F., Schwartz, H. G., and O'Leary, J. L. (1951). Experimental study of the spinothalamic and related tracts. *Acta Psychiat. Neurol.* **26**, 371–396.

Morin, F., Kitai, S. T., Portnoy, H., and Demirjian, C. (1963). Afferent projections to the
lateral cervical nucleus: a microelectrode study. *Amer. J. Physiol.*, **204**, 667–672.

Morrison, J. F. B. (1973). Splanchnic slowly adapting mechanoreceptors with punctate
receptive fields in the mesentery and gastrointestinal tract of the cat. *J. Physiol.* **233**,
349–361.

Morrison, J. F. B. (1977). The afferent innervation of the gastrointestinal tract. In: *Nerves
and the Gut*. pp. 297–322 (F. P. Brooks and P. W. Evers, eds.). C. B. Slack, Thorofare, New Jersey.

Mott, F. W. (1895). Experimental enquiry upon the afferent tracts of the central nervous
system of the monkey. *Brain* **18**, 1–20.

Mountcastle, V. B., Talbot, W. H., and Kornhuber, H. H. (1966). The neural transformation of mechanical stimuli delivered to the monkey's hand. In *Touch, Heat and Pain*.
pp. 325–345, (A. V. S. DeReuck and J. Knight, eds.). Ciba Foundation Symp., Little,
Brown, Boston.

Mountcastle, V. B., LaMotte, R. H., and Carli, G. (1972). Detection thresholds for stimuli
in humans and monkeys: comparison with threshold events in mechanoreceptive
afferent nerve fibers innervating the monkey hand. *J. Neurophysiol.* **35**, 122–136.

Müller, J. (1840-2). *Elements of physiology*. Transl. from German, with notes by W. Baly,

2nd ed., Vol. 2. London. Original German: (1838). *Handbuch der Physiologie des Menschen*, 2nd ed., Coblenz.

Müller, W. (1871). *Beitrage zu pathologischen Anatomie und Physiologie des menschlichen Ruckenmarks*. Leopold Voss, Leipzig.

Mullan, S. (1966). Percutaneous cordotomy for pain. *Surg. Clin. N. Amer.* **46**, 3–12.

Mullen, S., Harper, P. V. Hekmatpanah, J., Torres, H., and Dobbin, G. (1963). Percutaneous interruption of spinal-pain tracts by means of a Strontium[90] needle. *J. Neurosurg.* **20**, 931–939.

Munger, B. L. (1965). The intraepidermal innervation of the snout of the opossum. *J. Cell. Biol.* **26**, 79–97.

Munger, B. L. (1971). Patterns of organization of peripheral sensory receptors. In: *Handbook of Sensory Physiology*, Vol. 1, pp. 523–556. (W. R. Loewenstein, ed.). Springer, Berlin.

Murray, M. (1966). Degeneration of some intralaminar thalamic nuclei after cortical removals in the cat. *J. Compar. Neurol.* **127**, 341–368.

Myers, D. A., Hostetter, G., Bourassa, C. M., and Swett, J. E. (1974). Dorsal columns in sensory detection. *Brain Res.* **70**, 350–355.

Nadel, E. R., and Horvath, S. M. (1969). Peripheral involvement in thermoregulatory responses to an imposed heat debt in man. *J. Appl. Physiol.* **27**, 484–488.

Nafe, J. P. (1927). The psychology of felt experience. *Amer. J. Psychol.* **39**, 367–389.

Nafe, J. P. (1929). A quantitative theory of feeling. *J. Gen. Psychol.* **2**, 199–210.

Naka, K. I., and Rushton, W. A. H. (1966). S-potentials from colour units in the retina of fish (Cyprinidae). *J. Physiol.* **185**, 536–555.

Nashold, B. S., and Friedman, H. (1972). Dorsal column stimulation for control of pain. Preliminary report on 30 patients. *J. Neurosurg.* **36**, 590–597.

Nashold, B. S., Somjen, G., and Friedman, H. (1972). Paresthesias and EEG potentials evoked by stimulation of the dorsal funiculi in man. *Exp. Neurol.* **36**, 273–287.

Nathan, P. W. (1963). Results of antero-lateral cordotomy for pain in cancer. *J. Neurol. Neurosurg. Psychiat.* **26**, 353–362.

Nathan, P. W. (1976). The gate-control theory of pain: a critical review. *Brain* **99**, 123–158.

Nathan, P. W., and Smith, M. C. (1955). Spino-cortical fibres in man. *J. Neurol. Neurosurg. Psychiat.* **18**, 181–190.

Nathan, P. W., and Smith, M. C. (1959). Fasciculi proprii of the spinal cord in man: review of present knowledge. *Brain* **82**, 610–668.

Nauta, W. J. H., and Kuypers, H. G. J. M. (1958). Some ascending pathways in the brain stem reticular formation. In: *Reticular Formation of the Brain*, pp. 3–30 (H. H. Jasper *et al.*, eds.). Henry Ford Hosp. Internat. Symp., Little, Brown and Co., Boston.

Necker, R. (1975). Temperature-sensitive ascending neurons in the spinal cord of pigeons. *Pflügers Arch.* **353**, 275–286.

Netsky, M. G. (1953). Syringomyelia. A clinicopathologic study. *Arch. Neurol. Psychiat.* **70**, 741–777.

Nielson, K. D., Adams, J. E., and Hosobuchi, Y. (1975). Phantom limb pain. Treatment with dorsal column stimulation. *J. Neurosurg.* **42**, 301–307.

Nijensohn, D. E., and Kerr, F. W. L. (1975). The ascending projections of the dorsolateral funiculus of the spinal cord in the primate. *J. Compar. Neurol.* **161**, 459–470.

Noback, C. R. (1951). Morphology and phylogeny of hair. *Ann. N.Y. Acad. Sci.* **53**, 476–491.

Noordenbos, W. (1959). *Pain*. Elsevier, Amsterdam.

Noordenbos, W., and Wall, P. D. (1976). Diverse sensory functions with an almost totally divided spinal cord. A case of spinal cord transection with preservation of part of one anterolateral quadrant. *Pain* **2**, 185–195.

Nord, S. G. (1967). Somatotopic organization in the spinal trigeminal nucleus, the dorsal column nuclei and related structures in the rat. *J. Compar. Neurol.* **130**, 343–355.

Norrsell, U. (1966a). An evoked potential study of spinal pathways projecting to the cerebral somatosensory areas in the dog. *Exp. Brain Res.* **2**, 261–268.

Norrsell, U. (1966b). The spinal afferent pathways of conditioned reflexes to cutaneous stimuli in the dog. *Exp. Brain Res.* **2**, 269–282.

Norrsell, U., and Voorhoeve, P. (1962). Tactile pathways from the hindlimb to the cerebral cortex in cat. *Acta Physiol. Scand.* **54**, 9–17.

Norrsell, U., and Wolpow, E. R. (1966). An evoked potential study of different pathways from the hindlimb to the somatosensory areas in the cat. *Acta Physiol. Scand.* **66**, 19–33.

Nyberg-Hansen, R. (1965). Sites and mode of termination of reticulo-spinal fibers in the cat. *J. Compar. Neurol.* **124**, 71–100.

Nyberg-Hansen, R., and Brodal, A. (1963). Sites of termination of corticospinal fibers in the cat. An experimental study with silver impregnation methods. *J. Compar. Neurol.* **120**, 369–391.

O'Keefe, J., and Gaffan, D. (1971). Response properties of units in the dorsal column nuclei of the freely moving rat: changes as a function of behaviour. *Brain Res.* **31**, 374–375.

O'Leary, J. L., Heinbecker, P., and Bishop, G. H. (1932). Dorsal root fibers which contribute to the tract of Lissauer. *Proc. Soc. Exp. Biol.* **30**, 302–303.

Oliveras, J. L., Besson, J. M., Guilbaud, G., and Liebeskind, J. C. (1974a). Behavioral and electrophysiological evidence of pain inhibition from midbrain stimulation in the cat. *Exp. Brain Res.* **20**, 32–44.

Oliveras, J. L., Woda, A., Guilbaud, G., and Besson, J. M. (1974b). Inhibition of the jaw opening reflex by electrical stimulation of the periaqueductal gray matter in the awake, unrestrained cat. *Brain Res.* **72**, 328–331.

Oliveras, J. L., Redjemi, F., Guilbaud, G., and Besson, J. M. (1975). Analgesia induced by electrical stimulation of the inferior centralis nucleus of the raphe in the cat. *Pain* **1**, 139–145.

Oliveras, J. L., Hosobuchi, Y., Redjemi, F., Guilbaud, G., and Besson, J. M. (1977). Opiate antagonist, naloxone, strongly reduces analgesia induced by stimulation of a raphe nucleus (centralis inferior). *Brain Res.* **120**, 221–229.

Olszewski, J. (1954). The cytoarchitecture of the human reticular formation. In: *Brain Mechanisms and Consciousness*, pp. 54–76, (E. D. Adrian, F. Bremer and H. H. Jasper, eds.). Blackwell, Oxford.

Olszewski, J., and Baxter, D. (1954). *Cytoarchitecture of the Human Brain Stem*. Karger, New York.

Oscarsson, O. (1973). Functional organization of spinocerebellar paths. In: *Handbook of Sensory Physiology*. Vol. II. *Somatosensory System*, pp. 339–380 (A. Iggo, ed.). Springer-Verlag, New York.

Oscarsson, O., and Rosén, I. (1963). Projection to cerebral cortex of large muscle-spindle afferents in forelimb nerves of the cat. *J. Physiol.* **169**, 924–945.

Oscarsson, O., and Rosén, I. (1966). Short-latency projections to the cat's cerebral cortex from skin and muscle afferents in the contralateral forelimb. *J. Physiol.* **182**, 164–184.

Oscarsson, O., Rosén, I., and Uddenberg, N. (1964). A comparative study of ascending spinal tracts activated from hindlimb afferents in monkey and dog. *Arch. Ital. Biol.* **102**, 137–155.

Oswaldo-Cruz, E., and Kidd, C. (1964). Functional properties of neurons in the lateral cervical nucleus of the cat. *J. Neurophysiol.* **27**, 1–14.

Owman, C., and Santini, M. (1966). Adrenergic nerves in spinal ganglia of the cat. *Acta Physiol. Scand.* **68**, 127–128.

Pacini, F. (1840). Nuovi organi scoperti nel corpo umano. Ciro, Pistoja. Cited in: Pease and Quilliam (1957).

Paintal, A. S. (1957). Responses from mucosal mechanoreceptors in the small intestine of the cat. *J. Physiol.* **139**, 353–368.

Paintal, A. S. (1959). Intramuscular propagation of sensory impulses. *J. Physiol.* **148**, 240–251.

Paintal, A. S. (1960). Functional analysis of group III afferent fibres of mammalian muscles. *J. Physiol.* **152**, 250–270.

Palestini, M., Rossi, G. F., and Zanchetti, A. (1957). An electrophysiological analysis of pontine reticular regions showing different anatomical organization. *Arch. Ital. Biol.* **95**, 97–109.

Patrick, H. T. (1896). On the course and destination of Gowers' tract. *J. Nerv. Ment. Dis.* **21**, 85–107.

Pattle, R. E., and Weddell, G. (1948). Observations on electrical stimulation of pain fibres in an exposed human sensory nerve. *J. Neurophysiol.* **11**, 93–98.

Pearson, A. A. (1952). Role of gelatinous substance of spinal cord in conduction of pain. *Arch. Neurol. Psychiat.* **68**, 515–529.

Pease, D. C., and Quilliam, T. A. (1957). Electron microscopy of the Pacinian corpuscle. *J. Biophys. Biochem. Cytol.* **3**, 331–357.

Perl, E. R. (1968). Myelinated afferent fibres innervating the primate skin and their response to noxious stimuli. *J. Physiol.* **197**, 593–615.

Perl, E. R. (1971). Is pain a specific sensation? *J. Psychiat. Res.* **8**, 273–287.

Perl, E. R., and Whitlock, D. G. (1961). Somatic stimuli exciting spinothalamic projections to thalamic neurons in cat and monkey. *Exp. Neurol.* **3**, 256–296.

Perl, E. R., Whitlock, D. G., and Gentry, J. R. (1962). Cutaneous projection to second-order neurons of the dorsal column system. *J. Neurophysiol.* **25**, 337–358.

Pert, A., and Yaksh, T. (1974). Sites of morphine induced analgesia in the primate brain: relation to pain pathways. *Brain Res.* **80**, 135–140.

Pert, C. B., and Snyder, S. H. (1973). Opiate receptor: demonstration in nervous tissue. *Science* **179**, 1011–1014.

Peterson, B. W., and Felpel, L. P. (1971). Excitation and inhibition of reticulospinal neurons by vestibular, cortical and cutaneous stimulation *Brain Res.* **27**, 373–376.

Peterson, B. W., Anderson, M. E., and Filion, M. (1974). Responses of ponto-medullary reticular neurons to cortical, tectal and cutaneous stimuli. *Exp. Brain Res.* **21**, 19–44.

Peterson, D. F., and Brown, A. M. (1973). Functional afferent innervation of testis. *J. Neurophysiol.* **36**, 425–433.

Petit, D. (1972). Postsynaptic fibres in the dorsal columns and their relay in the nucleus gracilis. *Brain Res.* **48**, 380–384.

Petit, D., and Burgess, P. R. (1968). Dorsal column projection of receptors in cat hairy skin supplied by myelinated fibers. *J. Neurophysiol.* **31**, 849–855.

Petras, J. M. (1967). Cortical, tectal and tegmental fiber connections in the spinal cord of the cat. *Brain Res.* **6**, 275–324.

Petras, J. M. (1968). The substantia gelatinosa of Rolando. *Experientia* **24**, 1045–1047.

Petrén, K. (1902). Ein Beitrag zur Frage vom Verlaufe der Bahnen der Hautsinne im Rückenmarke. *Skand. Arch. Physiol.* **13**, 9–98.

Pickel, V. M., Reis, D. J., and Leeman, S. E. (1977). Ultrastructural localization of substance P in neurons of rat spinal cord. *Brain Res.* **122**, 534–540.

Pierau, F. K., Torrey, P., and Carpenter, D. O. (1975). Afferent nerve fiber activity responding to temperature changes of scrotal skin of the rat. *J. Neurophysiol.* **38**, 601–612.

Pin, C., Jones, B., and Jouvet, M. (1968). Topographie des neurones monoaminergiques du tronc cérébral du chat: étude par histofluorescence. *C. R. Soc. Biol.* **162**, 2136–2141.

Pinkus, H. (1964). Pinkus's Haarscheibe and tactile receptors in cats. *Science* **144**, 891.

Poggio, G. F., and Mountcastle, V. B. (1960). A study of the functional contributions of the lemniscal and spinothalamic systems to somatic sensibility. *Bull. Johns Hopkins Hosp.* **106**, 266–316.

Poggio, G. F., and Mountcastle, V. B. (1963). The functional properties of ventrobasal thalamic neurons studied in unanesthetized monkeys. *J. Neurophysiol.* **26**, 775–806.

Poirier, L. J., and Bertrand, C. (1955). Experimental and anatomical investigation of the lateral spino-thalamic and spino-tectal tracts. *J. Compar. Neurol.* **102**, 745–757.

Pomeranz, B. (1973). Specific nociceptive fibers projecting from spinal cord neurons to the brain: A possible pathway for pain. *Brain Res.* **50**, 447–451.

Pomeranz, B., Wall, P. D., and Weber, W. V. (1968). Cord cells responding to fine myelinated afferents from viscera, muscle and skin. *J. Physiol.* **199**, 511–532.

Pompeiano, O. (1973). Reticular formation. In: *Handbook of Sensory Physiology.* Vol. 2, *Somatosensory System*, pp. 381–488 (A. Iggo, ed.). Springer-Verlag, New York.

Pompeiano, O., and Barnes, C. D. (1971). Response of brain stem reticular neurons to muscle vibration in the decerebrate cat. *J. Neurophysiol.* **34**, 709–724.

Pompeiano, O., and Brodal, A. (1957). Spino-vestibular fibers in the cat. An experimental study. *J. Compar. Neurol.* **108**, 353–382.

Pompeiano, O., and Swett, J. E. (1963a). Actions of graded cutaneous and muscular afferent volleys on brain stem units in the decerebrate, cerebellectomized cat. *Arch. Ital. Biol.* **101**, 552–583.

Pompeiano, O., and Swett, J. E. (1963b). Cerebellar potentials and responses of reticular units evoked by muscular afferent volleys in the decerebrate cat. *Arch. Ital. Biol.* **101**, 584–613.

Pompeiano, O., Carli, G., and Kawamura, H. (1967). Transmission of sensory information through ascending spinal hindlimb pathways during sleep and wakefulness. *Arch. Ital. Biol.* **105**, 529–572.

Poulos, D. A. (1971). Temperature related changes in discharge patterns of squirrel monkey thermoreceptors. In: *Research in Physiology*, pp. 441–455, (F. F. Kao, K. Koizumi, and M. Vassalle (eds.). A. Gaggi, Bologna.

Poulos, D. A., and Benjamin, R. M. (1968). Response of thalamic neurons to thermal stimulation of the tongue. *J. Neurophysiol.* **31**, 28–43.

Poulos, D. A., and Lende, R. A. (1970a). Response of trigeminal ganglion neurons to thermal stimulation of oral–facial regions. I. Steady-state response. *J. Neurophysiol.* **33**, 508–517.

Poulos, D. A., and Lende, R. A. (1970b). Response of trigeminal ganglion neurons to thermal stimulation of oral–facial regions. II. Temperature change response. *J. Neurophysiol.* **33**, 518–526.

Price, D. D. (1972). Characteristics of second pain and flexion reflexes indicative of prolonged central summation. *Exp. Neurol.* **37**, 371–387.

Price, D. D., and Browe, A. C. (1973). Responses of spinal cord neurons to graded noxious and non-noxious stimuli. *Brain Res.* **64**, 425–429.

Price, D. D., and Dubner, R. (1977). Neurons that subserve the sensory–discriminative aspects of pain. *Pain* **3**, 307–338.

Price, D. D., and Mayer, D. J. (1974). Physiological laminar organization of the dorsal horn of *M. mulatta. Brain Res.* **79**, 321–325.

Price, D. D., and Mayer, D. J. (1975). Neurophysiological characterization of the anterolateral quadrant neurons subserving pain in *M. mulatta*. *Pain* **1**, 59–72.

Price, D. D., and Wagman, I. H. (1971). Characteristics of two ascending pathways which originate in spinal dorsal horn of *M. mulatta*. *Brain Res.* **26**, 406–410.

Price, D. D., Hull, C. D., and Buchwald, N. A. (1971). Intracellular responses of dorsal horn cells to cutaneous and sural nerve A and C fiber stimuli. *Exp. Neurol.* **33**, 291–309.

Price, D. D., Hu, J. W., Dubner, R., and Gracely, R. (1977). Peripheral suppression of first pain and central summation of second pain evoked by noxious heat pulses. *Pain* **3**, 57–68.

Proshansky, E., and Egger, M. D. (1977). Dendritic spread of dorsal horn neurons in cats. *Exp. Brain Res.* **28**, 153–166.

Proudfit, H. K., and Anderson, E. G. (1974). New long latency bulbospinal evoked potentials blocked by serotonin antagonists. *Brain Res.* **65**, 542–546.

Proudfit, H. K., and Anderson, E. G. (1975). Morphine analgesia: blockade by raphe magnus lesions. *Brain Res.* **98**, 612–618.

Provins, K. A. (1958). The effect of peripheral nerve block on the appreciation and execution of finger movements. *J. Physiol.* **143**, 55–67.

Pubols, L. M., and Pubols, B. H. (1973). Modality composition and functional characteristics of dorsal column mechanoreceptive afferent fibers innervating the raccoon's forepaw. *J. Neurophysiol.* **36**, 1023–1037.

Pubols, B. H., Welker, W. I., and Johnson, J. I. (1965). Somatic sensory representation of forelimb in dorsal root fibers of raccoon, coatimundi, and cat. *J. Neurophysiol.* **28**, 312–341.

Puletti, F., and Blomquist, A. J. (1967). Single neuron activity in posterior columns of the human spinal cord. *J. Neurosurg.* **27**, 255–259.

Putnam, J. E., and Whitehorn, D. (1973). Polarization changes in the terminals of identified primary afferent fibers at the gracile nucleus. *Exp. Neurol.* **41**, 246–259.

Quilliam, T. A. (1975). Neuro-cutaneous relationships in fingerprint skin. In: *The Somatosensory System*, pp. 193–199 (H. H. Kornhuber, ed.). Thieme, Stuttgart.

Quilliam, T. A., and Sato, M. (1955). The distribution of myelin on nerve fibres from Pacinian corpuscles. *J. Physiol.* **129**, 167–176.

Rabiner, A. M., and Browder, J. (1948). Concerning the conduction of touch and deep sensibilities through the spinal cord. *Trans. Amer. Neurol. Assoc.* **73**, 137–142.

Ralston, H. J. (1965). The organization of the substantia gelatinosa Rolandi in the cat lumbosacral cord. *Z. Zellforsch.* **67**, 1–23.

Ralston, H. J. (1968a). The fine structure of neurons in the dorsal horn of the cat spinal cord. *J. Compar. Neurol.* **132**, 275–302.

Ralston, H. J. (1968b). Dorsal root projections to dorsal horn neurons in the cat spinal cord. *J. Compar. Neurol.* **132**, 303–330.

Ralston, H. J. (1969). The synaptic organization of lemniscal projections to the ventrobasal thalamus of the cat. *Brain Res.* **14**, 99–115.

Ralston, H. J. (1971). The synaptic organization in the dorsal horn of the spinal cord and in the ventrobasal thalamus in the cat. In: *Oral–Facial Sensory and Motor Mechanisms*, pp. 229–250 (R. Dubner and Y. Kawamura, eds.). Appleton-Century-Crofts, New York.

Ralston, H. J. (1977). The synaptic organization of the dorsal horn of the monkey spinal cord. A quantitative electron microscopic study. *Soc. Neurosci. Abst.* **3**, 506.

Ramon y Cajal, S. (1909). Histologie du système nerveux de l'homme et des vertébrés, Vol. I. Inst. Cajal, Madrid. Reprinted in 1952.

Ramón-Moliner, E., and Nauta, W. J. H. (1966). The isodendritic core of the brain stem. *J. Compar. Neurol.* **126**, 311–335.

Randić, M., and Miletic, V. (1977). Effects of substance P and somatostatin in cat dorsal horn neurones activated by noxious stimuli. *Proc. Internat. Union Physiol. Sci.*, **13**, 619; *Abstr. 27th Internat. Congr.*

Randić, M., and Yu, H. H. (1976). Effects of 5-hydroxytryptamine and bradykinin in cat dorsal horn neurones activated by noxious stimuli. *Brain Res.* **111**, 197–203.

Ranieri, F., Mei, N., and Crousillat, J. (1973). Les afférences splanchniques provenant des mécanorécepteurs gastro-intestinaux et péritonéaux. *Exp. Brain Res.* **16**, 276–290.

Ranson, S. W. (1912). The structure of the spinal ganglia and of the spinal nerves. *J. Compar. Neurol.* **22**, 159–175.

Ranson, S. W. (1913a). The fasciculus cerebro-spinalis in the albino rat. *Am. J. Anat.* **14**, 411–424.

Ranson, S. W. (1913b). The course within the spinal cord of the non-medullated fibers of the dorsal roots: A study of Lissauer's tract in the cat. *J. Compar. Neurol.* **23**, 259–281.

Ranson, S. W. (1914). An experimental study of Lissauer's tract and the dorsal roots. *J. Compar. Neurol.* **24**, 531–545.

Ranson, S. W., and Billingsley, P. R. (1916). The conduction of painful afferent impulses in the spinal nerves. *Amer. J. Physiol.* **40**, 571–584.

Ranson, S. W., and Davenport, H. K. (1931). Sensory unmyelinated fibers in the spinal nerves. *Amer. J. Anat.* **48**, 331–353.

Ranson, S. W., and Hess, C. L. von (1915). The conduction within the spinal cord of the afferent impulses producing pain and the vasomotor reflexes. *Amer. J. Physiol.* **38**, 128–152.

Ranson, S. W., and Ingram, W. R. (1932). The diencephalic course and termination of the medial lemniscus and the brachium conjunctivum. *J. Compar. Neurol.* **56**, 257–275.

Ranson, S. W., Davenport, H. K., and Doles, E. A. (1932). Intramedullary course of the dorsal root fibers of the first three cervical nerves. *J. Compar. Neurol.* **54**, 1–12.

Rao, G. S., Breazile, J. E., and Kitchell, R. L. (1969). Distribution and termination of spinoreticular afferents in the brain stem of sheep. *J. Compar. Neurol.* **137**, 185–195.

Rasmussen, A. T., and Peyton, W. T. (1948). The course and termination of the medial lemniscus in man. *J. Compar. Neurol.* **88**, 411–424.

Repkin, A. H., Wolf, P., and Anderson, E. G. (1976). Non-GABA mediated primary afferent depolarization. *Brain Res.* **117**, 147–152.

Réthelyi, M. (1977). Preterminal and terminal axon arborizations in the substantia gelatinosa of cat's spinal cord. *J. Compar. Neurol.* **172**, 511–528.

Réthelyi, M., and Szentágothai, J. (1969). The large synaptic complexes of the substantia gelatinosa. *Exp. Brain Res.* **7**, 258–274.

Réthelyi, M., and Szentágothai, J. (1973). Distribution and connections of afferent fibres in the spinal cord. In: *Handbook of Sensory Physiology*. Vol. II. *Somatosensory System*. pp. 207–252 (A. Iggo, ed.). Springer-Verlag, New York.

Rexed, B. (1951). The nucleus cervicalis lateralis, a spinocerebellar relay nucleus. *Acta Physiol. Scand.* Suppl. **89**, 67–68.

Rexed, B. (1952). The cytoarchitectonic organization of the spinal cord in the cat. *J. Compar. Neurol.* **96**, 415–466.

Rexed, B. (1954). A cytoarchitectonic atlas of the spinal cord in the cat. *J. Compar. Neurol.* **100**, 297–380.

Rexed, B., and Brodal, A. (1951). The nucleus cervicalis lateralis. A spino-cerebellar relay nucleus. *J. Neurophysiol.* **14**, 399–407.

Rexed, B., and Ström, G. (1952). Afferent nervous connexions of the lateral cervical nucleus. *Acta Physiol. Scand.* **25**, 219–229.

Reynolds, D. V. (1969). Surgery in the rat during electrical analgesia induced by focal brain stimulation. *Science* **164**, 444–445.

Reynolds, P. J., Talbot, R. E., and Brookhart, J. M. (1972). Control of postural reactions in the dog: the role of the dorsal column feedback pathway. *Brain Res.* **40**, 159–164.

Riedel, W. (1976). Warm receptors in the dorsal abdominal wall of the rabbit. *Pflügers. Arch.* **361**, 205–206.

Rigamonti, D., and D. DeMichelle (1977). Visceral afferent projection to the lateral cervical nucleus. In: *Nerves and the Gut*, pp. 327–333 (F. P. Brooks and P. W. Evers, eds.). Charles B. Slack, Inc., Thorofare, New Jersey.

Rigamonti, D. D., and Hancock, M. B. (1974). Analysis of field potentials elicited in the dorsal column nuclei by splanchnic nerve A-beta afferents. *Brain Res.* **77**, 326–329.

Rinvik, E. (1968). A re-evaluation of the cytoarchitecture of the ventral nuclear complex of the cat's thalamus on the basis of corticothalamic connections. *Brain Res.* **8**, 237–254.

Rinvik, E., and Walberg, F. (1975). Studies on the cerebellar projections from the main and external cuneate nuclei in the cat by means of retrograde axonal transport of horseradish peroxidase. *Brain Res.* **95**, 371–381.

Robards, M. J., Watkins, D. W., and Masterton, R. B. (1976). An anatomical study of some somesthetic afferents to the intercollicular terminal zone of the midbrain of the opossum. *J. Compar. Neurol.* **170**, 499–524.

Roberts, P. J. (1974). The release of amino acids with proposed neurotransmitter function from the cuneate and gracile nuclei of the rat *in vivo*. *Brain Res.* **67**, 419–428.

Roberts, P. J., and Keen, P. (1974). Effect of dorsal root section on amino acids of rat spinal cord. *Brain Res.* **74**, 333–337.

Roberts, P. J., Keen, P., and Mitchell, J. F. (1973). The distribution and axonal transport of free amino acids and related compounds in the dorsal sensory neuron of the rat, as determined by the dansyl reaction. *J. Neurochem.* **21**, 199–209.

Rockel, A. J., Heath, C. J., and Jones, E. G. (1972). Afferent connections to the diencephalon in the marsupial phalanger and the question of sensory convergence in the "posterior group" of the thalamus. *J. Compar. Neurol.* **145**, 105–130.

Rosén I. (1967). Functional organization of group I activated neurones in the cuneate nucleus of the cat. *Brain Res.* **6**, 770–772.

Rosen, I. (1969a). Localization in caudal brain stem and cervical spinal cord of neurones activated from forelimb group I afferents in the cat. *Brain Res.* **16**, 55–71.

Rosén, I. (1969b). Afferent connexions to group I activated cells in the main cuneate nucleus of the cat. *J. Physiol.* **205**, 209–236.

Rosén, I., and Sjölund, B. (1973a). Organization of group I activated cells in the main and external cuneate nuclei of the cat: identification of muscle receptors. *Exp. Brain Res.* **16**, 221–237.

Rosén, I., and Sjölund, B. (1973b). Organization of group I activated cells in the main and external cuneate nuclei of the cat: convergence patterns demonstrated by natural stimulation. *Exp. Brain Res.* **16**, 238–246.

Rosomoff, H. L., Carroll, F., Brown, J., and Sheptak, P. (1965). Percutaneous radiofrequency cervical cordotomy: Technique. *J. Neurosurg.* **23**, 639–644.

Rosomoff, H. L., Sheptak, P., and Carroll, F. (1966). Modern pain relief: percutaneous chordotomy. *J.A.M.A.* **196**, 482–486.

Rossi, G. F., and Brodal, A. (1957). Terminal distribution of spinoreticular fibers in the cat. *Arch. Neurol. Psychiat.* **78**, 439–453.

Rossi, G. F., and Zanchetti, A. (1957). The brainstem reticular formation. Anatomy and physiology. *Arch. Ital. Biol.* **95**, 199–435.

Rozsos, I. (1958). The synapses of Burdach's nucleus. *Acta Morphol. Acad. Sci. Hung.* **8**, 105–109.

Ruch, T. C. (1947). Visceral sensation and referred pain. In: *Howell's Textbook of Physiology*, 15th ed., pp. 385–401 (J. F. Fulton, ed.). Saunders, Philadelphia.

Ruch, T. H., Patton, H. D., and Amassian, V. E. (1952). Topographical and functional determinants of cortical localization patterns. *Assoc. Res. Nervous Mental Dis. Proc.* **30**, 403–429.

Ruda, M. (1975). Autoradiographic study of the efferent projections of the midbrain central gray of the cat. Ph.D. Dissertation, Univ. Pennsylvania, Philadelphia.

Ruffini, A. (1894). Sur un nouvel organe nerveux terminal et sur la présence des corpuscles Golgi–Mazzoni dans le conjunctif sous-cutané de la pulpe des doigts de l'homme. *Arch. Ital. Biol.* **21**, 249–265.

Rustioni, A. (1973). Non-primary afferents to the nucleus gracilis from the lumbar cord of the cat. *Brain Res.* **51**, 81–95.

Rustioni, A. (1974). Non-primary afferents to the cuneate nucleus in the brachial dorsal funiculus of the cat. *Brain Res.* **75**, 247–259.

Rustioni, A., and Kaufman, A. B. (1977). Identification of cells of origin of non-primary afferents to the dorsal column nuclei of the cat. *Exp. Brain Res.* **27**, 1–14.

Rustioni, A., and Macchi, G. (1968). Distribution of dorsal root fibers in the medulla oblongata of the cat. *J.Compar. Neurol.* **134**, 113–126.

Rustioni, A., and Molenaar, I. (1975). Dorsal column nuclei afferents in the lateral funiculus of the cat: distribution pattern and absence of sprouting after chronic deafferentation. *Exp. Brain Res.* **23**, 1–12.

Rustioni, A., and Sotelo, C. (1974). Synaptic organization of the nucleus gracilis of the cat. Experimental identification of dorsal root fibers and cortical afferents. *J. Compar. Neurol.* **155**, 441–468.

Ryall, R. W., and Piercey, M. F. (1970). Visceral afferent and efferent fibers in sacral ventral roots in cats. *Brain Res.* **23**, 57–65.

Sadjapour, K., and Brodal, A. (1968). The vestibular nuclei in man. A morphological study in the light of experimental findings in the cat. *J. Hirnforsch.* **10**, 299–319.

Saito, K., Konishi, S., and Otsuka, M. (1975). Antagonism between Lioresal and substance P in rat spinal cord. *Brain Res.* **97**, 177–180.

Samanin, R., and Valzelli, L. (1971). Increase of morphine-induced analgesia by stimulation of the nucleus raphe dorsalis. *Eur. J. Pharmacol.* **16**, 298–302.

Samanin, R., Gumulka, W. and Valzelli, L. (1970). Reduced effect of morphine in midbrain raphe lesioned rats. *Eur. J. Pharmacol.* **10**, 339–343.

Sato, M., and Austin, G. (1961). Intracellular potentials of mammalian dorsal root ganglion cells. *J. Neurophysiol.* **24**, 569–582.

Schäfer, E. A. (1881). Note on the occurrence of ganglion cells in the anterior roots of the cat's spinal nerves. *Proc. Roy. Soc. London* **31**, 348.

Scheibel, M. E., and Scheibel, A. B. (1958). Structural substrates for integrative patterns in the brain stem reticular core. In: *Reticular Formation of the Brain*, pp. 31–55 (H. H. Jasper *et al.*, eds.). Henry Ford Hosp. Internat. Symp., Little, Brown & Co., Boston.

Scheibel, M. E., and Scheibel, A. B. (1966). Spinal motorneurons, interneurons and Renshaw cells. A Golgi study. *Arch. Ital. Biol.* **104**, 328–353.

Scheibel, M. E., and Scheibel, A. B. (1968). Terminal axonal patterns in cat spinal cord. II. The dorsal horn. *Brain Res.* **9**, 32–58.

Scheibel, M. E., Scheibel, A. B., Mollica, A., and Moruzzi, G. (1955). Convergence and interaction of afferent impulses on single units of reticular formation. *J. Neurophysiol.* **18**, 309–331.

Schmidt, R. F. (1963). Pharmacological studies on the primary afferent depolarization of the toad spinal cord. *Pflügers Arch.* **277**, 325–346.

Schmidt, R. F. (1971). Presynaptic inhibition in the vertebrate central nervous system. *Ergebn. Physiol.* **63**, 20–101.

Schmidt, R. F., and Weller, E. (1970). Reflex activity in the cervical and lumbar sympathetic trunk induced by unmyelinated somatic afferents. *Brain Res.* **24**, 207–218.

Schroeder, D. M., and Jane, J. A. (1971). Projection of dorsal column nuclei and spinal cord to brainstem and thalamus in the tree shrew, *Tupaia glis. J. Compar. Neurol.* **142**, 309–350.

Schwartz, A. S., Eidelberg, E., Marchok, P., and Azulay, A. (1972). Tactile discrimination in the monkey after section of the dorsal funiculus and lateral lemniscus. *Exp. Neurol.* **37**, 582–596.

Schwartz, H. G., and O'Leary, J. L. (1941). Section of the spinothalamic tract in the medulla with observations on the pathway for pain. *Surgery* **9**, 183–193.

Schwartzkroin, P. A., Duijn, H. van, and Prince, D. A. (1974a). Effects of projected cortical epileptiform discharges on field potentials in the cat cuneate nucleus. *Exp. Neurol.* **43**, 88–105.

Schwartzkroin, P. A., Duijn, H. van, and Prince, D. A. (1974b). Effects of projected cortical epileptiform discharges on unit activity in the cat cuneate nucleus. *Exp. Neurol.* **43**, 106–123.

Schwartzman, R. J., and Bogdonoff, M. D. (1968). Behavioral and anatomical analysis of vibration sensibility. *Exp. Neurol.* **20**, 43–51.

Schwartzman, R. J., and Bogdonoff, M. D. (1969). Proprioception and vibration sensibility discrimination in the absence of the posterior columns. *Arch. Neurol.* **20**, 349–353.

Segundo, J. P., Takenaka, T., and Encabo, B. (1967a). Electrophysiology of bulbar reticular neurons. *J. Neurophysiol.* **30**, 1194–1220.

Segundo, J. P., Takenaka, T., and Encabo, B. (1967b). Somatic sensory properties of bulbar reticular neurons. *J. Neurophysiol.* **30**, 1221–1238.

Seki, Y. (1962). Some aspects of the comparative anatomy of the spinal cord. *Recent Advan. Res. Nervous System (Tokyo)* **6**, 908–924. (In Japanese). Quoted in Mizuno *et al.* (1967).

Selzer, M., and Spencer, W. A. (1969). Convergence of visceral and cutaneous afferent pathways in the lumbar spinal cord. *Brain Res.* **14**, 331–348.

Sharpe, L. G., Garnett, J. E., and Cicero, T. J. (1974). Analgesia and hyperreactivity produced by intracranial microinjections of morphine into the periaqueductal gray matter of the rat. *Behav. Biol.* **11**, 303–313.

Shealy, C. N., Tyner, C. F., and Taslitz, N. (1966). Physiological evidence of bilateral spinal projections of pain fibers in cats and monkeys. *J. Neurosurg.* **24**, 708–713.

Shealy, C. N., Mortimer, J. T., and Reswick, J. B. (1967). Electrical inhibition of pain by stimulation of the dorsal columns. *Anesth. Anal.* **46**, 489–491.

Shealy, C. N., Mortimer, J. T., and Hagfors, N. R. (1970). Dorsal column electroanalgesia. *J. Neurosurg.* **32**, 560–564.

Sheehan, D. (1932). The afferent nerve supply of the mesentery and its significance in the causation of abdominal pain. *J. Anat.* **67**, 233–249.

Sherman, I. C., and Arieff, A. J. (1948). Dissociation between pain and temperature in spinal cord lesions. *J. Nervous Mental Dis.* **108**, 285–292.

Sherrington, C. S. (1893). Experiments in the examination of the peripheral distribution of the fibres of the posterior roots of some spinal nerves. *Phil. Trans. B.* **183**, 641–763.

Sherrington, C. S. (1894). On the anatomical constitution of nerves of skeletal muscles; with remarks on recurrent fibers in the ventral spinal nerve root. *J. Physiol.* **17**, 211–258.

Sherrington, C. S. (1898). Experiments in examination of the peripheral distribution of the fibres of the posterior roots of some spinal nerves. Part II. *Phil. Trans. B* **190**, 45–186.

Sherrington, C. S. (1906). *The Integrative Action of the Nervous System.* Yale Univ. Press, New Haven. 2nd ed., 1947.

Shriver, J. E., and Noback, C. R. (1967). Cortical projections to the lower brain stem and spinal cord in the tree shrew (*Tupaia glis*). *J. Compar. Neurol.* **130**, 25–54.

Shriver, J. E., Stein, B. M., and Carpenter, M. B. (1968). Central projections of spinal dorsal roots in the monkey. I. Cervical and upper thoracic dorsal roots. *Amer. J. Anat.* **123**, 27–74.

Silfvenius, H. (1970). Projections to the cerebral cortex from afferents of the interosseus nerves of the cat. *Acta Physiol. Scand.* **80**, 196–214.

Silvey, G. E., Gulley, R. L., and Davidoff, R. A. (1974). The frog dorsal column nucleus. *Brain Res.* **73**, 421–437.

Simantov, R., Kuhar, M. J., Pasternak, G. W., and Snyder, S. H. (1976). The regional distribution of a morphine-like factor enkephalin in monkey brain. *Brain Res.* **106**, 189–197.

Simon, E. (1972). Temperature signals from skin and spinal cord converging on spinothalamic neurons. *Pflügers. Arch.* **337**, 323–332.

Simon, E. (1974). Temperature regulation: the spinal cord as a site of extra-hypothalamic thermoregulatory functions. *Rev. Physiol. Biochem. Pharmacol.* **71**, 1–76.

Simon, E., and Iriki, M. (1971). Sensory transmission of spinal heat and cold sensitivity in ascending spinal neurons. *Pflügers. Arch.* **328**, 103–120.

Sinclair, D. C. (1955). Cutaneous sensation and the doctrine of specific energy. *Brain* **78**, 584–614.

Sinclair, D. (1967). *Cutaneous Sensation.* Oxford Univ. Press, New York.

Sinclair, D. C., Weddell, G., and Feindel, W. H. (1948). Referred pain and associated phenomena. *Brain* **71**, 184–212.

Sindou, M., Quoex, C., and Baleydier, C. (1974). Fiber organization at the posterior spinal cord–rootlet junction in man. *J. Compar. Neurol.* **153**, 15–26.

Skoglund, S. (1956). Anatomical and physiological studies of knee joint innervation in the cat. *Acta Physiol. Scand.* **36** (Suppl. 124), 1–101.

Skoglund, S. (1973). Joint receptors and kinaesthesis. In: *Handbook of Sensory Physiology.* Vol. II. *Somatosensory System*, pp. 111–136, (A. Iggo, ed.). Springer-Verlag, Berlin.

Smith, K. R. (1968). The structure and function of Haarscheibe. *J. Compar. Neurol.* **131**, 459–474.

Smith, K. R. (1970). The ultrastructure of the human Haarscheibe and Merkel cell. *J. Invest. Dermatol.* **54**, 150–159.

Smith, M. C. (1976). Retrograde cell changes in human spinal cord after anterolateral cordotomies. Location and identification after different periods of survival. In: *Advances in Pain Research and Therapy*, Vol. 1, pp. 91–98 (J. J. Bonica, and D. Albe-Fessard, eds.). Raven Press, New York.

Snow, P. J., Rose, P. K., and Brown, A. G. (1976). Tracing axons and axon collaterals of spinal neurons using intracellular injection of horseradish peroxidase. *Science* **191**, 312–313.

Snyder, R. (1977). The organization of the dorsal root entry zone in cats and monkeys. *J. Compar. Neurol.* **174**, 47–70.

Somjen, G. G., and Lothman, E. W. (1974). Potassium, sustained focal potential shifts, and dorsal root potentials of the mammalian spinal cord. *Brain Res.* **69**, 153–157.

Sotgiu, M. L., and Cesa-Bianchi, M. G. (1970). Primary afferent depolarization in the cuneate nucleus induced by stimulation of cerebellar and thalamic non-specific nuclei. *EEG Clin. Neurophysiol.* **29**, 156–165.

Sotgiu, M. L., and Cesa-Bianchi, M. G. (1972). Thalamic and cerebellar influence on single units of the cat cuneate nucleus. *Exp. Neurol.* **34**, 394–408.

Sotgiu, M. L., and Margnelli, M. (1976). Electrophysiological identification of pontomedullary reticular neurons directly projecting into dorsal column nuclei. *Brain Res.* **103**, 443–453.

Sotgiu, M. L., and Marini, G. (1977). Reticulo-cuneate projections as revealed by horseradish peroxidase axonal transport. *Brain Res.* **128**, 341–345.

Spiller, W. G. (1905). The occasional clinical resemblance between caries of the vertebrae and lumbothoracic syringomyelia, and the location with the spinal cord of the fibres for the sensations of pain and temperature. *Univ. Pennsylvania Med. Bull.* **18**, 147–154.

Spiller, W. G., and Martin, E. (1912). The treatment of persistent pain of organic origin in the lower part of the body by division of the anterolateral column of the spinal cord. *J.A.M.A.* **58**, 1489–1490.

Sprague, J. M., and Ha, H. (1964). The terminal fields of dorsal root fibers in the lumbosacral spinal cord of the cat and the dendritic organization of the motor nuclei. In: *Organization of the Spinal Cord, Progress in Brain Research, Vol. 11*, pp. 120–152 (J. C. Eccles and J. P. Schade, eds.). Elsevier, New York.

Stacey, M. J. (1969). Free nerve endings in skeletal muscle of the cat. *J. Anat.* **105**, 231–254.

Stein, B. E., and Arigbede, M. O. (1972). Unimodal and multimodal response properties of neurons in the cat's superior colliculus. *Exp. Neurol.* **36**, 179–196.

Steiner, F. A., and Meyer, M. (1966). Actions of L-glutamate, acetylcholine, and dopamine on single neurones in the nuclei cuneatus and gracilis of the cat. *Experientia* **22**, 58–59.

Sterling, P., and Kuypers, H. G. J. M. (1967). Anatomical organization of the brachial spinal cord of the cat. I. The distribution of dorsal root fibers. *Brain Res.* **4**, 1–15.

Sternbach, R. A., Ignelzi, R. J., Deems, L. M., and Timmermans, G. (1976). Transcutaneous electrical analgesia: a follow-up analysis. *Pain* **2**, 35–41.

Stevens, S. S. (1970). Neural events and the psychophysical law. *Science* **170**, 1043–1050.

Stolwijk, J. A. J., and Wexler, I. (1971). Peripheral nerve activity in response to heating the cat's skin. *J. Physiol.* **214**, 377–392.

Stookey, B. (1929). Further light on the transmission of pain and temperature within the spinal cord: human cordotomy to abolish pain sense without destroying temperature sense. *J. Nervous Mental Dis.* **69**, 552–557.

Straile, W. E. (1960). Sensory hair follicles in mammalian skin: the tylotrich follicle. *Amer. J. Anat.* **106**, 133–147.

Straile, W. E. (1961). The morphology of tylotrich follicles in the skin of the rabbit. *Amer. J. Anat.* **109**, 1–13.

Straile, W. E. (1969). Encapsulated nerve end-organs in the rabbit, mouse, sheep and man. *J. Compar. Neurol.* **136**, 317–336.

Straschill, M., and Hoffman, K. P. (1969). Functional aspects of localization in the cat's tectum opticum. *Brain Res.* **13**, 274–283.

Suda, I., Koizumi, K., and Brooks, C. McC. (1958). Reticular formation influences on neurons of spinal reflex pathway. *J. Neurophysiol.* **21**, 113–123.

Sugiura, Y. (1975). Three dimensional analysis of neurons in the substantia gelatinosa Rolandi. *Proc. Jpn. Acad.* **51**, 336–341.

Svaetichin, G. (1951). Electrophysiological investigations on single ganglion cells. *Acta Physiol. Scand.* **24** (Suppl. 86), 1–57.

Svaetichin, G. (1958). Component analysis of action potentials from single neurons. *Exp. Cell Res. Suppl.* **5**, 234–261.

Sweet, W. H., and Wepsic, J. G. (1968). Treatment of chronic pain by stimulation of fibers of primary afferent neuron. *Trans. Amer. Neurol. Assoc.* **93**, 103–105.

Sweet, W. H., White, J. C., Selverstone, B., and Nilges, R. (1950). Sensory responses from anterior roots and from surface and interior of spinal cord in man. *Trans. Amer. Neurol. Assoc.*, pp. 165–169.

Syková, E., Shirayev, B., Křiž, N., and Vyklický, L. (1976). Accumulation of extracellular potassium in the spinal cord of frog. *Brain Res.* **106**, 413–417.

Szentágothai, J. (1964). Neuronal and synaptic arrangement in the substantia gelatinosa Rolandi. *J. Compar. Neural.* **122**, 219–240.

Szentágothai, J., and Kiss, T. (1949). Projections of dermatomes on the substantia gelatinosa. *Arch. Neurol. Psychiat.* **62**, 734–744.

Szentágothai, J., and Réthelyi, M. (1973). Cyto- and neuropil architecture of the spinal cord. *New devel. Electromyogr. Clin. Neurophysiol.*, **3**, 20–37.

Taber, E. (1961). The cytoarchitecture of the brain stem of the cat. I. Brain stem nuclei of cat. *J. Compar. Neurol.* **116**, 27–70.

Taber-Pierce, E., Foote, W. E., and Hobson, J. A. (1976). The efferent connection of the nucleus raphe dorsalis. *Brain Res.* **107**, 137–144.

Takahashi, T., and Otsuka, M. (1975). Regional distribution of substance P in the spinal cord and nerve roots of the cat and the effect of dorsal root section. *Brain Res.* **87**, 1–11.

Talbot, W. H., Darian-Smith, I., Kornhuber, H. H., and Mountcastle, V. B. (1968). The sense of flutter–vibration: comparison of the human capacity with response patterns of mechanoreceptive afferents from the monkey hand. *J. Neurophysiol.* **31**, 301–334.

Tapper, D. N. (1965). Stimulus–response relationships in the cutaneous slowly-adapting mechanoreceptor in hairy skin of the cat. *Exp. Neurol.* **13**, 364–385.

Tapper, D. N. (1970). Behavioral evaluation of the tactile pad receptor system in hairy skin of the cat. *Exp. Neurol.* **26**, 447–459.

Tapper, D. N., and Mann, M. D. (1968). Single presynaptic impulse evokes postsynaptic discharge. *Brain Res.* **11**, 688–690.

Tapper, D. N., Brown, P. B., and Moraff, H. (1973). Functional organization of the cat's dorsal horn: connectivity of myelinated fiber systems of hairy skin. *J. Neurophysiol.* **36**, 817–826.

Taub, A. (1964). Local, segmental and supraspinal interaction with a dorsolateral spinal cutaneous afferent system. *Exp. Neurol.* **10**, 357–374.

Taub, A., and Bishop, P. O. (1965). The spinocervical tract: dorsal column linkage, conduction velocity, primary afferent spectrum. *Exp. Neurol.* **13**, 1–21.

Taub, E., and Berman, A. J. (1968). Movement and learning in the absence of sensory feedback. In: *The Neuropsychology of Spatially Oriented Behavior*, pp. 173–191. (S. J. Freedman, ed.). Dorsey, Homewood, Illinois.

Testa, C. (1964). Functional implications of the morphology of spinal ventral horn neurons of the cat. *J. Compar. Neurol.* **123**, 425–444.

Teuber, H. L. (1960). Perception. In: *Handbook of Physiology*. Section I. *Neurophysiology*, Vol. III, pp. 1595–1668 (J. Field, ed.). Amer. Physiological Soc., Washington, D.C.

Therman, P. O. (1941). Transmission of impulses through the Burdach nucleus. *J. Neurophysiol.* **4**, 153–166.

Thiele, F. H., and Horsley, V. (1901). A study of the degenerations observed in the central nervous system in a case of fracture dislocation of the spine. *Brain* **24**, 519–531.

Todd, J. K. (1964). Afferent impulses in the pudendal nerves of the cat. *Quart. J. Physiol.* **49**, 258–267.

Toennies, J. F. (1938). Reflex discharge from the spinal cord over the dorsal roots. *J. Neurophysiol.* **1**, 378–390.

Tomasulo, K. C., and Emmers, R. (1972). Activation of neurons in the gracile nucleus by two afferent pathways in the rat. *Exp. Neurol.* **36**, 197–206.

Torebjörk, H. E. (1974). Afferent C units responding to mechanical, thermal and chemical stimuli in human non-glabrous skin. *Acta Physiol. Scand.* **92**, 374–390.

Torebjörk, H. E., and Hallin, R. G. (1973). Perceptual changes accompanying controlled preferential blocking of A and C fibre responses in intact human skin nerves. *Exp. Brain Res.* **16**, 321–332.

Torebjörk, H. E., and Hallin, R. G. (1974). Identification of afferent C units in intact human skin nerves. *Brain Res.* **67**, 387–403.

Torvik, A., and Brodal, A. (1957). The origin of reticulospinal fibers in the cat. An experimental study. *Anat. Rec.* **128**, 113–138.

Towe, A. L. (1973). Somatosensory cortex: descending influences on ascending systems. In: *Handbook of Sensory Physiology. II. The Somatosensory System.* pp. 701–718 (A. Iggo, ed.). Springer, New York.

Towe, A. L., and Jabbur, S. J. (1961). Cortical inhibition of neurons in dorsal column nuclei of cat. *J. Neurophysiol.* **24**, 488–498.

Trevino, D. L. (1976). The origin and projections of a spinal nociceptive and thermoreceptive pathway. In: *Sensory Functions of the Skin in Primates, with Special Reference to Man*, pp. 367–376 (Y. Zotterman, ed.). Pergamon Press, New York.

Trevino, D. L., and Carstens, E. (1975). Confirmation of the location of spinothalamic neurons in the cat and monkey by the retrograde transport of horseradish peroxidase. *Brain Res.* **98**, 177–182.

Trevino, D. L., Maunz, R. A., Bryan, R. N., and Willis, W. D. (1972). Location of cells of origin of the spinothalamic tract in the lumbar enlargement of cat. *Exp. Neurol.* **34**, 64–77.

Trevino, D. L., Coulter, J. D., and Willis, W. D. (1973). Location of cells of origin of spinothalamic tract in lumbar enlargement of the monkey. *J. Neurophysiol.* **36**, 750–761.

Trotter, W., and Davies, H. M. (1909). Experimental studies in the innervation of the skin. *J. Physiol.* **38**, 134–246.

Truex, R. C., Taylor, M. J., Smythe, M. Q., and Gildenberg, P. L. (1965). The lateral cervical nucleus of cat, dog and man. *J. Compar. Neurol.* **139**, 93–104.

Tsou, K., and Jang, C. S. (1964). Studies on the site of analgesic action of morphine by intracerebral micro-injection. *Scientia Sinica* **13**, 1099–1109.

Uchida, Y., and Murao, S. (1974). Excitation of afferent cardiac sympathetic nerve fibers during coronary occlusion. *Amer. J. Physiol.* **226**, 1094–1099.

Uddenberg, N. (1968a). Differential localization in dorsal funiculus of fibres originating from different receptors. *Exp. Brain Res.* **4**, 367–376.

Uddenberg, N. (1968b). Functional organization of long, second-order afferents in the dorsal funiculus. *Exp. Brain Res.* **4**, 377–382.

Udo, M., and Mano, N. (1970). Discrimination of different spinal monosynaptic pathways converging onto reticular neurons. *J. Neurophysiol.* **33**, 227–238.

Valverde, F. (1961). Reticular formation of the pons and medulla oblongata. A Golgi study. *J. Compar. Neurol.* **116**, 71–99.

Valverde, F. (1966). The pyramidal tract in rodents. A study of its relations with the posterior column nuclei, dorsolateral reticular formation of the medulla oblongata, and cervical spinal cord. Golgi and electron microscopic observations. *Z. Zellforsch.* **71**, 297–363.

Van Hees, J., and Gybels, J. M. (1972). Pain related to single afferent C fibers from human skin. *Brain Res.* **48**, 397–400.

Vasilenko, D. A., and Kostyuk, P. G. (1965). Activation of various groups of spinal neurons on stimulation of cat sensorimotor cortex. *Zhur. Vyssh. Nervn. Deyat.* **15**, 695. Translation in *Federation Proc., Part II, Trans. Suppl.* **25**, T569–T573, 1966.

Vasilenko, D. A., and Kostyuk, P. G. (1966). Functional properties of interneurons monosynaptically activated by the pyramidal tract. *Zhur. Vyssh. Nervn. Deyat.* **16,** 1046–1054.

Vater, A. (1741). Dissertatio de consensu partium corporis humani. In: *Haller, Disputationum Anatomicarum selectarum.* Vol. II. *Gottingae,* pp. 953–972. Cited in Cauna and Mannan (1958).

Vierck, C. J. (1966). Spinal pathways mediating limb position sense. *Anat. Rec.* **154,** 437.

Vierck, C. J. (1973). Alterations of spatio-tactile discrimination after lesions of primate spinal cord. *Brain Res.* **58,** 69–79.

Vierck, C. J. (1974). Tactile movement detection and discrimination following dorsal column lesions in monkeys. *Exp. Brain Res.* **20,** 331–346.

Vierck, C. J., Hamilton, D. M., and Thornby, J. I. (1971). Pain reactivity of monkeys after lesions to the dorsal and lateral columns of the spinal cord. *Exp. Brain Res.* **13,** 140–158.

Vogt, M. (1974). The effect of lowering the 5-hydroxytryptamine content of the rat spinal cord on analgesia produced by morphine. *J. Physiol.* **236,** 483–498.

Volkmann, A. V. (1844). In: *Handwörterbuch der Physiologie,* Vol. 2, pp. 521–526 (R. Wagner, ed.), Braunschweig.

Voris, H. C. (1951). Ipsilateral sensory loss following chordotomy: Report of a case. *Arch. Neurol. Psychiat.* **65,** 95–96.

Voris, H. C. (1957). Variations in the spinothalamic tract in man. *J. Neurosurg.* **14,** 55–60.

Vyklický, L., Syková, E., Kříž, N., and Ujec, E. (1972). Post-stimulation changes of extracellular potassium concentration in the spinal cord of the rat. *Brain Res.* **45,** 608–611.

Vyklický, L., Syková, E., and Kříž, N. (1975). Slow potentials induced by changes of extracellular potassium in the spinal cord of the cat. *Brain Res.* **87,** 77–80.

Vyklický, L., Syková, E., and Mellerová, B. (1976). Depolarization of primary afferents in the frog spinal cord under high Mg^{2+} concentrations. *Brain Res.* **117,** 153–156.

Wagman, I. H., and Price, D. D. (1969). Responses of dorsal horn cells of *M. mulatta* to cutaneous and sural nerve A and C fiber stimuli. *J. Neurophysiol.* **32,** 803–817.

Walberg, F. (1957). Cortiofugal fibres to the nuclei of the dorsal columns. An experimental study in the cat. *Brain* **80,** 273–287.

Walberg, F. (1965). Axoaxonic contacts in the cuneate nucleus, probable basis for presynaptic depolarization. *Exp. Neurol.* **13,** 218–231.

Walberg, F. (1966). The fine structure of the cuneate nucleus in normal cats and following interruption of afferent fibres; An electron microscopical study with particular reference to findings made in Glees and Nauta sections. *Exp. Brain Res.* **2,** 107–128.

Walberg, F., Bowsher, D., and Brodal, A. (1958). The termination of primary vestibular fibers in the vestibular nuclei in the cat. *J. Compar. Neurol.* **110,** 391–419.

Waldeyer, H. (1888). Das Gorilla-Rückenmark. *Akad. Wissensch. Berlin,* pp. 1–147.

Waldron, H. A. (1969). The morphology of the lateral cervical nucleus in the hedgehog. *Brain Res.* **16,** 301–306.

Walker, A. E. (1938). The thalamus of the chimpanzee. I. Terminations of the somatic afferent systems. *Confinia Neurol.* **1,** 99–127.

Walker, A. E. (1940). The spinothalamic tract in man. *Arch. Neurol. Psychiat.* **43,** 284–298.

Walker, A. E. (1942a). Relief of pain by mesencephalic tractotomy. *Arch. Neurol. Psychiat.* **48,** 865–880.

Walker, A. E. (1942b). Somatotopic localization of spinothalamic and sensory trigeminal tracts in mesencephalon. *Arch. Neurol. Psychiat.* **48,** 884–889.

Walker, A. E., and Weaver, T. A. (1942). The topical organization and termination of the fibers of the posterior columns in *Macaca mulatta*. *J. Compar. Neurol.* **76**, 145–158.

Wall, P. D. (1958). Excitability changes in afferent fibre terminations and their relation to slow potentials. *J. Physiol.* **142**, 1–21.

Wall, P. D. (1959). Repetitive discharge of neurons. *J. Neurophysiol.* **22**, 305–320.

Wall, P. D. (1960). Cord cells responding to touch, damage, and temperature of skin. *J. Neurophysiol.* **23**, 197–210.

Wall, P. D. (1962). The origin of a spinal-cord slow potential. *J. Physiol.* **164**, 508–526.

Wall, P. D. (1964). Presynaptic control of impulses at the first central synapse in the cutaneous pathway. In: *Physiology of Spinal Neurons, Progress in Brain Research*, Vol. 12, pp. 92–115 (J. C. Eccles and J. P. Schade, eds.), Elsevier, New York.

Wall, P. D. (1967). The laminar organization of dorsal horn and effects of descending impulses. *J. Physiol.* **188**, 403–423.

Wall, P. D. (1970). The sensory and motor role of impulses travelling in the dorsal columns toward cerebral cortex. *Brain* **93**, 505–524.

Wall, P. D. (1973). Dorsal horn electrophysiology. In: *Handbook of Sensory Physiology*. Vol. II. *Somatosensory System*, pp. 253–270 (A. Iggo, ed.). Springer-Verlag, New York.

Wall, P. D., and Cronly-Dillon, J. R. (1960). Pain, itch and vibration. *Arch. Neurol.* **2**, 365–375.

Wall, P. D., and Dubner, R. (1972). Somatosensory pathways. *Ann. Rev. Physiol.* **34**, 315–336.

Wall, P. D., and Sweet, W. H. (1967). Temporary abolition of pain in man. *Science* **155**, 108–109.

Wall, P. D., and Taub, A. (1962). Four aspects of trigeminal nucleus and a paradox. *J. Neurophysiol.* **25**, 110–126.

Wall, P. D., Freeman, J., and Major, D. (1967). Dorsal horn cells in spinal and in freely moving rats. *Exp. Neurol.* **19**, 519–529.

Walsh, T. M., and Ebner, F. F. (1973). Distribution of cerebellar and somatic lemniscal projections in the ventral nuclear complex of the Virginia opossum. *J. Compar. Neurol.* **147**, 427–445.

Walshe, F. M. R. (1942). The anatomy and physiology of cutaneous sensibility: a critical review. *Brain* **65**, 48–112.

Weaver, T. A., and Walker, A. E. (1941). Topical arrangement within the spinothalamic tract of the monkey. *Arch. Neurol. Psychiat.* **46**, 877–883.

Webber, R. H., and Wemett, A. (1966). Distribution of fibers from nerve cell bodies in ventral roots of spinal nerves. *Acta Anat.* **65**, 579–583.

Weber, E. H. (1846). Der Tastsinn und das Gemeingefühl. In: *Wagner's Handwörterbuch der Physiologie*, Vol. III/2, pp. 481–588. Vieweg, Braunschweig. Quoted in Hensel *et al.* (1960).

Weddell, G. (1941). The pattern of cutaneous innervation in relation to cutaneous sensibility. *J. Anat.* **75**, 346–367.

Weddell, G. (1955). Somesthesis and the chemical senses. *Ann. Rev. Psychol.* **6**, 119–136.

Weddell, G., and Miller, S. (1962). Cutaneous sensibility. *Ann. Rev. Physiol.* **24**, 199–222.

Weddell, G., and Sinclair, D. C. (1953). The anatomy of pain sensibility. *Acta Neuroveg.* **7**, 135–146.

Weddell, G., Sinclair, D. C., and Feindel, W. H. (1948). An anatomical basis for alterations in quality of pain sensibility. *J. Neurophysiol.* **11**, 99–109.

Weight, F. F., and Salmoiraghi, G. C. (1966). Responses of spinal cord interneurons to acetylcholine, norepinephrine and serotonin administered by microelectrophoresis. *J. Pharmacal Exp. Therap.* **153**, 420–427.

Weinstein, E. A., and Bender, M. B. (1947). Dissociation of deep sensibility at different levels of the central nervous system. *Arch. Neurol. Psychiat.* **43**, 488–497.

Weisberg, J. A., and Rustioni, A. (1976). Cortical cells projecting to the dorsal column nuclei of cats. An anatomical study with the horseradish peroxidase technique. *J. Compar. Neurol.* **168**, 425–438.

Weisberg, J. A., and Rustioni, A. (1977). Cortical cells projecting to the dorsal column nuclei of Rhesus monkeys. *Exp. Brain Res.* **28**, 521–528.

Wen, C. Y., Tan, C. K., and Wong, W. C. (1977). Presynaptic dendrites in the cuneate nucleus of the monkey (*Macaca fascicularis*). *Neurosci. Lett.* **5**, 129–132.

Werner, G., and Mountcastle, V. B. (1965). Neural activity in mechanoreceptive cutaneous afferents: stimulus-response relations, Weber functions, and information transmission. *J. Neurophysiol.* **28**, 359–397.

Werner, G., and Mountcastle, V. B. (1968). Quantitative relations between mechanical stimuli to the skin and the neural responses evoked by them. In: *The Skin Senses.* pp. 112–137. (D. R. Kenshalo, ed.). Thomas, Springfield, Illinois.

Werner, G., and Whitsel, B. L. (1967). The topology of dermatomal projection in the medial lemniscal system. *J. Physiol.* **192**, 123–144.

West, D. C., and Wolstencroft, J. H. (1977). Location and conduction velocity of raphe-spinal neurones in nucleus raphe magnus and raphe pallidus in the cat. *Neurosci. Lett.* **5**, 147–151.

Westman, J. (1968a). The lateral cervical nucleus in the cat. I. A Golgi study. *Brain Res.* **10**, 352–368.

Westman, J. (1968b). The lateral cervical nucleus in the cat. II. An electron microscopical study of the normal structure. *Brain Res.* **11**, 107–123.

Westman, J. (1969). The lateral cervical nucleus in the cat. III. An electron microscopical study after transection of spinal afferents. *Exp. Brain Res.* **7**, 32–50.

Westman, J., and Bowsher, D. (1971). Ultrastructural observations on the degeneration of spinal afferents to the nucleus medullae oblongatae centralis (pars caudalis) of the cat. *Brain Res.* **26**, 395–398.

White, J. C. (1941). Spinothalamic tractotomy in the medulla oblongata: an operation for the relief of intractable neuralgias of the occiput, neck and shoulder. *Arch. Surg.* **43**, 113–127.

White, J. C., and Sweet, W. H. (1955). *Pain, Its Mechanisms and Neurosurgical Control.* Thomas, Springfield, Illinois.

White, J. C., and Sweet, W. H. (1969). *Pain and the Neurosurgeon.* Thomas, Springfield, Illinois.

White, J. C., and Sweet, W. H., Hawkins, R., and Nilges, R. G. (1950). Anterolateral cordotomy: Results, complications and causes of failure. *Brain* **73**, 346–367.

White, J. C., Richardson, E. P., and Sweet, W. H. (1956). Upper thoracic cordotomy for relief of pain: postmortem correlation of spinal incision with analgesic levels in 18 cases. *Ann. Surg.* **144**, 407–420.

Whitehorn, D., and Burgess, P. R. (1973). Changes in polarization of central branches of myelinated mechanoreceptor and nociceptor fibers during noxious and innocuous stimulation of the skin. *J. Neurophysiol.* **36**, 226–237.

Whitehorn, D., Morse, R. W., and Towe, A. L. (1969). Role of the spinocervical tract in production of the primary cortical response evoked by forepaw stimulation. *Exp. Neurol.* **25**, 349–364.

Whitehorn, D., Bromberg, M. B., Howe, J. F. Putnam, J. E., and Burgess, P. R. (1972). Activation of gracile nucleus: time distribution of activity in presynaptic and post-synaptic elements. *Exp. Neurol.* **37**, 312–321.

Whitehorn, D., Howe, J. F., Lessler, M. J., and Burgess, P. R. (1974). Cutaneous receptors supplied by myelinated fibers in the cat. I. Number of receptors innervated by a single nerve. *J. Neurophysiol.* **37**, 1361–1372.

Whitlock, D. G., and Perl, E. R. (1959). Afferent projections through ventrolateral funiculi to thalamus of cat. *J. Neurophysiol.* **22**, 133–148.

Whitlock, D. G., and Perl, E. R. (1961). Thalamic projections of spinothalamic pathways in monkey. *Exp. Neurol.* **3**, 240–255.

Whitsel, B. L., Petrucelli, L. M., and Sapiro, G. (1969). Modality representation in the lumbar and cervical fasciculus gracilis of squirrel monkeys. *Brain Res.* **15**, 67–78.

Whitsel, B. L., Petrucelli, L. M., Sapiro, G., and Ha, H. (1970). Fiber sorting in the fasciculus gracilis of squirrel monkeys. *Exp. Neurol.* **29**, 227–242.

Williams, W. J., Bement, S. L., Yin, T. C. T., and McCall, W. D. (1973). Nucleus gracilis responses to knee joint motion: a frequency response study. *Brain Res.* **64**, 123–140.

Willis, W. D., Grace, R. R., and Skinner, R. D. (1967). Ventral root afferent fibres and the recurrent inhibitory pathway. *Nature* **216**, 1010–1011.

Willis, W. D., Weir, M. A., Skinner, R. D., and Bryan, R. N. (1973). Differential distribution of spinal cord field potentials. *Exp. Brain Res.* **17**, 169–176.

Willis, W. D., Trevino, D. L., Coulter, J. D., and Maunz, R. A. (1974). Responses of primate spinothalamic tract neurons to natural stimulation of hindlimb. *J. Neurophysiol.* **37**, 358–372.

Willis, W. D., Maunz, R. A., Foreman, R. D., and Coulter, J. D. (1975). Static and dynamic responses of spinothalamic tract neurons to mechanical stimuli. *J. Neurophysiol.* **38**, 587–600.

Willis, W. D., Haber, L. H., and Martin, R. F. (1977). Inhibition of spinothalamic tract cells and interneurons by brain stem stimulation in the monkey. *J. Neurophysiol.* **40** 968–981.

Wilson, G., and Fay, T. (1929). Two cases of chordotomy, indicating the distinct separation of pain and temperature fibers in the anterolateral aspect of the spinal cord, as well as the relative position of these fibers supplying the trunk and lower extremity. *Arch. Neurol. Psychiat.* **22**, 638–641.

Windle, W. F. (1931). Neurons of the sensory type in the ventral roots of man and of other mammals. *Arch. Neurol. Psychiat.* **26**, 791–800.

Winter, D. L. (1965). N. gracilis of cat. Functional organization and corticofugal effects. *J. Neurophysiol.* **28**, 48–70.

Winter, D. L. (1971). Receptor characteristics and conduction velocities in bladder afferents. *J. Psychiat. Res.* **8**, 225–235.

Witt, I., and Hensel, H. (1959). Afferente impulse aus der Extremitätenhaut der Katze bie thermischer und mechanischer Reizung. *Pflügers Arch.* **268**, 582–596.

Wolstencroft, J. H. (1964). Reticulospinal neurones. *J. Physiol.* **174**, 91–108.

Woodbury, J. W., and Patton, H. D. (1952). Electrical activity of single spinal cord elements. *Cold Spring Harbor Symp. Quant. Biol.* **17**, 185–188.

Woudenberg, R. A. (1970). Projections of mechanoreceptive fields to cuneate-gracile and spinal trigeminal nuclear regions in sheep. *Brain Res.* **17**, 417–437.

Wünnenberg, W. and Brück, K. (1970). Studies on the ascending pathways from the thermosensitive region of the spinal cord. *Pflügers, Arch.* **321**, 233–241.

Yaksh, T. L., and Rudy, T. A. (1976). Analgesia mediated by a direct spinal action of narcotics. *Science* **192**, 1357–1358.

Yaksh, T. L., DuChateau, J. C., and Rudy, T. A. (1976a). Antagonism by methysergide and cinanserin of the antinociceptive action of morphine administered into the periaqueductal gray. *Brain Res.,* **104**, 367–372.

Yaksh, T. L., Yeung, J. C., and Rudy, T. A. (1976b). Systematic examination in the rat of brain sites sensitive to the direct application of morphine: observation of differential effects within the periaqueductal gray. *Brain Res.* **114**, 83–103.

Yaksh, T. L., Wall, P. D., and Merrill, E. G. (1977). Response properties of substantia gelatinosa neurones in the cat. *Soc. Neurosci. Abstr.* **3**, 495.

Yamamoto, S., and Miyajima, M. (1961). Unit discharges recorded from dorsal portion of medulla responding to adequate exteroceptive and proprioceptive stimulation in cats. *Jpn. J. Physiol.* **11**, 619–626.

Yamamoto, S., Sugihara, S., and Kuru, M. (1956). Microelectrode studies on sensory afferents in the posterior funiculus of cat. *Jpn. J. Physiol.* **6**, 68–85.

Yamamoto, T., Takahashi, K., Satomi, H., and Ise, H. (1977). Origins of primary afferent fibers in the spinal ventral roots in the cat as demonstrated by the horseradish peroxidase method. *Brain Res.* **126**, 350–354.

Yoss, R. E. (1953). Studies of the spinal cord. Part 3. Pathways for deep pain within the spinal cord and brain. *Neurology* **3**, 163–175.

Zimmermann, M. (1968). Dorsal root potentials after C-fiber stimulation. *Science* **160**, 896–898.

Zimmermann, M. (1976). Neurophysiology of nociception. *Internat. Rev. Physiol. Neurophysiol.* II, **10**, 179–221.

Zotterman, Y. (1939). Touch, pain and tickling: an electrophysiological investigation on cutaneous sensory nerves. *J. Physiol.* **95**, 1–28.

Index